Immune-Mediated Disorders of the Central Nervous System in Children

Fondazione Pierfranco e Luisa Mariani ONLUS
viale Bianca Maria 28
20129 Milan, Italy

Telephone: +39 02 795458
Fax: + 39 02 76009582
e-mail: info@fondazione-mariani.org
publications@fondazione-mariani.org
www.fondazione-mariani.org

Immune-Mediated Disorders of the Central Nervous System in Children

Edited by
Lucia Angelini, Maria Bardare and Alberto Martini

Mariani Foundation Paediatric Neurology Series: 10
Series Editor: Maria Majno

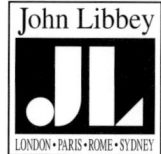

British Library Cataloguing in Publication Data

Immune-Mediated Disorders of the Central Nervous System in Children
– Mariani Foundation Paediatric Neurology Series: vol. 10

  1. Central nervous system – Diseases – Immunological aspects
  2. Pediatric neurology
  I. Angelini, Lucia   II. Bardare, Maria   III. Martini, Alberto
  IV. Mariani Foundation

  618.9' 28047
  ISSN: 0969-0301
  ISBN: 0 86196 631 7

Cover illustration: Image courtesy of Roberto Spreafico: *"Immunocytochemistry of CNS cells"*.

Published by

John Libbey & Company Ltd, PO Box 276, Eastleigh, SO50 5YS, England
Telephone: +44 (0)23 8065 0208; Fax: +44 (0)23 8065 0259; e-mail: johnlibbey@aol.com

© 2002 John Libbey & Company Ltd. All rights reserved.
Unauthorized duplication contravenes applicable laws.

Printed in Malaysia by Kum-Vivar Printing, 48000 Rawang, Selangor Darul Ehsan.

Contents

Chapter 1	Molecular mimicry and autoimmunity *Francesca Giannoni and Salvatore Albani*	1
Chapter 2	Interaction between immune system and central nervous system: peculiar aspects and relevance for the pathogenesis of immune-mediated diseases of the central nervous system *Renato Mantegazza and Pia Bernasconi*	19
Chapter 3	Inflammatory immune-mediated disorders of the central nervous system *Lucia Angelini, Federica Zibordi, Marianna Bugiani and Nicoletta Milani*	29
Chapter 4	Multiple sclerosis: a disease of many faces and many ages *Ari J. Green and Jorge R. Oksenberg*	39
Chapter 5	Multiple sclerosis in childhood: clinical aspects *Nicoletta Milani, Alex Gravante and Federica Zibordi*	53
Chapter 6	Acute disseminated encephalomyelitis *Marianna Bugiani, Chiara Conti, Elio Maccagnano and Lucia Angelini*	61
Chapter 7	Opsoclonus-myoclonus syndrome in children *Giovanna Zorzi, Nardo Nardocci, Anna Erba and Giovanni Lanzi*	69
Chapter 8	Rasmussen's syndrome *Tiziana Granata, Elena Freri, Carlo Antozzi, Renato Mantegazza, Marina Casazza, Flavio Villani, Federica Zibordi, Lucia Angelini, Francesca Ragona, Luisa Chiapparini and Roberto Spreafico*	75
Chapter 9	Rheumatic fever and its neurologic features *Maria Bardare*	85
Chapter 10	Neurological manifestations of rheumatic fever *Nardo Nardocci and Anna Erba*	93
Chapter 11	Systemic lupus erythematosus *Nicolino Ruperto and Alberto Martini*	99
Chapter 12	Neurological involvement in systemic lupus erythematosus *Andrea Salmaggi, Elena Lamperti, Silvana Zeni and Flavio Fantini*	113

Chapter 13	Pathogenetic mechanisms of the antiphospholipid syndrome *Marco Taglietti, Chiara Biasini, Micol Frassi, Massimo Cinquini,* *Genesio Balestrieri and Angela Tincani*	125
Chapter 14	The antiphospholipid syndrome in paediatrics: clinical aspects *Angelo Ravelli*	141
Chapter 15	Neurologic disorders associated with antiphospholipid antibodies *Federica Zibordi and Lucia Angelini*	153
Chapter 16	Endothelial cell role in the pathogenesis of the antiphospholipid syndrome *Cristina Luzzana, Elena Raschi, Luca Catelli, Paola Panzeri,* *Monica Riboni, Cinzia Testoni, Maria Orietta Borghi,* *Nicoletta Del Papa and Pier Luigi Meroni*	161
Chapter 17	Central nervous system vasculitis *Maurizia Rasura, Alexia Anzini and Cesare Fieschi*	171
Chapter 18	Neurological impairment in systemic vasculitides *Marina Cao, Marco Ferrari, Mario Beccia and Cesare Fieschi*	181
Chapter 19	Diagnostic and prognostic role of autoantibodies in connective tissue diseases *Fabrizia Corona and Mirella Scarazatti*	189
Chapter 20	Immune-mediated disorders of the CNS at paediatric age: neuroradiological findings *Elio Maccagnano and Mario Savoiardo*	201
Chapter 21	Use of magnetization transfer imaging to study multiple sclerosis and other immune-mediated disorders of the CNS *Marco Rovaris and Massimo Filippi*	215
Chapter 22	Corticosteroids *Maria Bardare*	225
Chapter 23	Intravenous immunoglobulins *Rosa Maria Dellepiane and Cristina Panisi*	231
Chapter 24	Cytotoxic and noncytotoxic immunosuppressive agents *Maria Grazia Sabbadini and Matteo Bellone*	245
Chapter 25	Immunomodulation by plasmapheresis and immunoadsorption for autoimmune neurological disorders in children *Carlo Antozzi*	261
Chapter 26	New perspectives in the treatment of childhood rheumatic diseases *Marina Vivarelli and Alberto Martini*	269
Chapter 27	Interferon beta and glatiramer acetate in multiple sclerosis *Giancarlo Comi and Bruno Colombo*	277

Chapter 1

Molecular mimicry and autoimmunity

Francesca Giannoni and Salvatore Albani*

Pediatric Department, University of California San Diego, 9500 Gilman Drive, *Androclous Therapeutics, La Jolla, CA 92093, USA

Summary

The term molecular mimicry has been initially used to indicate pathogens that escape the host immune system by mimicking host antigenic determinants. Pathogenic infections can lead to production of autoantibodies and activation of cross-reactive T-cells that recognize both foreign and related self-antigens. As a consequence, antigenic mimicry is considered as one of the potential mechanisms underlying the induction of autoimmune reactions.

Many infectious agents and major histocompatibility complex (MHC) haplotypes have been directly correlated with the susceptibility to develop autoimmune diseases both in animal models and humans. Recently a different role for MHC-derived antigenic determinants in positive selection and regulation of a repertoire of autoreactive T-cells has been proposed. These T-cell clones would be activated by encountering foreign antigens bearing epitopes also present in related MHC-derived self-proteins. The theory of the 'shared epitope' allows us to explain differently the aetiology of some autoimmune diseases, such as rheumatoid arthritis. The possibility to modulate the immune responses by using peptide ligands that share homologies with endogenous self-peptides is a promising tool in the therapy of autoimmune diseases.

Introduction

The term molecular mimicry was originally chosen to indicate how endocellular parasites could evade the immune response by mimicking determinants of the infected host, thus using the host self tolerance (Demian *et al.*, 1964; Demian, 1988). Successively, it has became clear that other infectious agents, such as viruses and bacteria, were able to overcome the host protective immunity by expressing antigens that are similar, or even identical, to host self-antigens and tolerated by the immune system. On the other hand, an immune response to the infectious agent can be directed against a related self-antigen, thus inducing an autoimmune reaction.

In this view, molecular mimicry can be considered as one of the mechanisms underlying the development of autoimmunity. Structural similarities between microbial and host constituents can lead to an antigenic cross-reactivity, exerted by both B-and T-cells, that generates transient autoimmune reactions to chronic autoimmune diseases.

Computer searches in protein databases have been performed to identify shared sequences between self-antigens and viral/bacterial proteins (Auger & Roudier, 1997). Relevant homologies between mammalian and pathogen sequences have been found and tested for the capacity to induce cross-reactivity in immunized animals.

Recently, a different type of molecular mimicry, regarding major histocompatibility complex (MHC)-derived determinants, has been postulated to be involved in autoimmunity. This model suggests that peptides derived from MHC class II molecules are naturally processed and presented by APC during the thymic development, thus inducing positive selection of peptide-specific CD4 T-cells. In the periphery these T-cell clones, activated by exogenous peptides similar to the MHC-derived peptides, could exert autoimmune responses against MHC-expressing cells or interfere with the regulatory activity of MHC system in the control of immune response.

This theory provides a more general explanation of the connection between infections, MHC haplotype and susceptibility to autoimmune disease.

An overview on how T-lymphocytes can generate autoimmune responses

A primary role of the immune system is to provide defence against infections; for this purpose, vertebrate hosts have evolved very large B-cell (BCR) and T-cell receptor (TCR) repertoires that should be able to recognize any invading infectious agent. The immune system has also developed a broad repertoire of antigen-presenting MHC molecules that should be able to present any foreign antigen to immunocompetent cells.

The cellular immunity exerted by T-lymphocytes plays a main role in the regulation of the immune system and in the induction of specific immune responses. A mature T-cell is activated by recognition of the antigen processed into peptides that are presented on the surface of an antigen-presenting cell (APC) in the context of the self MHC. T-cell activation also requires the interaction between costimulatory molecules expressed on APC surface and their receptors expressed on T-cell surface.

Traditionally, the induction of a T-cell response has been considered as highly specific for a defined antigen; this specificity depends on the fine structural interaction between the T-cell receptors and its antigenic ligand. Based on this concept was the idea that the immune system is able to discriminate finely between self and not self. During the thymic development, autoreactive T-cells would be deleted from the mature T-cell repertoire. Negative selection would occur in T-cell clones having high affinity for the specific self-antigen, presented by self-MHC in the thymic environment, whereas T-cell clones having low affinity for the same antigen would be positively selected and released in the peripheral circulation.

However, this self/not-self paradigm was insufficient to explain phenomena such as the occurrence of autoantibody-mediated reactions and the presence of autoreactive T-cell clones in healthy individuals in absence of autoimmunity symptoms. Furthermore, the immune system seems to tolerate foreign antigens present on mucosal surfaces of gastrointestinal and respiratory tract, and allo- and xenografts transplanted in immunologically privileged sites of the body are not rejected.

Several different theories have been proposed to explain these issues. The 'danger theory' (Matzinger, 1994, 1998) suggests that immune system activation is not necessarily affected by the origin of the recognized antigen, that could be self or not self, rather by the presence of endogenous molecular signals coming from distressed or damaged tissues that indicate a situation of danger for the body integrity. These molecules, typically released by necrotic but not by apoptotic cells, are able to increase the expression of MHC and costimulatory molecules on APC surface. In this context costimulation represents a second signal, being the interaction TCR-peptide, the first one essential for T-cell activation. This theory would explain why tumour cells are usually ignored by the immune system. As healthy cells they do not release alarm signals and are thus unable to induce a complete T-cell activation.

A different model (Zinkernagel, 1996, 2000) proposes that immune response is triggered if the antigen is able to reach the secondary lymphoid tissue. In this view, localization, dose and time of antigen exposure, but not costimulation, are critical in order to obtain a full T-cell activation.

Furthermore, many studies have recently provided the evidence that a single TCR, and consequently a single T-cell clone, can recognize and interact with multiple ligands (Kersh & Allen, 1996; Tallquist et al., 1996), including superantigens (Herman et al., 1991), antigen variant and related self-peptides (Hagerty & Allen, 1995; Nanda et al., 1995; Quaratino et al., 1995). X-ray analysis of the TCR/peptide/MHC complex crystal structure have also revealed a reduced number of peptide-specific interactions in the complex, indicating the possibility that TCR binds several peptide variants (Garcia et al., 1996).

Based on these findings, a modern concept about how T-cells can generate autoimmune reactions proposes that self-reactive T-cell clones, escaped by the thymic selection, are commonly present in the peripheral circulation; in normal conditions these T-cells are made unresponsive with different mechanisms, contributing to the maintenance of the peripheral tolerance to self-antigens. T-cells can be non-reactive for the unavailability and inaccessibility of the antigen or they can be anergized by the lack of the second signal of activation. Moreover, clonal deletion can be induced in these self-reactive T-cells by a Fas-dependent apoptosis, referred as activation-induced cell death (AICD).

During the course of a microbial infection peripheral T-cells, circulating in secondary lymphoid organs, encounter foreign antigens, coming from the pathogenic agent. These pathogen-derived antigens can encompass sequential or structural homologies with autologous related antigens. Based on TCR capacity to recognize and interact with different antigen variants, these T-cells might be activated by the microbial antigens and elicit a protective response for eliminating the pathogen. In this context, the inflammatory state and the cellular damage induced by the infection gives rise to the second signal required for a full T-cell activation through the release of stress molecules that act as alarm signals.

The activated T-cell clones could eventually exert an aggressive response against the self-antigen, thus inducing in the host an autoimmune reactivity that can persist after the resolution of the infection.

The inflammatory state consequent to the microbial infection can also reveal cryptic epitopes, which are potentially immunogenic components of self-antigens that evaded the thymic selection and might play a role in initiating or regulating the autoimmune process. Therefore, the occurrence of certain autoimmune responses would be ascribed to the presence of self-reactive T-cells that are maintained inactive in normal conditions and are activated by foreign antigens during infections.

The concept of cross-reactivity between endogenous and exogenous antigens suggests that the role of molecular mimicry in autoimmunity could be strictly related to the flexibility of the

TCR/peptide/MHC interactions and to the capacity of the system to adapt itself to the multiple variants of one antigenic determinant.

T-cell receptor functions in cellular immunity

The interaction of the T-cell receptors with a peptide, presented by an MHC molecule on antigen-presenting cell surfaces, is the initial event that leads to expansion and functional activation of antigen-specific T-lymphocytes. The TCR binds the peptide-MHC complex as part of a multicomponent signaling complex that includes CD3 chains and CD8 or CD4 coreceptors (Meuer et al., 1984; Clevers et al., 1988; Janeway, 1992; Jorgensen et al., 1992), so that while interacting with the peptide, the TCR is also able to trigger the signaling component of the system (Garcia & Teyton, 1998). The specificity of the response to the antigen is determined by the peptide primary sequence recognized by TCR (Babbitt et al., 1985; Townsend et al., 1986). On the other side of the complex, the MHC molecule, whose sequence variability is based on a broad genetic polymorphism, controls the size and diversity of the peptides presented, and the individual immune response can be thus considered as MHC-restricted (Zinkernagel & Doherty, 1974; Bevan 1977).

The possibility to recognize a wide array of antigenic determinants is based on what occurs through random rearrangements of gene segments within the TCR loci. A debated issue is whether specific interactions with self-peptides are needed for selecting the TCR repertoire, and in particular if a given self-peptide can select a limited number of different TCRs and generate the T-cell diversity during positive selection.

Several reports that analysed the selection of $CD4^+$ T-cells *in vivo* showed that the recognition of self-peptides during positive selection is a degenerate process (Ignatowicz et al., 1997; Surh et al., 1997; Tourne et al., 1997). However, a different study showed that it is possible to generate a raising number of $CD8^+$ T-cell clones by adding increasingly complex peptide mixtures to foetal thymic cultures (Hogquist et al., 1993). Moreover, an elevated diversity in the Va-Ja repertoire can be obtained by inducing T-cell selection with multiple self-peptides (Sant'Angelo et al., 1997). These latter observations clearly indicate that the degeneracy of selection is not unlimited.

Recently, an *in vivo* study confirmed that different populations of self-peptide MHC complexes are essential for T-cell positive selection (Barton & Rudensky, 1998), even if the peptides are present at very low concentration. The requirement for diverse, low-abundant peptides suggests that during the positive selection the specificity of the TCR-peptide interaction is fundamental to generate a complete and functional T-cell repertoire, and is possible that the complexity of the TCR repertoire reflects the diversity of self-peptides that mediated the positive selection.

It should be considered that all the T-cell clones that escaped the thymic negative selection are potentially self-reactive since their selective antigen is a self-derived one. Recognition of self can be then regarded as a physiologic process essential for the functionality of the mature immune system.

In the adult life, immunocompetent T-cells circulating in the periphery have to be able to respond to foreign and potentially pathogenic antigens and to tolerate the self-proteins.

Even if antigen recognition relies on T-cell specificity for a given peptide-MHC complex, there is a considerable level of cross-reactivity, such that one TCR can recognize different peptides with only marginal sequence homology (Bhardwaj et al., 1993; Reay et al., 1994; Wucherpfenning & Strominger, 1995; Kaliyaperumal *et al.*, 1996) and T-cells can be activated by peptides unrelated in sequence to the peptide on which they were selected (Ignotowicz *et al.*, 1997). The recognition of multiple peptides by one single T-cell clone could be necessary in order to ensure an adequate coverage of all the presented antigens; this might depend on the fact that the number of potential foreign antigens is greater than the number of the positively selected T-cell clones. On the other hand, an efficient protective immunity toward potentially pathogenic peptides might also require that each peptide-MHC complex be recognized by several different T-cells clonotypes (Mason, 1998).

In this view, cross-reactivity seems to be an intrinsic and necessary property of antigenic recognition and finally, of the protective immunity exerted by T-lymphocytes. The previously discussed data demonstrate that the T-cell receptor has evolved to have an optimal level of cross-reactivity, that is a compromise between a high number of T-cell clones responding at the same antigen and a high level of intrathymic clonal deletion (Mason, 1998). As a consequence of this elevated cross-reactivity level, we can expect that the T-cells' protective response to foreign antigens could lead to autoimmune response to self-related antigens.

Molecular basis of T-cell cross-reactivity: the TCR/peptide/MHC interaction

In the TCR/peptide/MHC trimolecular complex, a limited number of intramolecular interactions account for the specificity of binding, which controls the subsequent immune activation. Structural information derived from crystallographic analysis of TCR α and β chains (Garcia *et al.*, 1996) and of MHC-peptide complexes (Garcia *et al.*, 1998) permits us to envisage the molecular details of the trimolecular recognition event. In the trimolecular complex, the MHC helices dominate the TCR/pep/MHC interface, and the TCR seems to interact with the best conserved areas of MHC domains (Germain, 1990).

Mutagenesis studies and structural analysis (Danska *et al.*, 1990; Kasibhatla, 1993) indicate that the recognition area of the TCR α/β heterodimer is composed of three loops, denominated CDR1, CDR2, and CDR3 which are in both α and β chains (Bentley & Mariuzza, 1996; Michielin *et al.*, 2000). Conformational changes in CDR loops are an important mechanism for expanding TCR specificity and allowing for TCR recognition of multiple peptide ligands (Nanda *et al.*, 1995; Ausubel *et al.*, 1996).

The specificity of TCR recognition is determined by the primary sequence of short, linear peptides (Babbitt *et al.*, 1985; Townsend *et al.*, 1986) and is conferred by only a few peptide residues, as shown by the accessibility of only three to five aminoacids on the peptide chain (Sette *et al.*, 1987). More recently, it has been proposed that similar antigenic surfaces, rather than sequence homology, could be involved in antigen recognition by TCR (Quaratino *et al.*, 1995).

Many observations around TCR contact sites (Evavold *et al.*, 1993; Jameson & Bevan, 1995) revealed that peptide aminoacidic residues have a hierarchy of interaction and contribution to the resulting transduction of signal activation in the T-cell. Introducing aminoacid substitution, series of peptide analogs have been generated and tested in order to study T-cell responses in a panel of T-clones specific for the same epitope (Evavold *et al.*, 1993). From these studies, the presence of primary and secondary TCR interaction sites has emerged. The primary are the most critical aminoacidic residues in the TCR binding, the secondary residues being defined as other contact sites unique for a given TCR, which have a minor role in the binding. Analogs of immunogenic peptides, in which the TCR contact residues have been modified, have been defined as altered peptide ligands (APL) (Evavold *et al.*, 1993). Peptides having few primary sites shared with agonist ligands can either induce a state of partial activation (De Magistris *et al.*, 1992) or anergy (Sloane-Lancaster *et al.*, 1993) without necessarily stimulating T-cell clonal proliferation (Evavold *et al.*, 1995).

A repertoire of endogenous peptides acting as APL (Sloane-Lancaster & Allen, 1996) could have a significant role in shaping the immunoresponse to all different foreign antigens and thus indirectly influence the susceptibility to diseases.

These endogenous APLs could act either by a direct involvement in the positive selection during thymic maturation, as discussed previously, or following the interaction with mature T-cells, by an active participation in modulating immunoresponse in the periphery; these self-peptides might affect the response against related foreign antigens with different mechanisms such as antagonism (Hsu *et al.*, 1995), changes in T-cell phenotype (Windhagen *et al.*, 1995), and maintenance of memory T-cells (Sloane-Lancaster & Allen, 1996).

The observation that self-peptides can partially stimulate specific T-cells, although they do not have sequential or structural homologies with the natural agonist ligand, confirms the flexibility of a specific TCR in recognizing and binding of different unrelated antigenic determinants.

Based on data demonstrating that antigen processing generates either stimulatory or antagonistic peptides from a single immunogenic epitope, it is possible to consider the molecular mimicry of immunodominant epitopes as the result of TCR engagement by different peptide ligands that act like the agonist ligand, and thus are able to induce T-cell activation. These ligands could be derived from microbial antigens mimicking endogenous peptides.

A confirmation of this hypothesis came from a study analysing the ability of bacterial and viral peptides (with accommodating aminoacids for TCR and MHC) to stimulate several myelin basic protein (MBP)-specific T-clones derived from multiple sclerosis patients. Interestingly, both types of microbial antigens have been found able to stimulate three of these clones (Wucherpfenning & Strominger, 1995). Similar results have been recently obtained for experimental autoimmune encephalomyelitis (EAE) in a transgenic mice system (Grogan *et al.*, 1999).

Since other ligands have TCR antagonist properties, the possibility to utilize them as therapeutic tools in autoimmune diseases has been recently addressed. In one report, APL derived from papillomavirus and bacillus subtilis proteins, which contain sequence homologies with a major epitope of MBP, have been shown to suppress the development of EAE by modulation of the specific T-cell response (Ruiz *et al.*, 1999). In another report, inhibition of T-cell activation has been found related to peptide ligands, directly deriving from MBP, acting as TCR antagonist (Anderton *et al.*, 1999). In humans, some clinical trials have been recently applied to multiple sclerosis patients utilizing peptide ligands of MBP (Bielekova *et al.*, 2000; Kappos *et al.*, 2000).

Correlation between autoimmune diseases and infectious pathogens

Immunity to infections often has an immunopathological component, in that protective T-cell reactivity against infectious agents can imply destruction of the infected cell.

The association between infections and autoimmunity is well known, since the observation that the onset of an autoimmune reaction can follow an acute bacterial or viral infection.

There are many infectious agents, belonging to different categories of pathogens, that are considered to be directly involved in the development of autoimmune diseases in humans. These include parasites like trypanosoma cruzi as causal agent of Chaga's disease (Tanowitz *et al.*,

1992), bacteria like *Streptococcus pyogenes* inducing rheumatic fever (Stollerman, 1997) and viruses as coxsackie virus B3, causative agent of miocarditis (Rose et al., 1992) and involved in type I diabetes (Klemetti et al., 1999).

The likely role played by infections in generating autoimmune disease has been postulated by the observation that infections are commonly accompanied by high levels of circulating autoantibodies (Abs). These Abs have low affinity for non-accessible cellular antigens, and are usually not harmful for the host. On the other hand cross-reactive T-lymphocytes recognizing both host and infectious agent-derived antigens have also been detected during and after infections (Higuchi et al., 1997). It is then possible that cellular rather than humoral immunity is directly responsible for the pathogenic autoimmune reactions that follow the infection.

The involvement of cross-reactive T-cells in the autoimmune responses triggered by infections confirms the main role of molecular mimicry between microbial and self-antigens in the development of infection-related autoimmune diseases. However, it is also possible that a viral infection may induce autoimmune reactions through bystander activation of a pre-existing autoimmune state, overcoming the necessity of an antigen-specific activation (Benoist & Mathis, 1998).

Many relevant sequence homologies between mammalian and pathogens have been identified through protein database analysis, consisting in the alignment of primary aminoacidic sequences (Roudier et al., 1996).

One of the first applications of this method allowed the identification of a hepatitis B virus determinant sharing six aminoacids with an immunogenic epitope of the myelin basic protein (MBP) (Wucherpfenning & Strominger, 1995). Rabbits immunized with this viral epitope produced antibodies and T-cells recognizing MBP, and hystological analysis of animal brains showed lesions similar to those found in experimental allergic encephalomyelitis (Fujinami & Oldstone, 1985). In another report, herpes virus glycoprotein D showed a sequence homology with an immunodominant epitope of the α-chain acetylcholine receptor, and cross-reactivity has been found between the viral sequence and the related receptor peptide (Gebhardt, 2000). Autoantibodies against the α-chain acetylcholine receptor have been found in sera from myasthenia gravis patients, and they also react against herpes virus infected cells (Schwimmbeck et al., 1989).

Type I diabetes has been associated with diverse viral infections sustained by rubella, cytomegalovirus and coxsackie B virus, this latter virus being able to infect pancreatic cells. In NOD mice, which are mice strains susceptible to develop insulin-dependent diabetes mellitus (IDDM), early immune responses to self proteins seem to be against autoantigens like glutamic acid decarboxiylase (GAD), insulin, heat shock proteins and carboxipeptidase (Tisch et al., 1993). Cross-reactivity has been found between rubella virus capsid protein and a 52 K d islet antigen (Karounos et al., 1993). Sequence homology has been detected between human GAD65 and coxsackie B3 virus P2-C protein, which contains a T-cell epitope involved with GAD responses in human type I diabetes (Atkinson et al., 1994). NOD mice immunized with coxsackie B virus P2-C protein develop T-cell responses that cross-react with autologous GAD and GAD-derived peptides (Tian et al., 1994).

In susceptible mice and rat strains, adjuvant arthritis is induced by injection of complete Freund's adjuvant, containing mycobacterium T. Heat shock protein 60 (HSP60) has been proposed as a candidate self-antigen, expressed at the joint level, that is recognized by arthritogenic T-cell clones induced after adjuvant injection. Mycobacterial HSP proteins might induce activation of specific T-cells cross-reacting with endogenous HSP molecules, that are overexpressed by stressed cells during inflammation state (van Eden *et al.*, 1989). The cross-reactivity is here based on the elevated sequence homology between bacterial and mammalian HSP molecules, which is highly conserved during evolution. Table 1 shows several examples of molecular mimicry correlated with autoimmune diseases.

Table 1. Molecular mimicry in human autoimmune diseases

Disease	Self-antigen	Mimicking antigen	References
Rheumatoid arthritis	Human Heat shock protein 60	Mycobacterium Heat shock protein 65 *Escherichia coli*	Wilbrink *et al.*, 1993 Quayle *et al.*, 1992
	HLA-DR4	Heat shock protein dnaJ	Albani *et al.*, 1995
Juvenile rheumatoid arthritis	Human Heat shock protein 60	Mycobacterium Heat shock protein 65 *Escherichia coli* Heat shock protein dnaJ	Life *et al.*, 1993 Albani *et al.*, 1994
Juvenile dermatomyositis	Myosin	Streptococcal M5 protein	Albani *et al.*, 1994
Multiple sclerosis	Myelin basic protein	Hepatitis B virus protein	Wucherpfenning & Strominger, 1995
	α-chain acetylcholine Receptor	Herpes virus Glycoprotein D	Gebhardt, 2000
Chagas' disease	Cardiac myosin Heavy chain	Trypanosoma cruzi B13 protein	Tanowitz *et al.*, 1992
Insulin-dependent diabetes mellitus (IDDM)	GAD	Coxsackie virus P2-C protein	Atkinson *et al.*, 1994
	HLA-DQw8	Epstein-Barr virus BOLF 1 protein	Sairenji *et al.*, 1991
Rheumatic fever	Cardiac proteins	β-hemolytic streptococcus M protein	Stollerman, 1997
Ankylosing spondylitis	HLA-B27	*Klebsiella p.* Nitrogenase protein	Husby *et al.*, 1989
Myasthenia gravis	α-chain acetylcholine Receptor	Herpes virus Glycoprotein D	Schwimmbeck *et al.*, 1989
Myocarditis	Cardiac myosin	Coxsackie virus B3	Rose *et al.*, 1992

The role of the major histocompatibility complex

The role played by MHC in autoimmune diseases has been conventionally attributed either to the linkage disequilibrium with disease-susceptibility genes or to the MHC class I- and II-restricted presentation of pathogenic peptides.

Molecular mimicry between foreign antigens and MHC molecules has only been viewed in terms of cross-reacting antibodies, meaning that antibodies mapped to a viral or bacterial peptide would be able to cross-react with a conserved domain of an MHC molecule, with which the foreign peptide shares some sequence homologies.

Many of the previously cited animal experimental models of infection-induced autoimmune diseases have a genetic background that makes them susceptible to develop the disease as a consequence of the infection. This can depend on the expression of particular MHC haplotypes, and sometime the susceptible strain is transgenic for a human HLA allele.

In humans, genetic susceptibility to IDDM is closely related to the presence of HLA DQ 3.2 allele. The Epstein-Barr virus (EBV) protein BOLF 1 was found to include a sequence homologous to HLA-DQ 3.2 β chain, and anti EBV sera cross-react with the related DQ β chain (Sairenji et al., 1991). However, EBV infections do not seem to be correlated with diabetes onset (Elliot & Pilcher, 1995) indicating that the linkage between viral infection and MHC mimicry is not clear.

Another example consists in ankylosing spondilitis that is considered as strongly associated with HLA-B27 and *Klebsiella pneumoniae* infections. A common aminoacidic sequence has been detected in both B27 antigen and *Klebsiella* nitrogenase protein; this epitope is recognized in B27 by antibacterial antibodies specific for the shared sequence (Husby et al., 1989).

Finally, a shared sequence has been detected between EBV gp110 protein and the HLADR-0401 β chain allele, which is related to the susceptibility to develop rheumatoid arthritis (Roudier et al., 1989).

An alternative model of MHC mimicry has been recently proposed. This relies on the observation that a large proportion of self-peptides eluted from HLA class II αβ dimers derive from MHC class I and II molecules themselves, indicating that MHC molecules are normally processed and the deriving epitopes can be presented in the context of the same MHC, on antigen-presenting cells (Chicz et al., 1992; Bevan et al., 1994). The model suggests that during thymic development, MHC class II derived peptides are processed and presented by APCs to immature T-cells present in the cortical epithelium; different TCR affinities for these MHC-peptide complexes would determine the selection of mature thymocytes and thus define the CD4 T-repertoire of the pool of circulating naïve T-cells. In the periphery, different T-cell clonotypes can recognize various peptides that have a short sequential or structural homology with the MHC class II derived peptides. The recognized epitope can belong to an HLA molecule itself, to other self-antigens or to foreign antigens of microbial origin. Cross-reactive T-cells may be activated by encountering this epitope and may consequently trigger an autoimmune response. In this view, the MHC haplotype would determine the genetic susceptibility to develop autoimmune disease (Albani & Carson, 1996; Baum et al., 1996).

This model has been applied to explain in a different way the association between HLA and autoimmune diseases. One example is the strong correlation existing between rheumatoid arthritis and certain allelic variants of HLA-DR4.

Rheumatoid arthritis and the shared epitope hypothesis

Rheumatoid arthritis (RA) is a systemic autoimmune disease characterized by chronic synovial inflammation. The onset of the pro-inflammatory responses may depend on both environmental and genetic factors. Autoreactive T-cells are involved in the initial phase of the disease and more than one antigen could be the target of these abnormal immune responses.

It is widely accepted that there is a strong association between RA and several HLA class II alleles like DRB1*0401,*0404 and *0101 (Wallin et al., 1991).

Comparative analysis of the HLA-DR β chain proteins evidentiated an aminoacid conserved sequence that is present in most of the RA associated alleles. The motif LLEQ (K/R) RAA, defined as 'shared epitope' (Gregersen *et al.*, 1987; Auger & Roudier, 1997), is localized at position 67-74 in the third hypervariable region of the β chain, that is part of the rim of peptide-binding grove.

The presence of this epitope is predictive of a progressively destructive affection, acting in a dose-dependent manner, since individuals homozygous for a sequence-bearing allele have a higher risk to develop more serious disease (Gough *et al.*, 1994).

The shared sequence could be included in the self-peptides that determine selection of T-cells during the foetal time. Positive selection of T-cell clones requires that they have low affinity for the specific peptide. HLA-DR molecules purified from RA patients showed reduced affinity for peptides encompassing the shared epitope (Albani *et al.*, 1995; Roudier, 2000), indicating that this epitope could have positively selected a pool of specific T-lymphocytes which have low affinity for, and consequently are normally unresponsive to, the cognate self-antigen. However, during the adult life these T-cells might encounter exogenous antigens bearing the same epitope, and the high affinity binding with these antigens would induce the activation. Successively these clones, migrating in tissues as joints, cross-react with local self-antigens expressing the shared epitope and trigger the autoimmune reaction, thus breaking immunological tolerance toward the self (Baum *et al.*, 1995). Similar mechanisms could occur in other HLA-associated autoimmune diseases (Chicz *et al.*, 1993).

In RA patients, the presence of an HLA haplotype including the QKRAA sequence could provide the genetic background for producing the group of allele-specific peptides needed for selecting this pool of low affinity and potentially self-reactive T-cells (Albani & Carson, 1996).

Several human pathogens express the RA epitope inside immunogical-relevant proteins, as heat shock protein of *E. coli*, *Brucella ovis* and *Lactococcus lactis* or as gp110 external envelope protein of the EB virus. Immune responses to different antigens including the Q (K/ R) RAA shared epitope have been evaluated in RA patients (Albani, 1994; Albani *et al.*, 1995; La Cava *et al.*, 1997).

A relevant immunoreactivity has been evidentiated in RA patients but not in negative controls, toward a peptide derived from *E. coli* heat shock protein dnaJ and denominated dnaJP1 (QKRAAYDQGHAAFE). In the responsive patients, the T-cell proliferation measured after *in vitro* incubation with this peptide resulted positively correlated with the production of pro-inflammatory cytokines as IFNγ and TNFα (Albani *et al.*, 1995; La Cava *et al.*, 1997).

S1 (QKRAAVDTYCRHNYG) is a DR4-derived peptide homologous to dnaJP1 (Albani *et al.*, 1995; La Cava *et al.*, 1997). S1 and dnaJP1 could both be recognized in RA patients by dnaJ/S1 cross-reactive T-cells. Recognition of S1 may downregulate the T-cell activation previously induced by the high affinity interaction with the homologous peptide dnaJP1. The different effect of the two peptides on a T-cell is attributable to diversity in the primary sequence; indeed, both peptides include the shared epitope but differ in the portion of the aminoacidic chains that interact with the TCR (Fig.1).

The induction of inflammatory response upon stimulation with dnaJP1 has been considered, at the therapeutic level, as a target for modulating the immunoresponse by T-cells specific for dnaJP1.

In order to reduce the inflammation state in the synovium, a clinical trial has been performed on a group of 15 RA patients, by oral administration of a synthetic peptide encompassing the

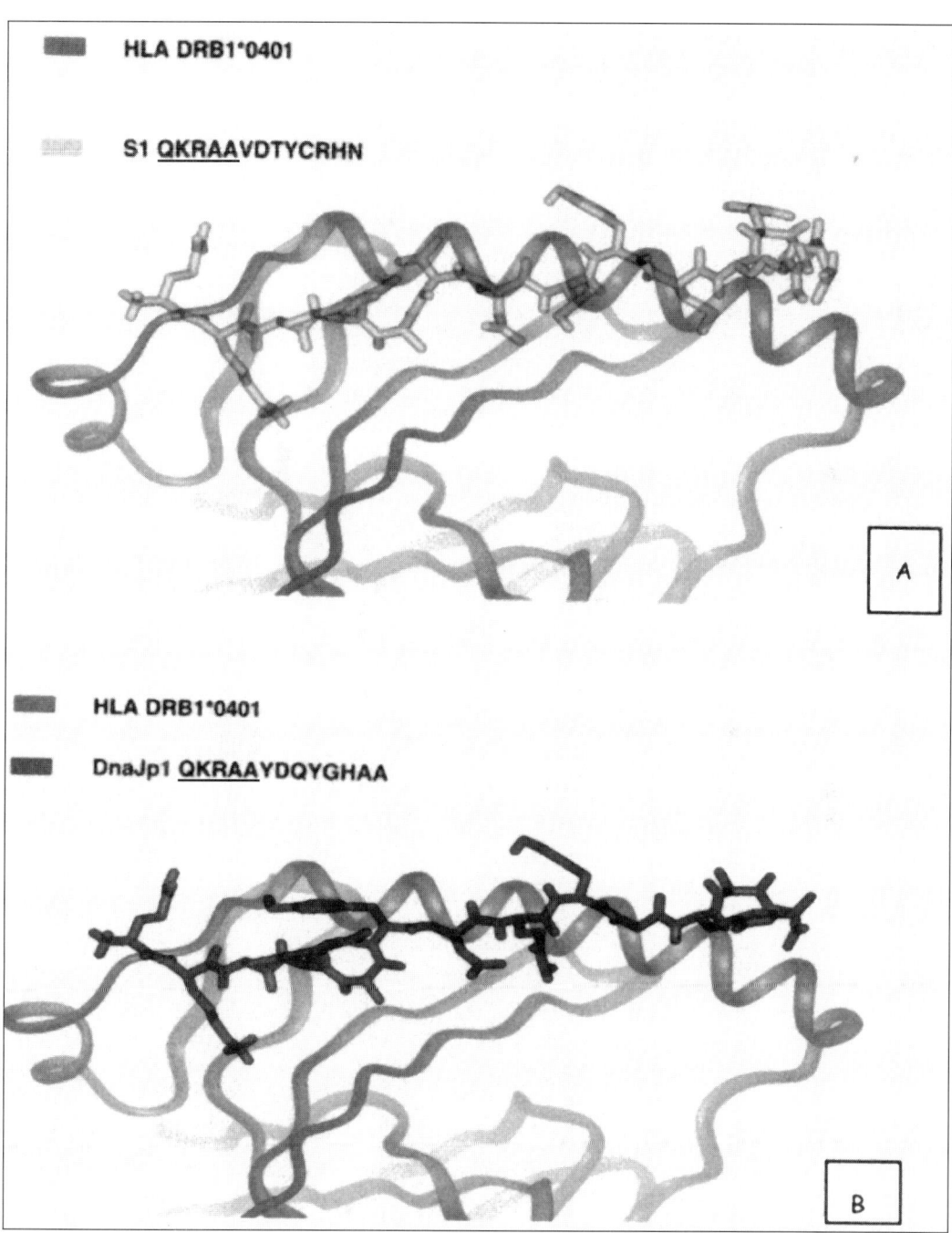

Fig. 1. A. S1 peptide sequence (top); B. DnaJP1 peptide sequence (bottom).
Both peptides encompass the shared epitope chain, but differ in the area of contact with the T-cell receptor (right side of the chain).
[Kindly provided by Marca Wauben.]

shared epitope in the context of dnaJP1 sequence, throughout a six months period. Preliminary results indicate that this treatment reduces T-cells proliferative response to dnaJP1, as well as production of IL2, IFNγ and TNFα by both bystander and dnaJP1 specific T-cells (Albani *et al.*, unpublished). These data supports the concept that it is possible to induce phenotypic changes and thus modulate bystander and antigen-specific T-cell responses involved in the RA inflammation state by using peptide analogs.

Other bacterial antigens have been proposed as potential targets of self-reactive T-cells involved in the development of disease. As previously reported, studies in animal models of arthritis showed that microbial and mammalian heat shock proteins 60 (HSP60) could be the target of autoreactive T-cell responses. Administration of purified mycobacterial hsp proteins induces activation of T-cells that cross-react with self-HSP molecules, which seems to protect the animal from the onset of arthritis (Van der Zee *et al.*, 1998). Responses to HSP60 have been also found in RA patients and correlated with the inflammation state (Wilkbrin *et al.*, 1993; Quayle *et al.*, 1992).

Based on these data, a set of homologous peptides derived from both human and mycobacterial HSP60 have been used for testing immunoreactivity in RA patients. Preliminary data indicate that RA patients are more reactive than healthy controls (Albani *et al.*, unpublished).

Rheumatoid arthritis can be therefore considered as an example of how autoimmune diseases are correlated with either the presence of a particular HLA haplotype or with a microbial infection. This linkage is based on the molecular homologies between self-proteins, HLA and microbial antigens.

Paediatric rheumatic diseases

The pathogenesis of childhood chronic autoimmune disease is in most cases unknown. Several factors can be involved in the loss of the self-tolerance to antigens that become the target of immune responses which generate the disease. The role of self-reactive T-cells has been demonstrated in juvenile idiopathic arthritis (JIA). T-cells infiltrating the synovial membrane bear markers of activation and produce cytokines. The association of particular subtypes of JIA with certain HLA class II alleles provides strong evidence in favour of T-cell involvement through an HLA-peptide-T-cell receptor complex (Sakkas & Platsoucas, 1995).

Even for paediatric rheumatic diseases, a molecular mimicry hypothesis has been proposed, since inflammatory reactions can be related to abnormal reactivity to common bacteria. Bacterial heat shock proteins (HSPs) are the likely candidates as potential antigens inducing cross-reactivity. Some evidence is provided from the analysis of the immunoresponse to bacterial HSP antigens in JRA patients (Boog *et al.*, 1992; Life *et al.*, 1993), even if immune responses to HSPs have been found in healthy individuals.

A more specific analysis of gut bacteria HSPs involved, revealed that *E. coli* heat shock protein dnaJ protein is able to induce immunoreactivity in RA patients but not in healthy controls (Albani, 1994). In one study, the reactivity toward dnaJ as been evaluated in children affected by JIA and other autoimmune diseases (Albani *et al.*, 1994). Interestingly, JIA patients were more reactive than patients with rheumatic fever, systemic lupus or dermatomyositis, and the disease activity was positively correlated with the intensity of cellular immune response.

As previously discussed, in adult RA a strong correlation exists between disease susceptibility and the presence of an HLA-DR4 allele encompassing the shared epitope QKRAA that is also included in dnaJP1. In JIA, activation of dnaJP1-specific T-cell clones could be initially triggered by gut bacteria and later perpetuated by a homologous, still undefined self-antigen (Albani et al., 1994).

Another childhood rheumatic disease, pauciarticular JIA (pJIA), is correlated with the presence of some HLA haplotypes: HLA DPw2.1, HLA DR5 and HLA DR w8. From a protein database search, shared sequences have been detected between these DR alleles and the Epstein-Barr virus BOLF 1 and BALF 2 proteins and pJRA patients bearing these alleles showed high titres of anti-EBV protein antibodies (Albani et al., 1994).

Juvenile dermatomyositis, a chronic autoimmune disease of the skin and the muscles, has been associated with streptococcal infections, and antistreptococcal M5 protein antibodies have been found to cross-react with cardiac myosin (Dale & Beachey, 1985). Recently susceptibility to dermatomyositis has been correlated with elevated serum level antibodies reactive for streptococcal M protein (Ichimiya et al., 1998). A molecular mimicry model has been proposed in which dermatomyositis could be derived from an immune response against myosin triggered by an abnormal reaction to *Streptococcus* infections (Albani et al., 1994).

Conclusions

Many studies on T-cell recognition have shown that a single TCR can recognize many different peptides, demonstrating the flexibility of the cellular immune system in recognizing a broad and variable spectrum of antigens. T-cells have a dynamic interaction with a network of homologous but not identical peptides, which can be of both self and foreign origin and can play different roles in the maintenance, activation and regulation of T-cells. Peptides containing a 'shared epitope' are an example of this network and molecular mimicry between them can be seen as an essential factor either for development and functionality of the immune system or for generation of pathogenic autoimmune responses.

Recently, this concept has been applied to the pharmacological therapy of human autoimmune diseases. The clinical trials have provided preliminary promising results.

Acknowledgements: We would like to thank Marca Wauben for producing Fig. 1. We would also like to thank Nicole Lewon for assistance in editing the manuscript. This study was supported in part by grants N01-AR-7-2232-0, N01-AR-9-2241-01, N01-AR-44850-03, N01-AR-40770, and N01-AR-41897.

References

Albani, S. (1994): Infection and molecular mimicry in autoimmune diseases of childhood. *Clin. Exp. Rheumatol.* **12** (Suppl. 10), S35–41.

Albani, S. & Carson, D.A. (1996): A multistep molecular mimicry hypothesis for the pathogenesis of rheumatoid arthritis. *Immunol. Today* **17** (10), 466–470.

Albani, S., Ravelli, A., Massa, M., De Benedetti, F., Andree, G., Roudier, J., Martini, A. & Carson, D.A. (1994): Immune responses to the *Escherichia coli* dnaJ heat shock protein in juvenile rheumatoid arthritis and their correlation with disease activity. *J. Pediatr.* **124** (4), 561–565.

Albani, S., Keystone, E.C., Nelson, J.L., Ollier, W.E., La Cava, A., Montemayor, A.C., Weber, D.A., Montecucco, C., Martini, A. & Carson, D.A. (1995): Positive selection in autoimmunity: abnormal immune responses to a bacterial dnaJ antigenic determinant in patients with early rheumatoid arthritis. *Nat. Med.* **1** (5), 448–452.

Anderton, S.M., Kissler, S., Lamont, A.G. & Wraith, D.C. (1999): Therapeutic potential of TCR antagonists is determined by their ability to modulate a diverse repertoire of autoreactive T-cells. *Eur. J. Immunol.* **29** (6), 1850–1857.

Atkinson, M.A., Bowman, M.A., Campbell, L., Darrow, B.L., Kaufman, D.L. & Maclaren, N.K. (1994): Cellular immunity to a determinant common to glutamate decarboxylase and coxsackie virus in insulin-dependent diabetes. *J. Clin. Invest.* **94** (5), 2125–2129.

Auger, I. & Roudier, J. (1997): HLA-DR and the development of rheumatoid arthritis. *Autoimmunity* **26** (2), 123–128.

Ausubel, L.J., Kwan, C.K., Sette, A., Kuchroo, V. & Hafler, D.A. (1996): Complementary mutations in an antigenic peptide allow for cross-reactivity of autoreactive T-cell clones. *Proc. Natl. Acad. Sci. USA* **93** (26), 15317–15322.

Babbit, B.P., Allen, P.M., Matsueda, G., Haber, E. & Unanue, E.R. (1985): Binding of immunogenic peptides to Ia histocompatibility molecules. *Nature* **317**, 359–361.

Barton, G.M. & Rudensky, A.Y. (1998): An altered invariant chain protein with an antigenic peptide in place of CLIP forms SDS-stable complexes with class II alphabeta dimers and facilitates highly efficient peptide loading. *Int. Immunol.* **10** (8), 1159–1165.

Baum, H., Wilson, C., Tiwana, H., Ahmadi, K. & Ebringer, A. (1995): HLA association with autoimmune disease: restricted binding or T-cell selection? *Lancet* **346** (8981), 1042–1043.

Baum, H., Davies, H. & Peakman, M. (1996): Molecular mimicry in the MHC: hidden clues to autoimmunity? *Immunol. Today* **17** (2), 64–70.

Benoist, C. & Mathis, D. (1998): Autoimmunity. The pathogen connection. *Nature* **394** (6690), 227–228.

Bentley, G.A. & Mariuzza, R.A. (1996): The structure of the T-cell antigen receptor. *Annu. Rev. Immunol.* **14**, 563–590.

Bevan, M.J. (1977): In a radiation chimaera, host H-2 antigens determine immune responsiveness of donor cytotoxic cells. *Nature* **269**, 417–419.

Bevan, M.J., Hogquist, K.A. & Jameson, S.C. (1994): Selecting the T-cell receptor repertoire. *Science* **264** (5160): 796–797.

Bhardwaj, V., Kumar, V., Geysen, H.M. & Sercarz, E.E. (1993): Degenerate recognition of a dissimilar antigenic peptide by myelin basic protein-reactive T-cells. Implication for thymic education and autoimmunity. *J. Immunol.* **151** (9), 5000–5010.

Bielekova, B., Goodwin, B., Richert, N., Cortese, I., Kondo, T., Afshar, G., Gran, B., Eaton, J., Antel, J., Frank, J.A., McFarland, H.F. & Martin, R. (2000): Encephalitogenic potential of the myelin basic protein peptide (amino acids 83-99) in multiple sclerosis: results of a phase II clinical trial with an altered peptide ligand. *Nat. Med.* **6** (10), 1167–1175.

Boog, C.J., de Graeff-Meeder, E.R., Lucassen, M.A., van der Zee, R., Voorhorst-Ogink, M.M., van Kooten, P.J., Geuze, H.J. & van Eden, W. (1992): Two monoclonal antibodies generated against human hsp60 show reactivity with synovial membranes of patients with juvenile chronic arthritis. *J. Exp. Med.* **175** (6), 1805–1810.

Chicz, R.M., Urban, R.G., Lane, W.S., Gorga, J.C., Stern, L.J., Vignali, D.A. & Strominger, J.L. (1992): Predominant naturally processed peptides bound to HLA-DR1 are derived from MHC-related molecules and are heterogeneous in size. *Nature* **358** (6389), 764–768.

Chicz, R.M., Urban, R.G., Gorga, J.C., Vignali, D.A., Lane, W.S. & Strominger, J.L. (1993): Specificity and promiscuity among naturally processed peptides bound to HLA-DR alleles. *J. Exp. Med.* **78** (1), 27–47.

Clevers, H., Alarcon, B., Wileman, T. & Terhorst, C. (1988): The T-cell receptor/CD3 complex: a dynamic protein ensemble. *Annu. Rev. Immunol.* **6**, 629–662.

Dale, J.B. & Beachey, E.H. (1985): Multiple, heart-cross-reactive epitopes of streptococcal M proteins. *J. Exp. Med.* **161** (1), 113–122.

Danska, J.S., Livingstone, A.M., Paragas, V., Ishihara, T. & Fathman, C.G. (1990): The presumptive CDR3 regions of both T-cell receptor alpha and beta chains determine T-cell specificity for myoglobin peptides. *J. Exp. Med.* **172** (1), 27–33.

De Magistris, M.T., Alexander, J., Coggeshall, M., Altman, A., Gaeta, F.C.A., Grey, H.M. & Sette, A. (1992): Antigen analog-major histocompatibility complexes act as antagonists of the T-cell receptor. *Cell* **68**, 625–634.

Demian, R.T. (1964): Molecular mimicry: antigen sharing by parasite and host and its consequences. *Am. Nat.* **98**, 129–149.

Demian, R.T. (1988): Parasites and molecular mimicry. In: *Molecular mimicry in health and disease*, eds. A. Lernmark, T. Dyrberg, L. Terenius & B. Hokfelt, pp. 211–221. Copenhagen: Elsevier Science.

Elliott, R.B. & Pilcher, C.C. (1995): Epstein-Barr virus infection is not associated with islet cell and insulin auto-antibody seroconversion. *Diabetologia* **38** (9), 1130.

Evavold, B.D., Sloane-Lancaster, J. & Allen, P.M. (1993): Tickling the TCR: selective T-cell functions stimulated by altered peptide ligands. *Immunol. Today* **14**, 602–609.

Evavold, B.D., Sloane-Lancaster, J., Wilson, K.J., Rothbard, J.B. & Allen, P.M. (1995): Specific T-cell recognition of minimally homologous peptides: evidence for multiple endogenous ligands. *Immunity* **2**, 655–663.

Fujinami, R.A. & Oldstone, M.B. (1985): Aminoacid homology between the encephalitogenic site of myelin basic protein and virus: mechanism for autoimmunity. *Science* **29**, 230 (4729), 1043–1045.

Garcia, K.C. & Teyton, L. (1998): T-cell receptor peptide-MHC interactions: biological lessons from structural studies. *Curr. Opin. Biotechnol.* **9** (4), 338–343.

Garcia, K.C., Degano, M., Stanfield, R.L., Brunmark, A., et al. (1996): An alpha beta T-cell receptor structure at 2.5 A and its orientation in the TCR-MHC complex. *Science* **274**, 209–219.

Garcia, K.C., Degano, M., Pease, L.R., Huang, M., Peterson, P.A., Teyton, L. & Wilson, I.A. (1998): Structural basis of plasticity in T-cell receptor recognition of a self peptide-MHC antigen. *Science* **279** (5354), 1166–1172.

Gebhardt B.M. (2000): Evidence for antigenic cross-reactivity between herpes virus and the acetylcholine receptor. *J. Neuroimmunol.* **105** (2), 145–153.

Germain, R.N. (1990): Immunology. Making a molecular match. *Nature* **344** (6261), 19–22.

Gough, A., Faint, J., Salmon, M., Hassell, A., Wordsworth, P., Pilling, D., Birley, A. & Emery, P. (1994): Genetic typing of patients with inflammatory arthritis at presentation can be used to predict outcome. *Arthritis Rheum.* **37** (8), 1166–1170.

Gregersen, P.K., Silver, J. & Winchester, R.J. (1987): The shared epitope hypothesis. An approach to understanding the molecular genetics of susceptibility to rheumatoid arthritis. *Arthritis Rheum.* **30** (11), 1205–1213.

Grogan, J.L., Kramer, A., Nogai, A., Dong, L., Ohde, M., Schneider-Mergener, J. & Kamradt, T. (1999): Cross-reactivity of myelin basic protein-specific T-cells with multiple microbial peptides: experimental autoimmune encephalomyelitis induction in TCR transgenic mice. *J. Immunol.* **163** (7), 3764–3770.

Hagerty, D.T. & Allen, P.M. (1995): Intramolecular mimicry identification and analysis of two cross-reactive T-cell epitopes within a single protein. *J. Immunol.* **155**, 2993–3001.

Herman, A., Kappler, J.W., Marrack, P. & Pullen, A.M. (1991): Superantigens: mechanism of T-cell stimulation and role in immune responses. *Annu. Rev. Immunol.* **13**, 459–486.

Higuchi, M.D., Riesm M.M., Aiello, V.D., Benvenuti, L.A., Gutierrez, P.S., Bellotti, G. & Pileggi, F. (1997): Association of an increase in $CD8^+$ T-cells with the presence of Trypanosoma cruzi antigens in chronic, human, chagasic myocarditis. *Am. J. Trop. Med. Hyg.* **56** (5), 485–489.

Hogquist, K.A., Gavin, M.A. & Bevan, M.J. (1993): Positive selection of $CD8^+$ T-cells induced by major histocompatibility complex binding peptides in fetal thymic organ culture. *J. Exp. Med.* **177** (5), 1469–1473.

Hsu, B.L., Evavold, B.D. & Allen, P.M. (1995): Modulation of T-cell development by an endogenous altered peptide ligand. *J. Exp. Med.* **181**, 805–810.

Husby, G., Tsuchiya, N., Schwimmbeck, P.L., Keat, A., Pahle, J.A., Oldstone, M.B. & Williams, R.C. Jr. (1989): Cross-reactive epitope with Klebsiella pneumoniae nitrogenase in articular tissue of HLA–B27$^+$ patients with ankylosing spondylitis. *Arthritis Rheum.* **32** (4), 437–445.

Ichimiya, M., Yasui, H., Hirota, Y., Ohmura, A. & Muto, M. (1998): Association between elevated serum antibody levels to streptococcal M12 protein and susceptibility to dermatomyositis. *Arch. Dermatol. Res.* **290** (4), 229–230.

Ignatowicz, L., Rees, W., Pacholczyk, R. et al. (1997): T-cells can be activated by peptides that are unrelated in sequence to their selecting peptide. *Immunity* **7**, 179–186.

Jameson, S.C. & Bevan, M.J. (1995): T-cell receptor antagonists and partial agonists. *Immunity* **2**, 1–11.

Janeway, C.A. Jr. (1992): The T-cell receptor as a multicomponent signalling machine: CD4/CD8 coreceptors and CD45 in T-cell activation. *Annu. Rev. Immunol.* **10**, 645–674.

Jorgensen, J.L., Reay, P.A., Ehrich, E.W. & Davis, M.M. (1992): Molecular components of T-cell recognition. *Annu. Rev. Immunol.* **10**, 835–873.

Kaliyaperumal, A., Mohan, C., Wu, W. & Datta, S.K. (1996): Nucleosomal peptide epitopes for nephritis-inducing T-helper cells of murine lupus. *J. Exp. Med.* **183** (6), 2459–2469.

Kappos, L., Comi, G., Panitch, H., Oger, J., Antel, J., Conlon, P., Steinman, L., Rae-Grant, A., Castaldo, J., Eckert, N., Guarnaccia, J.B., Mills, P., Johnson, G., Calabresi, P.A., Pozzilli, C., Bastianello, S., Giugni, E., Witjas, T., Cozzone, P., Pelletier, J., Pohlau, D. & Przuntek, H. (2000): Induction of a non-encephalitogenic type 2 T-helper-cell autoimmune response in multiple sclerosis after administration of an altered peptide ligand in a placebo-controlled, randomized phase II trial. *Nat. Med.* **6** (10), 1176–1182.

Karounos, D.G., Wolinsky, J.S. & Thomas, J.W. (1993): Monoclonal antibody to rubella virus capsid protein recognizes a beta-cell antigen. *J. Immunol.* **150** (7), 3080–3085.

Kasibhatla, S., Nalefski, E.A. & Rao A. (1993): Simultaneous involvement of all six predicted antigen binding loops of the T-cell receptor in recognition of the MHC/antigenic peptide complex. *J. Immunol.* **151** (6), 3140–3151.

Kersh, G.L. & Allen, P.M. (1996): Essential flexibility in the T-cells' recognition of antigen. *Nature* **380**, 495–498.

Klemetti, P., Hyoty, H., Roivainen, M., Ilonen, J., Savola, K., Knip, M., Akerblom, H.K. & Vaarala, O. (1999): Relation between T-cell responses to glutamate decarboxylase and coxsackie virus B4 in patients with insulin-dependent diabetes mellitus. *J. Clin. Virol.* **14** (2), 95–105.

La Cava, A., Nelson, J.L., Ollier, W.E., MacGregor, A., Keystone, E.C., Thorne, J.C., Scavulli, J.F., Berry, C.C., Carson, D.A. & Albani, S. (1997): Genetic bias in immune responses to a cassette shared by different microorganisms in patients with rheumatoid arthritis. *J. Clin. Invest.* **100** (3), 658–663.

Life, P., Hassell, A., Williams, K., Young, S., Bacon, P., Southwood, T. & Gaston, J.S. (1993): Responses to gram negative enteric bacterial antigens by synovial T-cells from patients with juvenile chronic arthritis: recognition of heat shock protein HSP60. *J. Rheumatol.* **20** (8), 1388–1396.

Mason, D. (1998): A very high level of cross-reactivity is an essential feature of the T-cell receptor. *Immunol. Today* **19**, 395–404.

Matzinger, P. (1994): Tolerance, danger and the extended family. *Annu. Rev. Immunol.* **12**, 991–1045.

Matzinger, P. (1998): An innate sense of danger. *Semin. Immunol.* **10**, 399–415.

Meuer, S.C., Acutom O., Hercend, T., Schlossman, S.F. & Reinherz, E.L. (1984): The human T-cell receptor. *Annu. Rev. Immunol.* **2**, 23–50.

Michielin, O., Luescher, I. & Karplus, M. (2000): Modeling of the TCR-MHC-peptide complex. *J. Mol. Biol.* **300** (5), 1205–1035.

Nanda, N.K., Arzoo, K.K., Geysen, H.M., Sette, A. & Sercarz, E.E. (1995): Recognition of multiple peptide cores by a single T-cell receptor. *J. Exp. Med.* **182**, 531–539.

Quaratino, S., Thorpe, C.J., Travers, P.J. & Londei, M. (1995): Similar antigenic surface, rather than sequence homology, dictates T-cell epitope molecular mimicry. *Proc.Natl. Acad. Sci. USA* **92**, 10398–10402.

Quayle, A.J., Wilson, K.B., Li, S.G., Kjeldsen-Kragh, J., Oftung, F., Shinnick, T., Sioud, M., Forre, O., Capra, J.D. & Natvig, J.B. (1992): Peptide recognition, T-cell receptor usage and HLA restriction elements of human heat-shock protein (hsp) 60 and mycobacterial 65-kDa hsp-reactive T-cell clones from rheumatoid synovial fluid. *Eur. J. Immunol.* **22** (5), 1315–1322.

Reay, P.A., Kantor, R.M. & Davis, M.M. (1994): Use of global aminoacid replacements to define the requirements for MHC binding and T-cell recognition of moth cytochrome c (93–103). *J. Immunol.* **152** (8), 3946–3957.

Rose, N.R., Neumann, D.A. & Herskowitz, A. (1992): Coxsackie virus myocarditis. *Adv. Intern. Med.* **37**, 411–429.

Roudier, J. (2000): Association of MHC and rheumatoid arthritis. Association of RA with HLA-DR4: the role of repertoire selection. *Arthritis Res.* **2** (3), 217–220.

Roudier, J., Petersen, J., Rhodes, G.H., Luka, J. & Carson, D.A. (1989): Susceptibility to rheumatoid arthritis maps to a T-cell epitope shared by the HLA-Dw4 DR beta-1 chain and the Epstein-Barr virus glycoprotein gp110. *Proc. Natl. Acad. Sci. USA* **86** (13), 5104–5108.

Roudier, C., Auger, I., Roudier, J. (1996): Molecular mimicry reflected through database screening: serendipity or survival strategy? *Immunol. Today* **17** (8), 357–358.

Ruiz, P.J., Garren, H., Hirschberg, D.L., Langer-Gould, A.M., Levite, M., Karpuj, M.V., Southwood, S., Sette, A., Conlon, P. & Steinman, L. (1999): Microbial epitopes act as altered peptide ligands to prevent experimental autoimmune encephalomyelitis. *J. Exp. Med.* **189** (8), 1275–1284.

Sairenji, T., Daibata, M., Sorli, C.H., Qvistback, H., Humphreys, R.E., Ludvigsson, J., Palmer, J. & Landin-Olsson, M. (1991): Relating homology between the Epstein-Barr virus BOLF1 molecule and HLA-DQw8 beta chain to recent onset type 1 (insulin-dependent) diabetes mellitus. *Diabetologia* **34** (1), 33–39

Sakkas, L.I. & Platsoucas, C.D. (1995): Immunopathogenesis of juvenile rheumatoid arthritis: role of T-cells and MHC. *Immunol. Res.* **14** (3), 218–236.

Sant'Angelo, D.B., Waterbury, P.G. & Cohen, B.E. *et al.* (1997): The imprint of intrathymic self-peptides on the mature T-cell receptor repertoire. *Immunity* **7**, 517–524.

Schwimmbeck, P.L., Dyrberg, T., Drachman, D.B. & Oldstone, M.B. (1989): Molecular mimicry and myasthenia gravis. An autoantigenic site of the acetylcholine receptor alpha-subunit that has biologic activity and reacts immunochemically with herpes simplex virus. *J. Clin. Invest.* **84** (4), 1174–1180.

Sette, A., Buus, S., Colon, S., Smith, J.A., Miles, C. & Grey, H.M. (1987): Structural characteristics of an antigen required for its interaction with Ia and recognition by T-cells. *Nature* **328**, 395–399.

Sloane-Lancaster, J. & Allen, P.M. (1996): Altered peptide ligand-induced partial T-cell activation: molecular mechanism and role in T-cell biology. *Annu. Rev. Immunol.* **14**, 1–27.

Sloane-Lancaster, J., Evavold, B.D., Hsu, B.L. & Allen, P.M. (1993): Induction of T-cell anergy by altered T-cell receptor ligand on live antigen presenting cells. *Nature* **363**, 156–159.

Stollerman, G.H. (1997): Rheumatic fever. *Lancet* **349** (9056), 935–942.

Surh, C.D., Lee, D.S., Fung Leung, W.P., Karlsson, L. & Sprent, J. (1997): Thymic selection by a single MHC/peptide ligand produces a semidiverse repertoire of CD4$^+$ T-cells. *Immunity* **7** (2), 209–219.

Tallquist, M.D., Yun, T.J. & Pease, L.R. (1996): A single T-cell receptor recognizes structurally distinct MHC/peptide complexes with high specificity. *J. Exp. Med.* **184**, 1017–1026.

Tanowitz, H.B., Kirchhoff, L.V., Simon, D., Morris, S.A., Weiss, L.M. & Wittner M. (1992): Chagas' disease. *Clin. Microbiol. Rev.* **5** (4), 400–419.

Tian, J., Lehmann, P.V. & Kaufman, D.L. (1994): T-cell cross-reactivity between coxsackie virus and glutamate decarboxylase is associated with a murine diabetes susceptibility allele. *J. Exp. Med.* **180**, 1979–1984.

Tisch, R., Yang, X.D., Singer, S.M., Liblau, R.S., Fugger, L. & McDevitt, H.O. (1993): Immune response to glutamic acid decarboxylase correlates with insulitis in non-obese diabetic mice. *Nature* **366** (6450), 72–75.

Tourne, S., Miyazaki, T., Oxenius, A., Klein, L., Fehr, T., Kyewski, B., Benoist C. & Mathis, D. (1997): Selection of a broad repertoire of CD4$^+$ T-cells in H-2Ma0/0 mice. *Immunity* **7** (2), 187–195.

Townsend, A.R.M., Rothbard, J., Gotch, F.M. *et al.* (1986): The epitopes of influenza nucleoprotein recognized by cytotoxic T-lymphocytes can be defined with short synthetic peptides. *Cell* **44**, 959–968.

van der Zee, R., Anderton, S.M., Prakken, A.B., Liesbeth Paul, A.G. & van Eden, W. (1998): T-cell responses to conserved bacterial heat-shock-protein epitopes induce resistance in experimental autoimmunity. *Semin. Immunol.* **10** (1), 35–41.

van Eden, W., Hogervorst, E.J., Hensen, E.J., van der Zee, R., van Embden, J.D. & Cohen, I.R. (1989): A cartilage-mimicking T-cell epitope on a 65K mycobacterial heat-shock protein: adjuvant arthritis as a model for human rheumatoid arthritis. *Curr. Topics Microbiol. Immunol.* **145**, 27–43.

Wallin, J., Hillert, J., Olerup, O., Carlsson, B. & Strom, H. (1991): Association of rheumatoid arthritis with a dominant DR1/Dw4/Dw14 sequence motif, but not with T-cell receptor beta chain gene alleles or haplotypes. *Arthritis Rheum.* **34** (11), 1416–1424.

Wilbrink, B., Holewijn, M., Bijlsma, J.W., van Roy, J.L., den Otter, W. & van Eden, W. (1993): Suppression of human cartilage proteoglycan synthesis by rheumatoid synovial fluid mononuclear cells activated with mycobacterial 60-kd heat-shock protein. *Arthritis Rheum.* **36** (4), 514–518.

Windhagen, A., Scholz, C., Hollsberg, P., Fukaura, H., Sette, A. & Hafler, D.A. (1995): Modulation of cytokine patterns of humans autoreactive T-cell clones by a single aminoacid substitution of their peptide ligand. *Immunity* **2**, 373–380.

Wucherpfenning, K.W & Strominger, J.L. (1995): Molecular mimicry in T-cell-mediated autoimmunity: viral peptides activate human T-cell clones specific for myelin basic protein. *Cell* **80**, 695–705.

Zinkernagel, R.M. (1996): Immunology taught by viruses. *Science* **271**, 173–178.

Zinkernagel, R.M. (2000): Localization dose and time of antigens determine immune reactivity. *Semin. Immunol.* **12**, 163–171.

Zinkernagel, R.M. & Doherty, P.C. (1974): Restriction of *in vitro* T-cell-mediated cytotoxicity in lymphocytic choriomeningitis. *Nature* **248**, 701–702.

Chapter 2

Interaction between immune system and central nervous system: peculiar aspects and relevance for the pathogenesis of immune-mediated diseases of the central nervous system

Renato Mantegazza and Pia Bernasconi

Myopathology & Immunology Unit, Department of Neuromuscular Diseases, Istituto Nazionale Neurologico 'C. Besta', via Celoria 11, 20133 Milan, Italy

Summary

The central nervous system is frequently the target of immune-mediated reactions which may have an autoimmune or an infectious aetiology. For many years the central nervous system has been considered an immune privileged site because of the presence of the blood-brain barrier. The recent great improvement in the understanding of the basic functions of the immune system has considerably expanded our knowledge on how the effector or regulatory cells of the immune system interact with the cells or the structures of the central nervous system. Here, we review the particular and peculiar interactions between T-lymphocytes and glial cells of the central nervous system; specifically, we focused on the expression of major histocompatibility complex and accessory molecules by glial cells residing in the central nervous system, on their ability to behave as antigen-presenting cells, on their ability to express soluble factors such as cytokines and chemokines, and on the possible relevance of this information for the understanding of the immunopathology of the diseases of the central nervous system.

The central nervous system (CNS) is considered an immune privileged site since alloengraftment within CNS induced a poor alloreactivity (Barker & Billingham, 1977). Several elements contribute to maintaining this characteristic: (a) tight endothelial junctions of the blood-brain barrier (BBB); (b) lack or low expression of proteins of the immune system [major histocompatibility complex (MHC) class I and II, co-stimulatory and accessory molecules] on cells of the CNS (glial cells, neurons, astrocytes); (c) lack of lymphatic drainage. The BBB is relatively impermeable to proteins, ions, small peptides and aminoacids. The selective permeability of the barrier is due to the interactions between microvessel endothelial cells and the underlying basement membrane and associated cells, as smooth muscle/pericytes and astrocytes (Fabry et al., 1994). Tight junctions, present in the endothelial cells, possess an extremely high electrical resistance, thus limiting the paracellular diffusion. Moreover, the brain endothelial cells possess a relatively slow rate of fluid-phase endocytosis, limiting the transcellular influx, while pericytes possess a high phagocytic capacity (Fabry et al., 1994). The BBB is considered a stringent gatekeeper for haematopoietic cells, e.g. naïve T-cells – cells that have never been stimulated – do not cross the barrier. Nevertheless, inflammatory processes or autoimmune diseases involve the CNS, often leading to irreversible neurological impairment; activated, but not resting, T-lymphocytes can cross the BBB (Wekerle et al., 1986; Wekerle, 1992); a lymphatic-like system is present in the brain; glial cells can behave as cells of the immune system in certain conditions. It has been demonstrated that, once activated against neurotrophic pathogens or CNS autoantigen in lymphoid organs, T-cells can readily cross the BBB and be restimulated by local antigen-presenting cells (APCs) which present on their surface the target antigen (Shrikant & Benveniste, 1996). However, it is not completely clear whether CNS cells can present the antigen to naïve T-lymphocytes within CNS or whether they sequester the antigens and then present them to already activated immune cells, which are migrated from the periphery into the brain.

In this chapter we will focus on the synthesis of the molecules, generally involved in an immune reaction, by the different cell populations present in the CNS, and on the functional capacity of CNS cells to act as APCs.

MHC and accessory molecule expression

There are two distinct types of APC: those with the capacity to initiate a primary immune response by presenting the antigen to naïve T-cells ['professional' APCs, e.g. dendritic cells (DC), the most potent APCs (Steinman, 1991)]; and those able to stimulate a secondary response presenting the antigen to already activated T-cells ('facultative' APCs) (Germain & Margulies, 1993). T-cell activation requires: (a) the interaction between T-cell receptor (TCR) and the antigen-MHC complex; (b) the cooperation in the intercellular adhesion between accessory molecules, such as intercellular adhesion molecule-1 (ICAM-1), and the corresponding receptors, such as leukocyte function-associated molecule 1 (LFA-1) (Springer et al., 1987); (c) the interaction between CD28 (a molecule expressed on T-surface) and B7.1 and B7.2 (termed as co-stimulatory molecules) expressed on target cells, which delivers the second signal necessary to activate T-cells, in particular naïve T-lymphocytes (Germain & Margulies, 1993; Reiser & Stadecker, 1996; Janeway & Bottomly, 1994). The cellular interactions between an APC and a T-cell and the immunological consequences are schematically illustrated in Fig. 1.

MHC class I molecules are constitutively expressed on all cell types, while MHC class II are expressed on professional or facultative APCs only after proper stimulation (Germain & Margulies, 1993). In normal brain, MHC class II molecules are readily detectable on smooth muscle cells of pericapillary arterioles and capillary pericytes (Pardridge et al., 1989). Moreover, MHC class II molecules are constitutively expressed on perivascular cells (Graeber et al., 1992), meninges and within the stroma of the choroid plexus (Matyszak et al., 1992). The perivascular macrophages are located close to the BBB and are considered the first cells that T-lymphocytes crossing the BBB encounter within the CNS. The constitutive expression of MHC class II is

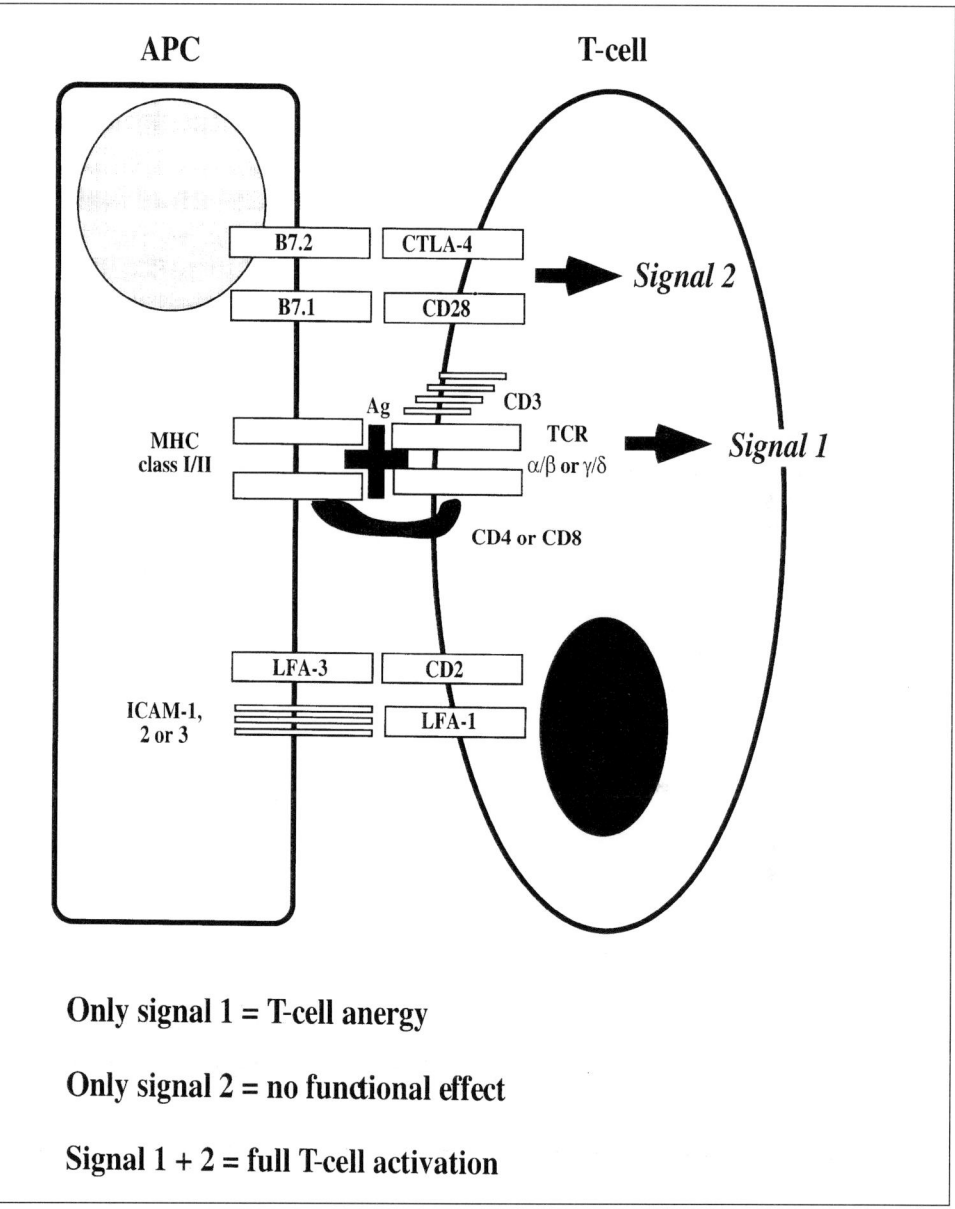

Fig. 1. Schematic representation of some of the cell surface molecules involved in antigen-presenting cell (APC)-T-cell interactions. The T-cell receptor (TCR), expressed on T-cell surface, recognizes specifically the antigenic peptide (Ag) bound to major histocompatibility complex (MHC) class I or class II molecule on APC and, together with CD4 or CD8 co-receptors, delivers the primary signal (Signal 1) which induces T-cell anergy, a reversible antiproliferative state. For a full T-cell activation, along with signal 1, a costimulatory signal (Signal 2) is necessary. This signal is provided by the interaction between CD28/CTLA-4, on T-cell surface, and B7.1/B7.2, on APC surface. Intercellular adhesion molecule (ICAM)-1, -2 and -3, leukocyte function-associated molecule (LFA)-1 and-3, CD2 are nonantigen-specific adhesion molecules, which stabilize the interaction between the T-cell and the APC, promoting T-cell activation by prolonging signal transduction events.

up-regulated by pro-inflammatory cytokines (Graeber *et al.*, 1992) or after injury (Streit *et al.*, 1989); however, the perivascular cells are continuously replaced by bone marrow-derived cells (Hickey *et al.*, 1992; Lassmann *et al.*, 1993) and it is not clear whether perivascular cells migrate to regional lymph node and prime T-cells (Perry, 1998; Aloisi *et al.*, 2000a). Perivascular macrophages are positive for B7.1 only after a proper stimulus (De Simone *et al.*, 1995), while no data on B7.2 expression are available.

MHC class II molecules are expressed on some microglia, particularly in human white matter (Aloisi *et al.*, 2000a). Resident microglia represent about 10 per cent of the non-neuronal cells in the CNS parenchyma (Lawson *et al.*, 1990) and, with astrocytes, are regularly distributed throughout the grey and white matter, constituting the main intraparenchymal cell type (Aloisi *et al.*, 2000a). Microglia, when activated by systemic delivery (Steiniger & van der Meide, 1988) or intracranial injection of pro-inflammatory cytokines, as interferon (IFN)-γ (Vass & Lassmann, 1990), become more readily positive for MHC class II molecules than other cells. In several CNS diseases, such as multiple sclerosis (MS), experimental allergic encephalomyelitis (EAE, an animal model which represents the effector phase of MS), AIDS dementia complex, Alzheimer's and Parkinson's diseases, a strong expression of MHC class II molecules can be observed on microglia (McGeer *et al.*, 1993; Dickson *et al.*, 1993; Hofman *et al.*, 1986). This induced phenotype together with the up-regulation of adhesion molecules, such as LFA-1 and ICAM-1, is typical of activated microglia (Kreutzberg, 1996). *In vitro* cultured microglia express low levels of B7/BB-1 but, when stimulated with IFN-γ or co-cultured with CD4$^+$ T-cells, become positive (Williams *et al.*, 1994; De Simone *et al.*, 1995; Satoh *et al.*, 1995). *In vivo* in sections of MS brain, B7/BB-1 expression was found on activated microglia in correspondence of the parenchymal lesions, on the perivascular cells and infiltrating monocytes (Williams *et al.*, 1994; De Simone *et al.*, 1995). These data suggest that microglia can play an important role in maintaining the immune response within CNS. This role is further supported by the observations that in EAE and in MS active lesions microglia is positive for CD40 expression (Carson *et al.*, 1998; Kreutzberg, 1996; Issazadeh *et al.*, 1998; Gerritse *et al.*, 1996) and co-localized with activated helper T-cells, positive for CD40 ligand (CD40L) expression. The interaction between CD40 and CD40L induces B-cell proliferation, differentiation and IgG production as well as cytokine production by APCs (Noelle, 1996). In EAE model treatment of mice with antibodies, anti-CD40L prevented development of the disease and suppressed clinical signs when treatment started after onset of the disease (Gerritse *et al.*, 1996), suggesting that CD40/CD40L interaction might play an important role in extravasation and accumulation of activated T-lymphocytes into target tissue/organ. Moreover, interfering in this interaction might provide a therapeutic approach to several CNS diseases.

In healthy parenchyma, expression of MHC class II and ICAM-1 on astrocytes, the major neuroectoderm-derived glial cell type and an important cellular component in the control of the specialization of the BBB endothelium (Girard & Springer, 1995), is almost undetectable (Weber *et al.*, 1994). Conversely, in MS lesions astrocytes present in the edges of demyelinated plaques are positive for MHC class II-DR and ICAM-1, suggesting that astrocytes may play a role in antigen presentation in pathological conditions. However, *in vitro* studies have demonstrated that incubation of astrocytes with pro-inflammatory stimuli [IFN-γ, tumour necrosis factor (TNF)-α, interleukin (IL)-1] up-regulates the expression of MHC class II, ICAM-1 and LFA-3 but not of B7/BB-1 molecules (Shrikant & Benveniste, 1996; Weber *et al.*, 1994; Williams *et al.*, 1994; Satoh *et al.*, 1995). These results indicate that astrocytes are only partially competent cells and that they may play a role only in secondary responses (Perry, 1998).

APC function in the CNS

Besides the analysis of the expression of molecules, antigen presentation has to be demonstrated functionally. Selected cells, isolated from tissue and treated or not with pro-inflammatory cytokines, must be able to stimulate T-cell lines in the presence of the specific antigen or in primary and secondary mixed lymphocyte reactions (MLR). Perivascular cells, CD45^{high} positive, isolated from adult rat brain, induce proliferation of T-cell lines and secretion of Th1-type cytokines (i.e. IL-2, IFN-γ, TNF-α) by stimulated T-cells (Ford *et al.*, 1995; Ford *et al.*, 1996). However, these cells are present in low number in the CNS and, thus, it is not known about the importance of perivascular cells in acting as APCs in pathological conditions (Aloisi *et al.*, 2000a).

Microglia can be isolated from newborn rodent and adult human brains and cultured *in vitro* in the presence of astrocytes. Microglia can be separated from other CNS cells, in particular from perivascular cells, by flow cytometric sorting on the basis of CD45 low expression (CD45^{low}) and MHC class II molecules positivity (Ford *et al.*, 1995). CD45^{low+} microglia weakly stimulate CD4$^+$ myelin basic protein (MBP)-specific T-lymphocytes and secrete low levels of IL-2 (Ford *et al.*, 1995; Carson *et al.*, 1998). When stimulated with IFN-γ, microglia can prime naïve T-cells and restimulate memory T-cells specific for viral or bacterial antigens (Williams *et al.*, 1993; Dhib-Jalbut *et al.*, 1996). To better understand the contribution of local and recruited cells within CNS in stimulating and maintaining the activated state of intracerebral T-cells, recent studies have compared the APC activity of microglia and astrocytes with that of DC and B-cells, the 'professional' APCs. Microglia, isolated from neonatal mouse brain and pre-treated with IFN-γ, were able to activate naïve CD4$^+$ T-cells, to induce secretion of IL-2 and IFN-γ from naïve T-cells, to promote the maturation of CD4$^+$ naïve T-cells into Th1, but not Th2, cells and to restimulate Th1/Th2 lymphocytes. The efficiency of all these functions was lower than that exerted by DC but higher than that of large and small B-cells and astrocytes; this suggests that activated microglia may effectively contribute to Th1 response leading to CNS inflammation and tissue damage (Aloisi *et al.*, 1999a).

Preactivated T-cells seem to be important in inducing maturation of resting microglia into competent APCs. In a rat model, in which the expression of MHC class II molecules on microglia has been induced by systemic graft versus host disease (GVHD), after infiltration in the CNS of T-cell blasts, microglia proliferate, become CD45^{high+}/MHC class II$^+$, process the antigen, induce IFN-γ and TNF-α secretion by T-cell lines but do not express B7.1-B7.2 molecules, do not induce T-cell proliferation and IL-2 secretion. On the contrary, T-cells in the presence of activated microglia undergo apoptosis, suggesting that microglia may act to protect the brain from the immune attack and to ensure a rapid elimination of infiltrating lymphocytes (Ford *et al.*, 1996; Sedgwick *et al.*, 1998).

Cocultures of resting microglia acutely isolated from adult mouse CNS, with Th1 and Th2 cell lines from transgenic mice where 95–100 per cent of CD4$^+$ T-cells were Vβ8.1.2$^+$ and express a TCR specific for ovalbumin peptide 323-339 presented by MHC I-A^d, demonstrated that microglia interact directly with Th1, but not Th2 cells. Th1-derived IFN-γ up-regulated APC molecules on microglia and induced maturation of microglia into an APC capable of T-cell restimulation (Aloisi *et al.*, 2000b). Altogether these data suggest that CNS infiltrating Th1 cells, already activated in the periphery and recognizing viral or self-antigens expressed in the brain, may induce local resting microglia to mature into competent APCs and to sustain CD4$^+$ T-cell responses within CNS.

Other soluble factors present in CNS microenvironment seem to influence microglia APC activity: local ion fluxes, secretion of neurotransmitters, as neurotrophins, and neuronal damage seem to be involved in the regulation of MHC class II expression (Neumann & Wekerle, 1998). Astrocytes seem to play an important role in the regulation of microglia and T-cell activation and in T-cell apoptosis by secreting factors such as macrophage colony-stimulating factor (M-CSF), prostaglandin E_2 (PGE_2), transforming growth factor (TGF)-β and granulocyte-macrophage CSF (GM-CSF) (Eddleston & Mucke, 1993; Streit *et al.*, 1999; Hailer *et al.*, 1998; Matsumoto *et al.*, 1993: Meinl *et al.*, 1994). Recent studies on factors promoting microglia maturation have demonstrated that GM-CSF, secreted also by T-cells, increased the capacity of microglia to activate Th1, but not Th2, cells without enhancing MHC class II, CD40 and ICAM-1 expression, indicating that GM-CSF render microglia more responsive to Th1-derived signals without inducing on microglia an APC phenotype (Aloisi *et al.*, 2000b). Altogether, these data indicate that CNS microenvironment has a potent influence on resident cell populations and their capacity to initiate or sustain an immune response.

Data on APC activity of astrocytes are conflicting: cytokine-treated astrocytes can act as inefficient or efficient APCs in processing the antigen, in stimulating naïve or primed T-lymphocytes and in releasing cytokines, such as IL-12. The discrepancy depends on the source of astrocytes, neonatal or adult brains, the use of immortalized astrocyte cell lines or astrocyte cultures contaminated by microglia, the type of responding cells, Th1 versus Th2 (Williams *et al.*, 1993; Aloisi *et al.*, 1998; Matsumoto *et al.*, 1993; Aloisi *et al.*, 1999a; Fontana *et al.*, 1984; Meinl *et al.*, 1994; Nikcevich *et al.*, 1997; Soos *et al.*, 1998). It has been demonstrated that astrocytes, in the presence of a specific peptide, activate Th2 cells with an equal efficiency to that demonstrated by microglia, suggesting that astrocytes have a defective antigen processing machinery and may restimulate Th2 cells only in the presence of peptides obtained during CNS damage (Aloisi *et al.*, 1998).

Cytokine and chemokine expression

T-lymphocyte features (proliferation, phenotype differentiation and Th1 versus Th2 typing) depend on cytokine production, as IL-1, IL-2, IL-4, IL-6, IL-10, IFN-γ, TNF-α etc. (Paul & Seder, 1994). Cytokines are soluble peptides released by cells of the immune system and by many other cell types, that bind high-affinity receptors expressed on target cells and induce biochemical signals within those cells (for review see Hohlfeld, 1997). IL-1α and IL-1β, the best characterized cytokines within CNS, produced by astrocytes, are able to alter neuroendocrine activity, slow-wave sleep and induce fever (Gwosdow *et al.*, 1990; Malipiero *et al.*, 1990). TNF-α is a critical inflammatory cytokine which stimulates the release of IL-1 and other cytokines, induces and enhances the expression of adhesion molecules on endothelial cells, thus influencing leukocyte traffic within the inflamed area (for review see Hohlfeld, 1997). Transgenic mice expressing mutant transmembrane TNF on astrocytes, but not neurons, develop chronic CNS inflammation (Akassoglou *et al.*, 1997). TNF-α is associated with $CD3^+$ T-cells, microglia and astrocytes in MS lesions and it is cytotoxic for oligodendrocytes *in vitro* (Hohlfeld, 1997). IL-12, an heterodimeric protein composed by two chains, p35 and p40, plays an crucial role in cell-mediated immune responses (Gately *et al.*, 1998). Recently, it has been demonstrated that IL-12 is important in inducing a protective immune response against neurotropic viruses (Bi *et al.*, 1995) and in the immunopathology of CNS induced by viruses (Sato *et al.*, 1997). Upon CNS inflammation and, *in vitro*, upon antigen-dependent interaction with Th1, but not Th2 cell lines, microglia secrete IL-12. On the contrary astrocytes, in the same experimental conditions, do not secrete IL-12 but inhibit IL-12 production by *in vitro*-activated microglia (Aloisi *et al.*, 1999b). These data further support the role of astrocytes in regulating CNS inflammation.

Besides proinflammatory cytokines, during CNS inflammation anti-inflammatory cytokines can be produced. IL-10 and TGF-β have been found associated with astrocytes and activated microglia in EAE and MS lesions (Kennedy *et al.*, 1992; Aloisi *et al.*, 2000a). TGF-β has been demonstrated to have a wide ranging influence on glial response during and after CNS inflammation (Fabry *et al.*, 1994, 1995; Issazadeh *et al.*, 1998).

Chemokines are chemotactic cytokines that induce the directional migration of several cell types, including neutrophils, monocytes, T-lymphocytes, into immunologically active sites (Luster, 1998). The chemokines are divided into three families, which differ for the position of highly conserved cysteine aminoacid residues. The β-chemokines, or C-C chemokines due to the position of two cysteine residues adjacent to each other, together with the α-chemokines are the largest and best-characterized families, and function primarily as activators and chemoattractors of T- and B-lymphocytes and monocytes (Luster, 1998). MCP-1, as well as macrophage inflammatory protein (MIP)-1α, MIP-1β and RANTES, belong to the family of β-chemokines. Activated microglia produce MIP-1α, a potent chemoattractant of Th1 cells and a stimulator of Th1 response *in vitro* (Karpus & Kennedy, 1997). Astrocytes synthesize MCP-1, a β-chemokine which favours Th2 responses (Karpus & Kennedy, 1997), in chronic relapsing EAE and in MS lesions (Ransohoff, 1997).

Conclusions

Microglia, once activated to mature by the interaction with Th1 T-cells, by pathogens and CNS damage, together with perivascular macrophages can act as efficient APCs; once activated, microglia are also able to regulate a Th2 response, and together with astrocytes contribute to limit the intracerebral expansion of T-cells by inducing apoptosis of T-cells and by releasing anti-inflammatory factors, which down-regulate the expression of an APC phenotype on microglia. The balance between the activity of microglia, perivascular macrophages and astrocytes in the CNS parenchyma seems to be a crucial factor in initiating and maintaining the inflammation state within CNS.

References

Akassoglou, K., Probert, L., Kontogeorgos, G. & Kollias, G. (1997): Astrocyte-specific but not neuron-specific transmembrane TNF triggers inflammation and degeneration in the central nervous system of transgenic mice. *J. Immunol.* **158**, 438–445.

Aloisi, F., Ria, F., Penna, G. & Adorini, L. (1998): Microglia are more efficient than astrocytes in antigen processing and in Th1 but not Th2 cell activation. *J. Immunol.* **160**, 4671–4680.

Aloisi, F., Ria, F., Columba-Cabezas, S., Hess, H., Penna, G. & Adorini, L. (1999a): Relative efficiency of microglia, astrocytes, dendritic cells and B-cells in naive CD4+ T-cell priming and Th1/Th2 cell restimulation. *Eur. J. Immunol.* **29**, 2705–2714.

Aloisi, F., Penna, G., Polazzi, E., Minghetti, L. & Adorini, L. (1999b): CD40-CD154 interaction and IFN-γ are required for IL-12 but not prostaglandin E_2 secretion by microglia during antigen presentation to Th1 cells. *J. Immunol.* **162**, 1384–1391.

Aloisi, F., Ria, F. & Adorini, L. (2000a): Regulation of T-cell response by CNS antigen-presenting cells: different roles for microglia and astrocytes. *Immunol. Today* **21**, 141–147.

Aloisi, F., De Simone, R., Columba-Cabezas, S., Penna, G. & Adorini, L. (2000b): Functional maturation of adult mouse resting microglia into an APC is promoted by granulocyte-macrophage colony-stimulating factor and interaction with Th1 cells. *J. Immunol.* **164,** 1705–1712.

Barker, C.F. & Billingham, R.E. (1977): Immunologically privileged sites. *Adv. Immunol.* **25,** 1–54.

Bi, Z., Quandt, P., Komatsu, T., Barna, M. & Reiss, C.S. (1995): IL-12 promotes enhanced recovery from vesicular stomatitis virus infection of the central nervous system. *J. Immunol.* **155,** 5684–5689.

Carson, M.J., Reilly, C.R., Sutcliffe, J.G. & Lo, D. (1998): Mature microglia resemble immature antigen-presenting cells. *Glia* **22,** 72–85.

De Simone, R., Giampaolo, A., Giometto, B., Gallo, P., Levi, G., Peschle, C. & Aloisi, F. (1995): The costimulatory molecule B7 is expressed on human microglia in culture and in multiple sclerosis acute lesions. *J. Neuropathol. Exp. Neurol.* **54,** 175–187.

Dhib-Jalbut, S., Gogate, N., Jiang, H., Eisenberg, H. & Bergey, G. (1996): Human microglia activate lymphoproliferative responses to recall viral antigens. *J. Neuroimmunol.* **65,** 67–73.

Dickson, D.W., Lee, S.C., Mattiace, L.A., Yen, S.-H. & Brosnan C. (1993): Microglia and cytokines in neurological disease, with special reference to AIDS and Alzheimer's disease. *Glia* **7,** 75–83.

Eddleston, M. & Mucke, L. (1993): Molecular profile of reactive astrocytes – implications for their role in neurologic disease. *Neuroscience* **54,** 15–36.

Fabry, Z., Raine, C.S. & Hart, M.N. (1994): Nervous tissue as an immune compartment: the dialect of the immune response in the CNS. *Immunol. Today* **15,** 218–224.

Fabry, Z., Topham, D.J., Fee, D., Herlein, J., Carlino, J.A., Hart, M.N. & Sriram, S. (1995): TGF-beta 2 decreases migration of lymphocytes *in vitro* and homing of cells into the central nervous system *in vivo*. *J. Immunol.* **155,** 325–332.

Fontana, A., Fierz, W. & Wekerle, H. (1984): Astrocytes present myelin basic protein to encephalitogenic T-cell lines. *Nature* **307,** 273–275.

Ford, A.L., Goodsall, A.L., Hickey, W.F. & Sedgwick, J.D. (1995): Normal adult ramified microglia separated from other central nervous system macrophages by flow cytometric sorting. Phenotypic differences defined and direct *ex vivo* antigen presentation to myelin basic protein-reactive CD4[+] T-cells compared. *J. Immunol.* **154,** 4309–4321.

Ford, A.L., Foulcher, E., Lemkert, F.A. & Sedgwick, J.D. (1996): Microglia induce CD4 T-lymphocyte final effector function and death. *J. Exp. Med.* **184,** 1737–1745.

Gately, M.K., Renzetti, L.M., Magram, J., Stern, A.S., Adorini, L., Gubler, U. & Presky, D.H. (1998): The interleukin-12/interleukin-12 receptor system: role in normal and pathologic immune responses. *Annu. Rev. Immunol.* **16,** 495–521.

Germain, R.N. & Margulies, D.H. (1993): The biochemistry and cell biology of antigen processing and presentation. *Annu. Rev. Immunol.* **11,** 403–450.

Gerritse, K., Laman, J.D., Noelle, R.J., Aruffo, A., Ledbetter, J.A., Boersma, W.J.A. & Claassen, E. (1996): CD40-CD40 ligand interactions in experimental allergic encephalomyelitis and multiple sclerosis. *Proc. Natl. Acad. Sci. USA* **93,** 2499–2504.

Girard, J-P. & Springer, T.A. (1995): High endothelial venules (HEVs): specialized endothelium for lymphocyte migration. *Immunol. Today* **16,** 449–457.

Graeber, M.B., Streit, W.J., Buringer, D., Sparks, D.L. & Kreutzberg, G.W. (1992): Ultrastructural location of major histocompatibility complex (MHC) class II perivascular cells in histologically normal human brain. *J. Neuropathol. Exp. Neurol.* **51,** 303–311.

Gwosdow, A.R., Kumar, M.S. & Bode, H.H. (1990): Interleukin-1 stimulation of the hypothalamic-pituitary-adrenal axis. *Am. J. Physiol.* **258,** E65-E70.

Hailer, N.P., Heppner, F.L., Haas, D. & Nitsch, R. (1998): Astrocytic factors deactivate antigen-presenting cells that invade the central nervous system. *Brain Pathol.* **8,** 459–474.

Hickey, W.F., Vass, K. & Lassmann, H. (1992): Bone marrow-derived elements in the central nervous system: an immunohistochemical and ultrastructural survey of rat chimeras. *J. Neuropathol. Exp. Neurol.* **51**, 246–256.

Hofman, F.M., von Hanwehr, R.I., Dinarello, C.A., Mizel, S.B., Hinton, D. & Merrill, J.E. (1986): Immunoregulatory molecules and IL 2 receptors identified in multiple sclerosis brain. *J. Immunol.* **136**, 3239–3245.

Hohlfeld, R. (1997): Biotechnological agents for the immunotherapy of multiple sclerosis. Principles, problems and perspectives. *Brain* **120**, 865–916.

Issazadeh, S., Navikas, V., Schaub, M., Sayegh, M. & Khoury, S. (1998): Kinetics of expression of costimulatory molecules and their ligands in murine relapsing experimental autoimmune encephalomyelitis *in vivo*. *J. Immunol.* **161**, 1104–1112.

Janeway, C.A. & Bottomly, K. (1994): Signals and signs for lymphocyte responses. *Cell* **76**, 275–285.

Karpus, W.J. & Kennedy, J.K. (1997): MIP-1α and MCP-1 differentially regulate acute and relapsing autoimmune encephalomyelitis as well as Th1/Th2 lymphocyte differentiation. *J. Leukoc. Biol.* **62**, 681–687.

Kennedy, M.K., Torrance, D.S., Picha, K.S. & Mohler, K.M. (1992): Analysis of cytokine mRNA expression in the central nervous system of mice with experimental autoimmune encephalomyelitis reveals that IL-10 mRNA expression correlates with recovery. *J. Immunol.* **149**, 2496–2505.

Kreutzberg, G.W. (1996): Microglia: a sensor for pathological events in the CNS. *Trends Neurosci.* **19**, 312–318.

Lassmann, H., Schmied, M., Vass, K. & Hickey, W.F. (1993): Bone marrow-derived elements and resident microglia in brain inflammation. *Glia* **7**, 19–24.

Lawson, L.J., Perry, V.H., Dri, P. & Gordon, S. (1990): Heterogeneity in the distribution and morphology of microglia in the normal adult mouse brain. *Neuroscience* **39**, 151–170.

Luster, A.D. (1998): Chemokines. Chemotactic cytokines that mediate inflammation. *N. Engl. J. Med.* **338**, 436–445.

Malipiero, U.V., Frei, K. & Fontana, A. (1990): Production of hemopoietic colony-stimulating factors by astrocytes. *J. Immunol.* **144**, 3816–3821.

Matsumoto, Y. Hanawa, H., Tsuchida, M. & Abo, T. (1993): In situ inactivation of infiltrating T-cells in the central nervous system with autoimmune encephalomyelitis. The role of astrocytes. *Immunology* **79**, 381–390.

Matyszak, M.K., Lawson, L.J., Perry, V.H. & Gordon, S. (1992): Stromal macrophages of the choroid plexus situated at an interface between the brain and peripheral immune system constitutively express major histocompatibility class II antigens. *J. Neuroimmunol.* **40**, 173–181.

McGeer, P.L., Kawamata, T., Walker, D.G., Akiyama, H., Tooyama, I. & McGeer, E.G. (1993): Microglia in degenerative neurological disease. *Glia* **7**, 84–92.

Meinl, E., Aloisi, F., Ertl, B., Weber, F., de Waal Malefyt, R., Wekerle, H. & Hohlfeld, R. (1994): Multiple sclerosis. Immunomodulatory effects of human astrocytes on T-cells. *Brain* **117**, 1323–1332.

Neumann, H. & Wekerle, H. (1998): Neuronal control of the immune response in the central nervous system: linking brain immunity to neurodegeneration. *J. Neuropathol. Exp. Neurol.* **57**, 1–9.

Nikcevich, K.M., Gordon, K.B., Tan, L., Hurst, S.D., Kroepfl, J.F., Gardinier, M., Barratt, T.A. & Miller, S.D. (1997): IFN-γ activated primary murine astrocytes express B7 costimulatory molecules and prime naive antigen-specific T-cells. *J. Immunol.* **158**, 614–621.

Noelle, R.J. (1996): CD40 and its ligand in host defense. *Immunity* **4**, 415–419.

Pardridge, W.M., Yang, J., Buciak J. & Tourtellotte, W.W. (1989): Human brain microvascular DR-antigen. *J. Neurosci. Res.* **23**, 337–341.

Paul, W.E. & Seder, R.A. (1994): Lymphocyte responses and cytokines. *Cell* **76**, 241–251.

Perry, V.H. (1998): A revised view of the central nervous system microenvironment and major histocompatibility complex class II antigen presentation. *J. Neuroimmunol.* **90**, 113–121.

Ransohoff, R.M. (1997): Chemokines in neurological disease models: correlation between chemokine expression patterns and inflammatory pathology. *J. Leukoc. Biol.* **62,** 645–652.

Reiser, H. & Stadecker, M.J. (1996): Costimulatory B7 molecules in the pathogenesis of infectious and autoimmune diseases. *N. Engl. J. Med.* **335,** 1369–1377.

Sato, S., Reiner, S.L., Jensen, M.A. & Roos, R.P. (1997): Central nervous system cytokine mRNA expression following Theiler's murine encephalomyelitis virus infection. *J. Neuroimmunol.* **76,** 213–223.

Satoh, J., Lee, Y.B. & Kim, S.U. (1995): T-cell costimulatory molecules B7-1 (CD80) and B7-2 (CD86) are expressed in human microglia but not in astrocytes in culture. *Brain Res.* **704,** 92–96.

Sedgwick, J.D., Ford, A.L., Foulcher, E. & Airriess, R. (1998): Central nervous system microglia cell activation and proliferation follows direct interaction with tissue-infiltrating T-cell blasts. *J. Immunol.* **160,** 5320–5330.

Shrikant, P. & Benveniste, E.N. (1996): The central nervous system as an immunocompetent organ: role of glial cells in antigen presentation. *J. Immunol.* **157,** 1819–1822.

Soos, J.M., Morrow, J., Ashley, T.A., Szente, B.E., Bikoff, E.K. & Zamvil, S.S. (1998): Astrocytes express elements of the class II endocytic pathway and process central nervous system autoantigen for presentation to encephalitogenic T-cells. *J. Immunol.* **16,** 5959–5966.

Springer, T.A., Dustin, M.L., Kishimoto, T.H. & Marlin, S.D. (1987): The lymphocyte function-associated LFA-1, CD2 and LFA-3 molecules: cell adhesion receptors of the immune system. *Annu. Rev. Immunol.* **5,** 223–252.

Steiniger, B. & van der Meide, P.H. (1988): Rat ependyma and microglia cells express class II MHC antigens after intravenous infusion of recombinant gamma interferon. *J. Neuroimmunol.* **19,** 111–118.

Steinman, R.M. (1991): The dendritic cell system and its role in immunogenicity. *Annu. Rev. Immunol.* **9,** 271–296.

Streit, W.J., Graeber, M.B. & Kreutzberg, G.W. (1989): Expression of Ia antigen on perivascular and microglial cells after sublethal and lethal motor neuron injury. *Exp. Neurol.* **105,** 115–126.

Streit, W.J., Walter, S.A. & Pennell, N.A. (1999): Reactive microgliosis. *Prog. Neurobiol.* **57,** 563–581.

Vass, K. & Lassmann, H. (1990): Intrathecal application of interferon gamma. Progressive appearance of MHC antigens within the rat nervous system. *Am. J. Pathol.* **137,** 789–800.

Weber, F., Meinl, E., Aloisi, F., Nevinny-Stickel, C., Albert, E., Wekerle, H. & Hohlfeld, R. (1994): Human astrocytes are only partially competent antigen-presenting cells. Possible implications for lesion development in multiple sclerosis. *Brain* **117,** 59–69.

Wekerle, H., Linington, C., Lassmann, H. & Meyermann, R. (1986): Cellular immune reactivity within the CNS. *Trends Neurosci.* **9,** 271–277.

Wekerle, H. (1992): Myelin specific, autoaggressive T-cell clones in the normal immune repertoire: their nature and their regulation. *Int. Rev. Immunol.* **9,** 231–241.

Williams, K., Ulvestad, E., Cragg, L., Blain, M. & Antel, J.P. (1993): Induction of primary T-cell responses by human glial cells. *J. Neurosci. Res.* **36,** 382–390.

Williams, K., Ulvestad, E. & Antel, J.P. (1994): B7/BB-1 antigen expression on adult human microglia studied *in vitro* and *in situ*. *Eur. J. Immunol.* **24,** 3031–3037.

Chapter 3

Inflammatory immune-mediated disorders of the central nervous system

Lucia Angelini, Federica Zibordi, Marianna Bugiani and Nicoletta Milani

Department of Child Neurology, Istituto Nazionale Neurologico 'C. Besta', via Celoria 11, 20133 Milan, Italy

Summary

The inflammatory immune-mediated disorders of the central nervous system are a group of diseases caused by an inflammatory reaction, triggered by foreign or self-antigens, associated or not with demyelination. In spite of the historical concept of 'immune privilege' of the central nervous system, it is now established that antigen presentation to the brain by macrophages-microglia is similar to that of other tissues and that the blood-brain barrier can be crossed by activated T-cells. The peculiarity of the immunoresponse, however, explains why the immunologic events are relatively rare and confined to the central nervous system.

The clinical classification distinguishes between the immune-mediated disorders confined to the brain (multiple sclerosis, acute disseminated encephalomyelitis and related forms) and immune-mediated disorders secondary to systemic immunologic disease (central nervous system complications of connective tissue disease and vasculitis).

The group of the purely central nervous system-immunomediated diseases is the topic of this chapter, while the relationships between the main demyelinating disorders affecting children and multiple sclerosis are underlined. The pathogenetic conclusions call attention to the synergism of both cellular and humoral immune responses in determining the immune-mediated damage to the central nervous system.

Introduction

The disorders included in this definition are characterized by an inflammatory reaction of the central nervous system (CNS) with perivascular and/or parenchymal lymphomononuclear and oligoglial infiltrates, associated or not associated with perivascular demyelination (Aicardi, 1998).

The inflammatory reaction derives from an immunologic response to different antigens, some of which are foreign, in the autoimmune processes represented by CNS components. In both conditions, the immunological response itself, independently from the aetiology, is responsible for the neuronal damage and the therapeutic approach must therefore be targeted against it.

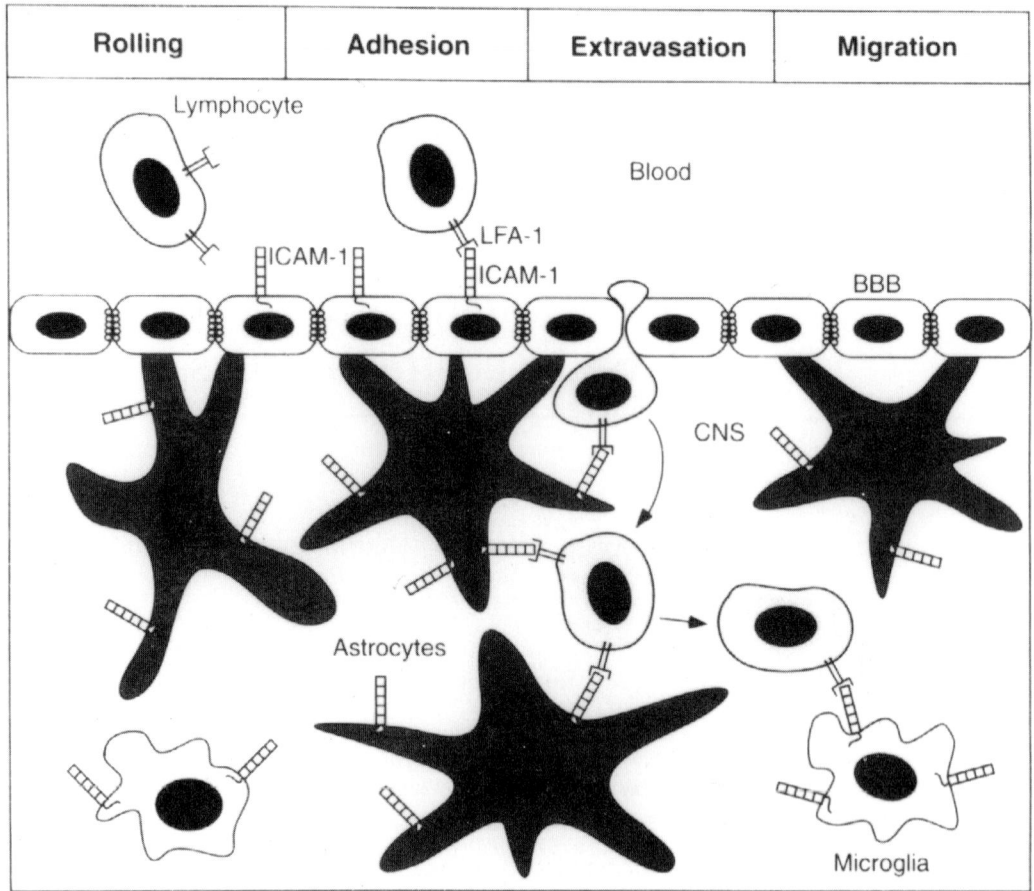

Fig. 1. T-cell migration through the BBB. [Reprinted from Trends in Neurosciences, *Vol. 19, Merrill J.E. & Benveniste E.N., Cytokines in inflammatory brain lesions: helpful and harmful, 331–338, copyright 1996, with permission from Elsevier Science.]*

This chapter will be divided in three parts: in the first one attention will be called to some basic aspects of the immunological response in the CNS; the second part will be devoted to the nosography; in the third, pathogenetic aspects will be briefly considered.

CNS antigen presentation

The knowledge of how and where antigen presentation occurs within the CNS may improve the understanding of pathogenetic mechanisms involved in the immunologic disorders confined to the CNS.

For antigen presentation to occur within the CNS there have to be both antigen-presenting cells (APC) and T-lymphocytes (T-cells) which can be specifically activated in the CNS parenchyma.

Microglia and resident macrophages have the requirements to be considered professional antigen-presenting cells: they express intrinsically or by induction the major histocompatibility complex (MHC) class II molecules plus a group of co-stimulatory molecules and have the

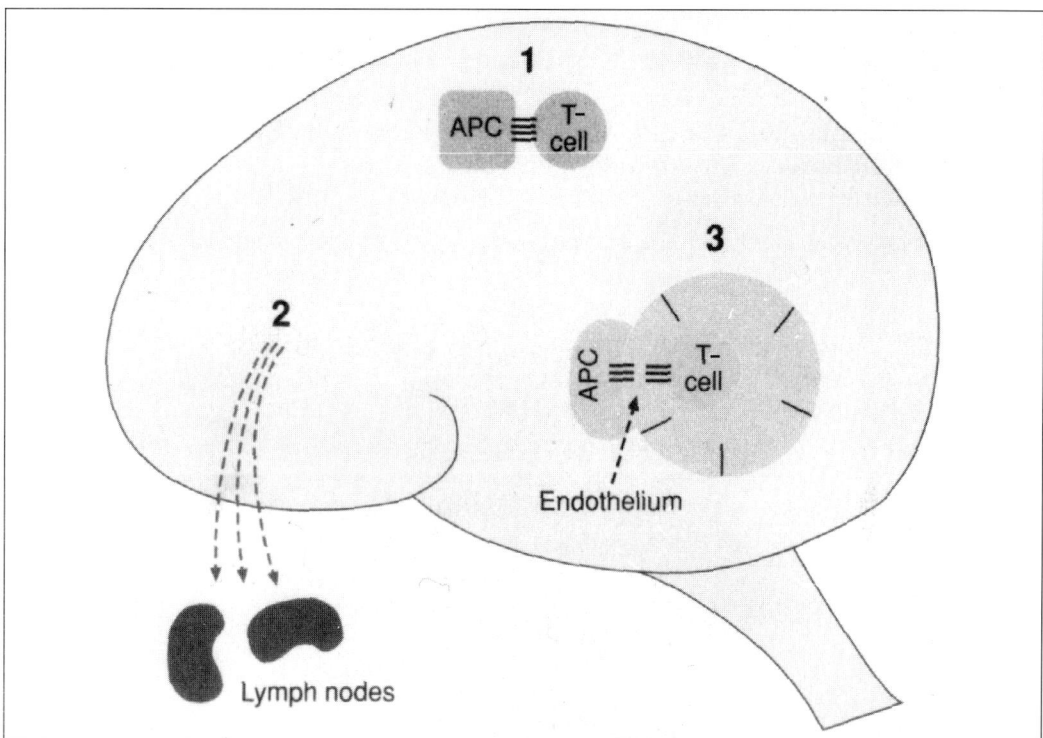

Fig. 2. Three possible ways that CNS antigens can be presented to T-cells. [Reprinted from Trends in Neurosciences, *Vol. 18, Hart M.N. & Fabry Z., CNS antigen presentation, 475–481,copyright 1995, with permission from Elsevier Science.]*

capability to process and present antigens *in vitro*. They represent the interfaces between the nervous and the immune systems (Kreutzberg, 1996).

T-cells previously activated cross the blood-brain barrier (BBB) and become reactivated in an antigen-specific manner (Fig. 1).

If presentation of antigens takes place in the brain, the macrophages, due to their strategic perivascular location between the venule and the parenchyma (the site regarded as the point of exit from vascular system for migrating leukocytes), are the best APC candidates (Fig. 2.3). Another possible way of antigen presentation is to be presented by a resident CNS APC, through the microvessel endothelium, to a specifically activated T-cell, which is wandering through the parenchyma (Fig. 2.1). Lastly, the occurrence of antigen presentation outside the CNS, in cervical lymph nodes, has been hypothesized (Fig. 2.2). This way of presentation is followed by transport of the CNS antigen through a lymphatic-like drainage system, recently described in humans. In this case effector T-cells would need to cross the BBB and encounter the antigen in a secondary recognition event.

Occurrences of CNS antigens inside and outside the CNS are likely not to be mutually exclusive (Hart & Fabry, 1995).

The concept of *immune privilege* was historically based on the following paradigms: (1) self or foreign antigen sequestration within the CNS; (2) lack of communication between CNS and the immune system; and (3) impossibility for the effector lymphocytes to cross the BBB. It is now well known that antigen presentation to CNS is common to that of other tissues. Under appropriate conditions, in fact, the immune system does react to CNS specific antigens and activated T-cells migrated into CNS parenchyma through the BBB (Archelos *et al.*, 1999).

However, the presence of peculiar APC, the restrictive properties of BBB and the possible dominance of suppressor mechanisms argue strongly for unique CNS antigen-presentation, with the consequence of relatively rare and confined immunological events in the brain.

As to potential antigens in the CNS which can trigger autoimmune demyelination, they may be myelin-associated (oligodendroglial) antigens including myelin basic protein, proteolipid protein, myelin-associated glycoproteins or astrocyte-associated proteins such as S-100. Furthermore, attention has been recently called to neuronal glutamate receptors as possible targets of autoimmune disease (Rogers *et al.*, 1994). Thus, the three most important neuroectodermal cells in the CNS (neurons, astrocytes and oligodendroglia) all have antigens potentially targeted in inflammatory-autoimmune diseases.

Non-endogenous antigens, such as numerous viruses (rubella, measles, varicella) might also elicit CNS autoimmune disease when presented under special circumstances.

Nosography

Several disorders may be included among the inflammatory immune-mediated conditions. The nosography proposed here distinguishes between immune-mediated disorders confined to the CNS and immune-mediated disorders secondary to systemic immunologic diseases.

Table 1. Immune-mediated neurologic disorders confined to the central nervous system

Multiple sclerosis (MS)
Acute disseminated encephalomyelitis and related disorders
• Acute disseminated encephalomyelitis (ADEM)   Uniphasic parainfectious or postvaccination inflammatory demyelinating disorder of the CNS
• Acute haemorrhagic leukoencephalitis   Hyperacute form of ADEM, occurring after respiratory infections, with more tissue-destructive pathology

• Site-restricted forms of uniphasic acute inflammatory demyelinating disorders that may occur after viral illness or vaccination
   Transverse myelitis
   Optic neuritis
   Cerebellitis
   Brainstem encephalitis

• Chronic or recurrent forms of parainfectious or postvaccination encephalomyelitis
   Subacute sclerosing panencephalitis
   Human immunodeficiency virus encephalopathy
   Rubella panencephalitis
   Protracted chronic encephalitis of unknown origin (? relationship with MS)

Disorders of presumed viral cause (Rasmussen's encephalitis)
Parainfectious of paraneoplastic disorders (opsoclonus-myoclonus syndrome)
Primary CNS vasculitis

Chapter 3   Inflammatory immune-mediated disorders of the central nervous system

The neurologic presentation depends on which component of CNS is predominantly or exclusively targeted by immune reaction: the myelin as in demyelinating diseases, neuronal parts as in rheumatic chorea and in myoclonic encephalopathy of Kinsbourne, or receptors as in Rasmussen's encephalitis according to recent pathogenetic hypotheses. Furthermore, the endothelium may be the target of the autoimmune process as in vasculitis and, with a different pathogenetic mechanism, in the antiphospholipid syndrome (Angelini *et al.*, 1994; Lie, 1996).

This chapter is dedicated to the group of the purely CNS immune diseases and particularly to demyelinating disorders. Their classification is reported in Tables 1 and 2.

Diseases involving CNS myelin may be classified as those in which normal myelin is disrupted, termed *demyelinating*, and in those in which a biochemical abnormality exists, termed *dysmyelinating* (Table 3).

Table 2. Immune-mediated neurologic disorders secondary to systemic immunopathologic disease

Secondary to rheumatic and connective tissue diseases
• Sydenham chorea
• Neurolupus
• Polyarteritis nodosa
• CNS complications of rheumatoid arthritis, Schoenlein-Henoch purpura and Kawasaki disease
Neurosarcoidosis
Neuro-Behçet
CNS involvement secondary to systemic vasculitis and antiphospholipid syndrome

Table 3. Diseases of myelin

Immune-mediated
Acute disseminated encephalomyelitis (ADEM)
Acute haemorrhagic leukoencephalopathy (AHLE)
Multiple sclerosis (MS)
Infectious
Progressive multifocal leukoencephalopathy (PML)
Toxic/metabolic
Carbon monoxide intoxication
Vitamin B_{12} deficiency
Mercury intoxication
Central pontine myelinolysis
Hypoxia
Radiation
Hereditary disorders of myelin metabolism
Adrenoleukodystrophy
Metachromatic leukodistrophy
Krabbe's disease
Alexander's disease
Canavan-van Bogaert disease
Van Der Knaap' disease
CACH (childhood ataxia with diffuse CNS hypomyelination)
Pelizaeus-Merzbacher disease
Phenylketonuria (PKU)

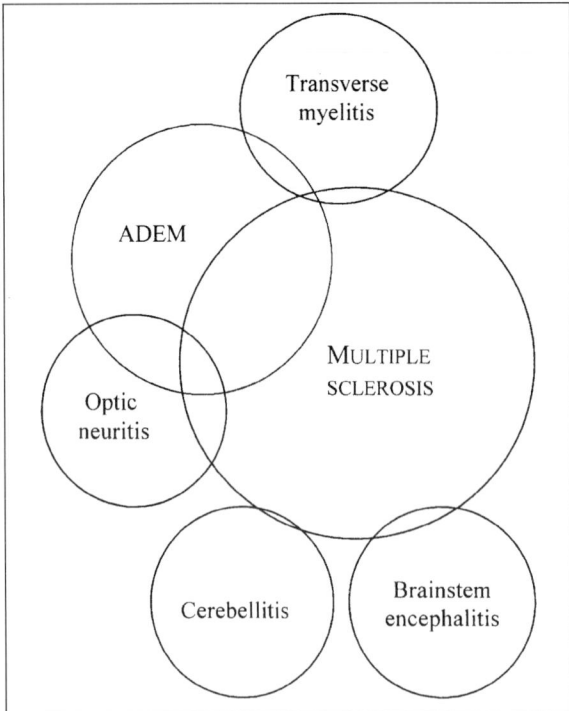

Fig. 3. Nosological relationships between multiple sclerosis and other demyelinating diseases of the central nervous system.

The knowledge of these different conditions is particularly important for the diagnostic approach to demyelinating diseases with onset in childhood.

Instead of treating singularly the demyelinating disease, we will focus on the relationships between each of them and multiple sclerosis (MS). Differential diagnosis in childhood in fact is often a challenge to the diagnostic and prognostic workup.

Figure 3 shows the parainfectious disease on the left, represented by acute disseminated encephalomyelitis (ADEM) and related disorders, such as site-restricted forms of uniphasic acute inflammatory demyelinating disease possibly due to viral illness or immunization. On the right MS is represented, differently overlapping with each disorder of the previous group.

In Table 4 MS and ADEM are compared and distinguished. The clinical aspects of ADEM will be extensively treated in the chapter on ADEM.

Table 4. Comparison and distinction between multiple sclerosis (MS) and acute disseminated encephalomyelitis (ADEM)

MS	ADEM
Both are inflammatory demyelinating diseases	
Prototype of inflammatory demyelinating disease, chronic, multiphasic	Acute, uniphasic
Immunogenetic predisposition triggered by additional factors due to environmental exposure	Association with systemic viral infection or immunization/vaccination. Immunogenetic predisposition has been hypothesized
Both are diseases of the CNS mediated by an aberrant immunoresponse	
Rare in childhood (2.5–5 per cent)	Frequent in childhood (?). More frequent than primary viral infections of CNS
Perivascular infiltration of T-cells, demyelination mediated by macrophages-microglia, and axonal loss	Perivascular inflammation and surrounding demyelination within the CNS

The differential diagnosis between MS and ADEM may be particularly difficult in cases of acute encephalomyelitis occurring in the background of unspecific viral illness, the so-called idiopathic forms. Diagnosis is also difficult when onset is atypic and the course is protracted or chronic-recurrent. On the basis of revised reported data (Francis *et al.*, 1996; Kesselring *et al.*,

1990) and according to the study of our patient population we have selected clinicoradiological and CSF criteria that could establish the differential diagnosis between MS and ADEM (Table 5).

Table 5. ADEM and MS

ADEM	MS
CLINICAL FEATURES	
Multifocal neurologic signs and symptoms involving the brain, spinal cord and optic nerve	Focal neurologic signs and symptoms
Optic neuritis, usually simultaneously bilateral	Unilateral optic neuritis
	Diplopia
Epileptic seizures	
Decreased tendon reflexes with retained abdominal reflexes and positive Babinski	Hyperactive tendon reflexes
Loss of consciousness	Preserved awareness
Shooting limb pains	
Headache	
Rapid recovery (days) possible recurrence for up to 18 months	Slow recovery (weeks), recurrence
CSF FINDINGS	
Mild pleiocytosis	
IgG band possible, but transient	IgG band persistent
MRI FINDINGS	
Extensive and relatively symmetric alterations in the cerebral and cerebellar white matter, and also in basal ganglia, all showing the same enhancing	Asymmetric, multifocal alterations in the white matter of variable size, showing a mixture of enhancing and non-enhancing
Appearance of new alterations within one month from the onset	
Resolution of alterations within 18 months without appearance of new lesions	Persistent visualization of abnormalities and appearance of new lesions
Rare persistence of life-long alterations	

Optic neuritis consists of inflammatory-demyelinating attack to the optic nerve with consequent impairment of function. Signs and symptoms are represented by unilateral or bilateral reduction of visual acuity sometime preceded by headache and/or painful eye movements. The blurred vision which characterizes onset rapidly progresses, within a few days, to partial or total blindness. From the ophthalmologic point of view the acute phase may be characterized either by retrobulbar neuritis (with normal fundoscopic examination) or by neuropapillitis (with swollen optic disc) which occurs in three quarters of children. Visual field examination reveals central scotomas, and the study of visual evoked potential demonstrates a delay which usually lasts longer than clinical symptoms.

Aetiology includes the following causes: parainfectious (measles, rubella, mumps), isolated or associated with ADE/ADEM; immunization; Miller-Fisher syndrome; first attack of MS.

The reported risk of MS after monosymptomatic episodes, based on clinical criteria, depends on:

- Age at onset: the risk ranges between 60–75 per cent in adults and 15–25 per cent in children.
- Unilateral involvement of the optic nerve has greater predictive risk of developing MS than bilateral involvement; the latter usually has good prognosis in children.
- MRI signal alterations in periventricular regions are indicative of a risk of developing MS and so are pleyocitosis and intrathecal IgG production.

Acute transverse myelitis consists of acute involvement of motor and sensory tracts on both sides on the spinal cord, often preceded by back pain and/or paraesthesias and more frequently by weakness and urinary retention. Fever and meningeal signs are also frequent.

Exclusion of cord compression (neoplasm, abscess, arterovenous malformation) is mandatory by mean of spinal MRI. Asymptomatic demyelinating lesions should be also ruled out by cerebral MRI.

Aetiology includes different causes: parainfectious (several viruses may be responsible: measles, mumps, rubella, varicella, influentia, HSV1 and 2, EBV, coxsackie; other infectious agents: Borrelia, mycoplasma pneumoniae); post immunization; primary infectious (HIV-HTLV); vascular (LES, APL syndrome); secondary to meningitis: sarcoidosis, Bchçct's syndrome.

The risk of MS after an acute transverse myelitis is cited as low (5–10 per cent) and particularly in childhood:

- Partial or incomplete myelitis bears more relevance to MS;
- Cranial MRI abnormalities and intrathecal IgG production may also be taken into account as to a higher risk of developing MS in respect to the absence of these findings.

Brainstem encephalitis. This disorder occurs in adolescents and young men while it is exceptional in childhood. It is characterized by subacute brainstem dysfunction (ophthalmoplegia, facial palsy, sensory loss, dysarthria, deafness and ataxia). Fever may be present.

Aetiology includes the following conditions: parainfectious syndromes and true viral infections (EBV in both conditions must be carefully considered in childhood; Angelini *et al.*, 2000); paraneoplastic syndromes; initial manifestation of MS (adult onset, acellular CSF with positive intrathecal IgG production are suggestive).

Cerebellitis consists of cerebellar dysfunction with sudden onset and time-relation with a specific varicella or aspecific viral infections. Cerebellitis is the most common restricted form of parainfectious CNS disease in children, commonly occurring during the second year of life.

Signs and symptoms consist of trunk ataxia and gait disturbances often associated with nystagmus (45 per cent of cases) and sometime with action tremor.

CSF pleiocytosis and late increase in protein content have been described. Recovery is usually

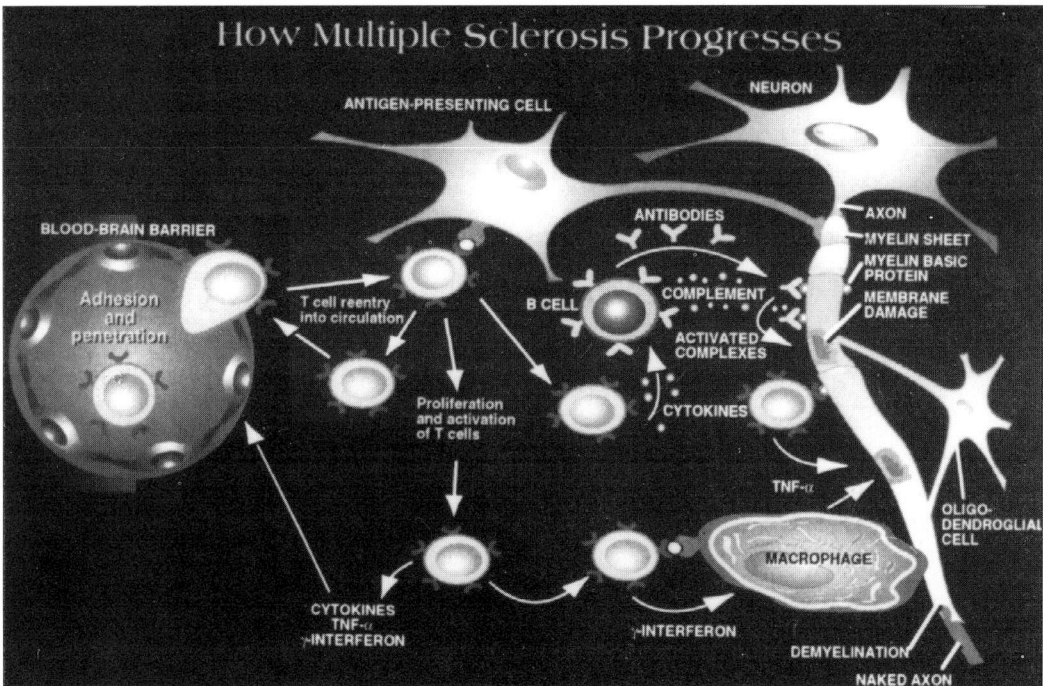

Fig. 4. A coordinated immunological attack against myelin in the central nervous system. [Reprinted from Cell, *Vol 85, Steiman L., Multiple sclerosis: a coordinated immunological attack against myelin in the central nervous system, 299–302, 1996: copyright is held by Cell Press.]*

spontaneous within a few weeks or months notwithstanding the possibility of residual cerebellar atrophy (25–30 per cent of children).

Aetiology includes parainfectious (varicella virus and other viruses of exanthematic illnesses) and possibly also true infectious conditions.

The relationship and even the overlapping of cerebellitis and opsoclonus-myoclonus syndrome as well as paraneoplastic syndrome must be stressed. In spite of the differences between these diseases both under the pathogenetic and clinical aspects, some common findings may be described:

- Both cerebellitis and opsoclonus-myoclonus syndrome may be related, in childhood, with a viral infection (EBV, coxsackie, enterovirus).
- Cerebellar ataxia may offer the clinical presentation of a neuroblastoma in children.
- Opsoclonus (or ocular flutter) may be the revealing symptom of a paraneoplastic cerebellar degeneration in adults (i.e. ovarian tumours, lung mycrocytoma with anti-YO and anti-HU autoantibodies) and it is the main symptom, together with myoclonus, of the typical paraneoplastic form of childhood, neuroblastoma.

Immunopathogenetic remarks

The aetiology of CNS demyelinating disorders remains enigmatic. Experimental autoimmune encephalomyelitis (EAE), the animal model of human disorders of CNS mediated by an aberrant immune response, is induced either by sensitization with a central myelin antigen or by intravenous injection of myelin-specific CD4 cells previously activated *in vitro*. In spite of its inadequacy to explain the clinical complexity of ADEM and particularly of MS, EAE is indispensable to investigation, and helps understand the basic mechanisms of the immune attack to the CNS. Its sequence may be schematically divided into an induction and an effector phase (Archelos *et al.*, 1999).

Induction phase: the injected autoantigen is presented to 'naïve' T-cells by professional APC, resulting in T-cell activation. The activated T-cells then circulate in the blood, attach to the endothelium in the CNS and cross the BBB.

Effector phase. The transendothelial migration gives rise to the effector phase. In the CNS the autoantigen is presented by microglia to T-cells. The reactivated CD4 cells amplify the immune response by recruiting further T-cells and macrophages by mean of chemokines and cytokines which determine the breakdown of the BBB. The passage of circulating autoantibodies is then allowed. Autoantibodies in all likelihood synergize with T-cells to initiate demyelination (Steinmann, 1996).

It must be underlined, for the therapeutic implications, that both cellular and humoral immune responses contribute to the complete expression of immune-mediated CNS damage.

References

Aicardi, J. (1998): Parainfectious and other inflammatory disorders of immunological origin. In: *Diseases of nervous system in childhood*, ed. J. Aicardi, pp. 438–459. London: MacKeith Press.

Angelini, L., Ravelli, A., Caporali, R., Rumi, V., Nardocci, N. & Martini A. (1994): High prevalence of antiphospholipid antibodies in children with idiopathic cerebral ischemia. *Pediatrics* **94**, 500–503.

Angelini, L., Bugiani, M., Zibordi, F., Bizzi, A. & Cinque, P. (2000). Brainstem encephalitis resulting from EBV mimicking an infiltrating tumor in a children. *Pediatr. Neurol.* **22**, 130–132.

Archelos, J.J., Previtali, S.C. & Hartung, H.-P. (1999): The role of integrins in immune-mediated disease of the nervous system. *Trends Neurosci.* **22**, 30–38.

Francis, G.S., Duquette, P. & Antel, J.P. (1996): Inflammatory demyelinating diseases of the central nervous system. In: *Neurology in clinical practice,* eds. W.G. Bradley, R.B. Daroff, G.M. Fenichel & C.D. Marsden, pp. 1307–1343. Boston: Butterworth-Heinemann.

Hart, M.N. & Fabry, Z. (1995): CNS antigen presentation. *Trends Neurosci.* **18**, 475–481.

Kesselring, J., Miller, D.H., Robb, S.A., Kendall, B.E., Moseley I.F., Kingsley D., Du Boulay, G.H. & McDonald, W.I. (1990): Acute disseminated encephalomyelitis. MRI findings and the distinction from multiple sclerosis. *Brain* **113**, 291–302.

Kreutzberg, G.W. (1996): Microglia: a sensor for pathological events in the CNS. *Trends Neurosci.* **19**, 312–318.

Lie, J.T. (1996): Angiitis of the central nervous system. In: *The vasculitides*, eds. B.M. Ansell, P.A. Bacon, J.T. Lie & H. Yazici, pp. 246–263. London: Chapman & Hall Medical.

Rogers, S.W., Andrews, P.I., Gahring, L.C., Whisenand, T., Cauley, K., Crain, B., Hughes, T.E., Heinemann, S.F. & McNamara, J.O. (1994): Autoantibodies to glutamate receptor GluR3 in Rasmussen's encephalitis. *Science* **265**, 648–651.

Steinman, L. (1996): Multiple sclerosis: a coordinated immunological attack against myelin in the central nervous system. *Cell* **85**, 299–302.

Chapter 4

Multiple sclerosis: a disease of many faces and many ages

Ari J. Green and Jorge R. Oksenberg

Department of Neurology, School of Medicine, University of California, San Francisco, CA 94143-0435, USA

Summary

A large body of immunologic, epidemiologic, and genetic data indicates that tissue injury in multiple sclerosis (MS) results from an abnormal immune response directed against one or more myelin antigens. The most widely accepted models propose that the disease develops in genetically susceptible individuals after exposure to an as-yet undefined causal agent. High incidence rates for this disorder are found in Scandinavia, Iceland, the British Isles and the countries settled by their descendants, where it is the leading cause of acquired neurological disability in young adults. However, because MS is considered a disease of young adults, it has probably been underdiagnosed in the paediatric population. It is estimated that one in ten MS patients develop clinical symptoms before 18, although their disease may initially go unrecognized.

A genetic component in MS is indicated by an increased relative risk to siblings compared to the general population, and an increased concordance rate in monozygotic compared to dizygotic twins. The past few years have seen real progress in defining the genetic basis of MS. Whole genome screens conducted in different populations identified discrete chromosomal regions potentially harbouring MS susceptibility genes, including the major histocompatibility complex (MHC) locus in chromosome 6p21. This has set the stage for the final characterization of the genes involved in MS susceptibility and pathogenesis. These results suggest a complex genetic aetiology, including multiple genes of small to moderate effect and probable genetic heterogeneity. The identification and characterization of MS susceptibility genes and their correlation with disease phenotypes is likely to define the basic aetiology of the disease, improve risk assessment and influence therapeutics.

Introduction

Multiple sclerosis (MS) is a common neuroinflammatory disorder, associated with an autoimmune response directed against myelin proteins within the central nervous system (CNS) (Table 1). Demyelination results in brain atrophy and impaired transmission of action potentials along exposed axons, producing a multiplicity of neurologic deficits such as sensory loss, weakness, visual loss, vertigo, incoordination, sphincter disturbances and altered cognition. MS pathogenesis is complex and multifactorial, with an underlying genetic susceptibility acting in concert with undefined environmental agents. MS is the most common cause of acquired neurological dysfunction arising in early and mid-adulthood. Prevalence rates in the Western hemisphere are 15–145/100,000 in the population. No curative therapy for MS is currently available, and approximately 90 per cent of afflicted individuals are ultimately disabled. The socio-economic consequences of this long-lasting disease are staggering, as 75–85 per cent of patients are eventually unemployed and at high risk for social isolation. MS is estimated to be the second most costly neurological disorder in the industrialized world (after Alzheimer's disease).

Table 1. Putative autoantigens in MS

Myelin basic protein (MBP)
Proteolipid protein (PLP)
Myelin oligodendrocyte glycoprotein (MOG)
Myelin-associated glycoprotein (MAG)
Heat shock proteins
β-arrestin and arrestin
Glial fibrillary acidic protein
Astrocyte-derived calcium-binding protein
Transaldolase

The disease is typically characterized by the rapid onset of neurological impairments followed by a period of clinical improvement with or without residual symptoms after the relapses (relapsing-remitting). After 10 years, about 50 per cent of the relapsing-remitting patients transition to a secondary progressive course, which is characterized by gradual progression of disability with or without superimposed relapses. The primary progressive course of MS involves about 10 per cent of patients, who experience gradual progression of disability from onset and never experience relapses. Fewer than 5 per cent of MS patients experience a primary progressive onset and later have exacerbations. This relatively uncommon pattern is called progressive relapsing MS.

Pathology

The pathological hallmark of MS is the plaque – a discrete area of demyelination that appears pink-gray on gross examination. In addition to the loss of myelin and oedema, plaques are histologically characterized by inflammation and gliosis (Hauser & Goodkin, 1998). MS patients frequently exhibit multiple plaques in an asymmetric distribution. However, their location does not appear random. They are preferentially located in the periventricular white matter, corpus callosum, optic nerves and tracts, corticomedullary junction and the cervical spinal cord. It has been recently recognized that MS plaques are heterogeneous in their structural and immunopathological patterns. In Asians for example, one form of MS ('Western-type') is characterized by disseminated CNS, whereas more restricted forms of disease in which optic nerve and or spinal cord involvement predominate ('Asian-type'), are frequently more severe and necrotizing than in the disseminated form (Kira et al., 1996).

Plaques are probably initiated by a breakdown in the blood-brain barrier (BBB) followed by the infiltration of T-cells activated in the periphery (Hauser et al., 1986; Kermode, 1990). A common finding in an acute plaque is T-cells and macrophages in a perivascular distribution (Raine, 1994). Lymphocytes activated in the periphery home to the CNS, become attached to receptors on endothelial cells, and then proceed to pass across the BBB, through the endothelium and the subendothelial basal lamina into the interstitial matrix. After traversing the BBB, pathogenic T-cells are reactivated by fragments of myelin antigens presented in the framework of MHC class II molecules on the surface of antigen-presenting cells (macrophages, microglia, and perhaps astrocytes). The high expression of MHC class II molecules in MS brains suggests that the local microenvironment may be enriched in MHC-activating factors such as interferon (IFN)-γ, and that antigen is possibly presented to T-cells (Bo et al., 1994; Sanders et al., 1993; Traugott, 1987). Reactivation induces release of proinflammatory cytokines and chemokines that further compromise the BBB and stimulate chemotaxis, resulting in a second larger wave of inflammatory cell recruitment and leakage of antibody and other plasma proteins into the nervous system. Pathogenic T-cells may not be capable of producing or inducing tissue injury in the absence of the secondary leukocyte recruitment (Sorensen & Ransohoff, 1998). Following the breach in the BBB, myelin appears to be the primary target of the pathogenic immune reaction (Lassman et al., 1994; Lucchinetti et al., 1998). The most convincing mechanisms of myelin damage involve (1) antibody binding and complement activation, (2) T-cell-mediated myelinosis secondary to the release of cytokines, (3) T-cell-directed cytolysis, and (4) macrophage/microglia activation followed by myelin phagocytosis and the release of toxic factors mediators – including free radicals (nitric oxide and superoxid anion), vasoactive amines, complement, proteases, cytokines (IL-1, TNF-α) and eicosanoids (Raine, 1994; Oksenberg & Hauser, 1999). Vesicular disruption of the myelin membrane is an early pathologic feature, a finding that can be simulated *in vitro* by the application of cytokines, autoantibodies, or calcium ionophores. As lesions evolve, axons traversing the plaque show marked irregular beading, astrocytes proliferate, and lipid-laden macrophages containing myelin debris become prominent. Progressive fibrillary gliosis ensues and mononuclear cells gradually disappear. In some MS lesions, proliferation of oligodendrocytes appears to be present initially, but these cells are apparently destroyed as the gliosis progresses. In chronic MS lesions, complete or nearly complete demyelination, dense gliosis (more severe than in most other neuropathologic conditions), and loss of oligodendroglia are all found. In some chronic active MS lesions, gradations in the histologic findings from the centre to the lesion edge suggest that lesions expand by concentric outward growth.

Preservation of axon cylinders in the presence of demyelination is characteristic, although this finding is relative rather than absolute; in approximately 10 per cent of lesions there is significant axonal destruction, and in rare cases, complete destruction of the neuropil and cavitation occur. Long-term disability has been correlated with the degree of axonal damage, and radiographic measures of neuronal loss (Mag transfer) may become the mainstay of assessing disease severity (De Stefano et al., 1998; Trapp et al., 1998). Oligodendrocytes are frequently conserved in an acute lesion and oligodendrocyte precursors sometimes appear to proliferate (Ozawa et al., 1994; Prineas et al., 1993; Wu & Raine, 1992). This probably underlies the early effort to remyelinate the stripped axons, as remyelination appears dependent on at least a single mitosis of oligodendrocytes. The efficacy of this remyelination is unclear and it is unlikely that it explains the tendency of most MS attacks to remit. In fact it has been implied that remission is better correlated with the expansion of sodium channels in the demyelinated axon (McDonald, 1994). As a lesion ages it often evidences a relative absence of oligodendrocytes; however, this finding is highly variable between patients (Rodriguez et al., 1993). In addition it is unclear whether oligodendrocyte destruction is immunologically mediated or is caused by loss of trophic support and exposure to the toxic microenvironment of the plaque (Bonetti & Raine, 1997).

Paediatric MS

MS primarily affects young adults, with a peak incidence between the ages of 20 and 40, and is a leading cause of acquired neurological disability in this population in industrialized countries. However, it has been diagnosed in patients from age 2 to age 80. Because of overly strict adherence to age guidelines, MS has probably been underdiagnosed in the paediatric population. Some observers have reported that one in 10 MS patients develop clinical symptoms before 18 (Poser *et al.*, 1982; Riser *et al.*, 1971; McAlpine, 1973) although their disease may initially go unrecognized. A significant confounding factor is the clinical overlap between certain paediatric neurological disorders and MS. The adrenoleukodystrophies, certain post-infectious conditions and rare mitochondrial disorders (e.g. Leber's hereditary optic neuropathy), all can mimic MS symptomatology. In addition, other diseases can demonstrate a similar capacity to 'relapse' and 'remit' (e.g. moyamoya disease). In fact, Hauser *et al.* (1982) suggested that misdiagnoses have led to the false impression that paediatric MS was more virulent than its adult counterpart. Additional reports underscore the potential for MS misdiagnosis in paediatric patients. Two recently published cases centred on the early misdiagnosis of a large demyelinating lesion as a neoplasm (Stein *et al.*, 1998; Kumar *et al.*, 1998). Although the severity of disease course for these cases was atypical, they highlight the tendency of paediatricians to overlook MS in their differential. The pathologic and phenotypic similarity between these two cases may even reflect a clinically distinct MS sub-type that warrants further study. The wider availability of paraclinical studies that are used to support an MS diagnosis (i.e. MRI, evoked potentials, LP) reflects in more reliable reports of paediatric MS, particularly in very young patients (Bauer *et al.*, 1990; Boutin *et al.*, 1988, Brandt *et al.*, 1981; Bye *et al.*, 1985; Cole & Stuart, 1995; Ghezzi *et al.*, 1997; Glasier *et al.*, 1995; Haas *et al.*, 1987; Hanefeld *et al.*, 1991; Hauser *et al.*, 1982; Izquierdo *et al.*, 1986; Lucchinetti *et al.*, 1997; Pinhas-Hamiel *et al.*, 1998; Ruggieri *et al.*, 1999; Scaioli *et al.*, 1991; Sindern *et al.*, 1992). Altogether, the most reliable data indicates that more than 10 per cent of MS patients develop their first symptoms in adolescence (before age 20) and one in 20 to one in 40 before age 15. MS before age 10 is generally considered to be rare comprising only somewhere between 0.2 per cent and 1 per cent of all cases (Adams *et al.*, 1999; Duquette *et al.*, 1987; Eraksvoy *et al.*, 1998; Muller, 1949; Poser *et al.*, 1982; Riser *et al.*, 1971; Ruggieri *et al.*, 1999; Sindern *et al.*, 1992).

There appear to be two relatively distinct age-related subsets of paediatric MS patients. No official classification has been developed, but relevant clinical studies appear to divide the paediatric population into two subgroups. These might best be described as juvenile MS (onset before age 21) and childhood MS (onset before age 10) (Bauer *et al.*, 1990; Boutin *et al.*, 1988; Izquierdo *et al.*, 1986; Pinhas-Hamiel *et al.*, 1998; Sindern *et al.*, 1992). The exact age for distinction is somewhat arbitrary and may reflect the importance of pubescence and sex hormones in MS pathogenesis. Juvenile MS appears very similar to adult MS except in regard to its sex distribution. Male patients appear relatively more common in the juvenile population (1.4 females: 1 male) than among adults. Juvenile onset has not been correlated with accelerated progression of the disease. Most juvenile patients exhibit only mild neurologic disability and impairment is related to length of time with disease (Pinhas-Hamiel *et al.*, 1998). This correlates with the observation by Poser and coworkers that early onset of MS is a good prognostic sign with regard to course of disease (Poser *et al.*, 1982).

Childhood MS appears to be somewhat different. Overall, childhood MS appears less aggressive than either adult or juvenile MS with few patients exhibiting disability. Most symptoms are transitory and remit more quickly than in adults. The distribution of certain clinical findings is also different. Children are more likely to present with seizures and/or ataxia than adults (Brandt et al., 1981; Bye et al., 1985; Izquierdo et al., 1986; Ruggieri et al., 1999). These differences may simply reflect the different impact of demyelination on the developing CNS or they may highlight important immunological differences between children and adults. Paradoxically, extremely early onset of MS (younger than age 2) appears associated with a very poor prognosis, although the small number of observed cases makes extrapolation unreliable (Cole et al., 1995; Ruggieri et al., 1999). Finally, a similar sex distribution has been reported for childhood MS as for juvenile MS (1.4:1). This provides further evidence of the role of female sex hormones in MS pathogenesis, as the female prevalence is also relatively decreased among patients with middle age MS onset.

Some clinical studies have provided evidence for ethnic variability in paediatric MS incidence and course. A large (256 patients) series of MS patients from China found that 3.5 per cent of Chinese MS patients developed symptoms before the age of 10 and 22 per cent developed symptoms before the age of 20 (Baoxun et al., 1982). Other smaller series from Asia have seemed to support the contention that Asian MS patients are more likely to have onset before 20 (Kim et al., 1982; Higa et al., 1982; Hung, 1982; Navarro et al., 1982; Gourie-Devi & Nagaraja, 1982; Vejjajiva, 1982). This is particularly interesting considering the reported phenotypic differences between 'Asian' and 'Western' MS (Kira et al., 1996). There has also been the intriguing observation that MS in African-American and West Indian children may follow a more debilitating course than in Caucasians (Elian & Dean, 1987; Shermata et al., 1981; Zelnik et al., 1991). Finally, Cole et al.'s (1995) observation that only 1.8 per cent of patients presented before age 16 at single hospital in Aberdeen, might be evidence that the prevalence of paediatric MS is different in varying population groups. Still, efforts to identify unique genetic factors in paediatric MS have been largely unsuccessful. In particular, a complete evaluation of polymorphisms in mitochondrial DNA (mtDNA) known to be associated with Leber's hereditary optic neuropathy (LHON) revealed no association with MS (Kalman et al., 1996; Kellar-Wood et al., 1994; Ohlenbusch et al., 1998). Anecdotal information and case reports seem to indicate that both juvenile and childhood MS are responsive to beta-interferon. In addition, steroid therapy is commonly and effectively used in the treatment of MS exacerbations in children. However, some observers have reported a tendency for children's symptoms to remit rapidly without treatment (Adams et al., 1999; Ruggieri et al., 1999). Double-blind placebo-controlled trials need to be conducted in children before we can determine the appropriate role for immunomodulatory drugs in the treatment of paediatric MS.

MS genetics

A genetic component in MS pathogenesis is primarily indicated by the increased relative risk to siblings of affected individuals compared with the general population. This familial aggregation (λ_s) can be determined by estimating the ratio of the prevalence in siblings (K_s) versus the population prevalence (K) of the disease. For MS, λ_s is between 20 (0.02/0.001) and 40 (0.04/0.001) (Risch, 1992). Half-sibling (Sadovnick et al., 1996) and adoption (Ebers et al., 1995) studies confirm that genetic, and not environmental factors, are responsible for familial aggregation. Twin studies from different populations consistently indicate that a monozygotic twin of an MS patient is at higher risk (25–30 per cent concordance) for MS than is a dizygotic twin (2–5 per cent) (Sadovnick et al., 1993; Mumford et al., 1994), providing additional evidence for a significant, but complex, genetic aetiology (Table 2). The frequent occurrence of

MS in some ethnic populations (particularly those of northern European origin) compared with others (African and Asian groups), irrespective of geographic location also provides evidence for a complex genetic aetiology (Ebers & Sadovnick, 1994; Oksenberg et al., 1996; Poser, 1995; Compston, 1997). The observation of resistant ethnic groups residing in high risk regions – for example the Romani (Gypsies) in Bulgaria (Milanov et al., 1999) – suggests that the relatively low risk in some ethnic groups results primarily from genetic resistance.

Table 2. Multiple sclerosis as a genetic disease

1. Racial clustering of MS cases. Resistant ethnic groups residing in high risk regions

2. Familial aggregation of MS cases
    Increased relative risk to sibs (λ_S = 20–40)
    Low incidence of conjugal MS
    MS sibling pairs tend to cluster by age of onset, rather than year of onset
    No detectable effect of shared environment on MS susceptibility in first-degree non-biological relatives (spouses, adoptees, half siblings)

3. High disease concordance in monozygotic twins (25–30 per cent) compared with dizygotic twins and non-twin siblings (3–5 per cent)
4. Suggestive correlations between certain polymorphic loci and disease susceptibility

The genetic component of MS aetiology is believed to result from the action of several susceptibility genes with common alleles (polymorphisms) of weak, but cumulative effects and penetrance. The incomplete penetrance of MS susceptibility alleles probably reflects interactions with other genes, post-transcriptional regulatory mechanisms, and significant nutritional and environmental influences (Table 3).

Table 3. Confounding factors in genetic studies of multiple sclerosis

1. Aetiologic and genetic heterogeneity

2. Unknown genetic parameters
    Single vs. multiple genes
    Dominant vs. recessive mode of inheritance
    Incomplete penetrance

3. Epistatic gene interactions (additive vs. multiplicative)
4. Post-genomic mechanisms
5. Unidentified nonheritable (environmental) factors

The genetic analysis of MS has traditionally focused on association studies of candidate polymorphic genes, in which the frequencies of marker alleles in groups of patients and healthy controls are compared, and the difference is subjected to statistical analysis. Candidate genes are defined as genes that are logical possibilities based on their biological activity; for MS candidate genes might encode cytokines, immune-receptors, and proteins involved in viral clearance. The association is often expressed as the relative risk that an individual will develop the disorder if he/she carries the particular allele or marker, compared to an individual who does not carry the allele or marker. With the notable exception of the major histocompatibility complex (MHC or HLA in humans) locus on chromosome 6p21 (Fig. 1), genetic studies in MS have met with only moderate success in identifying disease-causing or disease-modifying genes (Seboun et al., 1997; http://www.ucsf.edu/msdb/r_ms_candidate_genes.html). This is due in

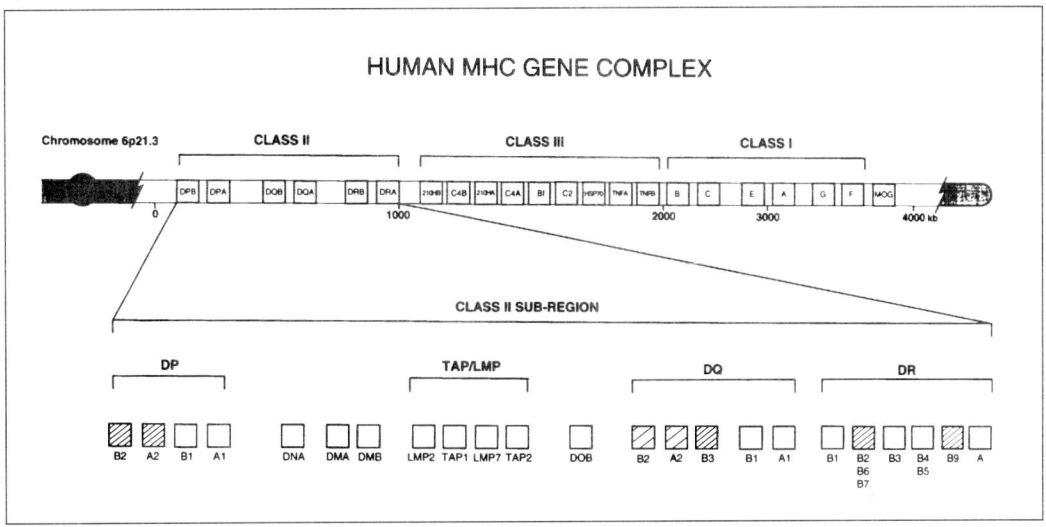

Fig. 1. Genomic organization of the MHC.
The diagram shows the relative positions of the major class I and class II loci involved in antigen presentation, as well as other examples of the more than 250 genes encoded within this 4 million base pair complex. There are three classic class I genes: HLA-A, B and C. Class I molecules consist of a heavy chain, noncovalently associated with the chromosome 17-encoded β2-microglobulin. The classic class II genes (DR, DQ, DP) are arranged in a block centromeric to HLA-B, each containing one or more genes, although not all are expressed (////), coding for heterodimer glycoproteins. Other genes mapped in the MHC region include complement proteins, genes for the 21-hydroxylase, tumour necrosis factor and heat-shock proteins, collectively known as class III.

part to limitations in study-design (case-control and small sample sizes), the difficulty in selecting from among the many candidate disease gene possibilities, and the modest effect of any single MS susceptibility gene.

The genetic effect of the HLA locus on MS susceptibility has been consistently associated with the class II HLA-DRB1*1501-DQA1*0102-DQB1*0602 haplotype (the molecular designation for the serologically defined 'DR2' haplotype) (Olerup & Hillert, 1991). The mechanism(s) underlying linkage and association of HLA-DRB1*1501-DQA1*0102-DQB1*0602 with MS is not yet fully understood. These MHC molecules may fail to negatively select (delete) autoreactive T-cells within the embryonic thymic microenvironment. Alternatively, HLA-DRB1*1501 and/or DQA1*0102-DQB1*0602 genes may encode a class II recognition molecule with a propensity to bind peptide antigens of myelin and stimulate encephalitogenic T-cells. Attempts to further localize the MS susceptibility gene within the DR or DQ regions of the MHC have not provided consensus. The strong linkage disequilibrium (LD) across the DR DQ region has prevented so far a clear resolution of the relative contribution of each gene. Because patterns of genomic disequilibrium across the MHC region may differ among different ethnic groups due to infrequent recombination events during evolution, studies of contrasting ethnic cohorts may prove especially informative in identifying MS predisposing genes within the HLA region.

An alternative strategy to the analysis of candidate genes selected according to their biological function involves first determining the chromosomal region of the genomic defect by genetic linkage analysis, and then isolating the disease gene (Fig. 2). This approach for gene localization

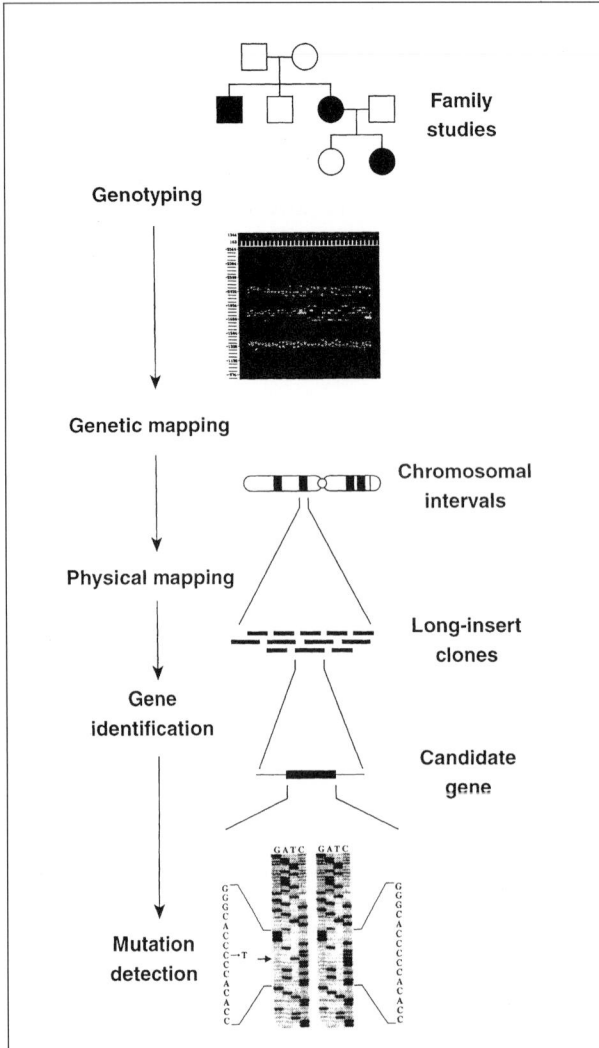

Fig. 2. Steps in positional cloning.
Large collections of informative polymorphic markers are use to position disease loci to discrete chromosomal segments. Genetic linkage is established by tracking the inheritance of discrete chromosomal segments that co-segregate with the disease. Once these regions are identified and confirmed, the process of disease gene characterization can be initiated.

requires the collection of pedigrees with more than one affected member and the establishment of linkage by tracking the inheritance of discrete chromosomal segments that co-segregate with the disease. In contrast to monogenic diseases, for complex disorders such as MS, with no evidence of gross chromosomal aberrations, linkage analysis must be performed on an extremely large group of individuals if small genetic effects are to be detected and/or if genetic heterogeneity is present. Genetic heterogeneity means that different genes influence susceptibility to the same phenotype in different individuals. The smaller the genetic contribution, the greater the required sample size, and more stringent the inclusion criteria to minimize effects of clinical heterogeneity. Indeed, analysis of candidate genes in small familial cohorts have been largely uninformative (http://www.ucsf.edu/msdb/r_ms_candidate_genes.html). In 1996, three groups completed and reported whole genome screens in familial MS in an attempt to localize genomic loci that may contain MS susceptibility genes (Ebers *et al.*, 1996; The MS Genetic Group, 1996; Sawcer *et al.*, 1996). A fourth study concentrated on a genetically isolated region of Finland but was based on only 15 families (Kuokkanen *et al.*, 1997). The data was analysed using a combination of parametric (model-based) and nonparametric (model-free) statistical methods. This multi-analytical strategy identified several potential susceptibility regions including the MHC on 6p21 (Table 4). Meta-analysis of all data obtained from genome screening (Lewis *et al.*, 1998), comparison of the linkage results to other human and experimental immune-mediated diseases (Becker *et al.*, 1998), direct analysis of candidate genes mapped to these regions (The MS Genetic Group, 1998), and follow-up screenings in larger datasets of multiplex families (Chataway *et al.*, 1998) are currently in progress.

A model of inheritance for multiple sclerosis

A simple model of inheritance for all MS is unlikely and cannot account for the nonlinear decrease in disease risk in families with increasing genetic distance from the MS proband (Table 5). Taken together, the available data is compatible with a complex multifactorial aetiology in MS, including both genetic and environmental factors. Recurrence risk estimates in first, second, and third degree relatives, combined with twin data, predict that the MS-prone genotype results from multiple independent or interacting genes, each exerting small or moderate effect.

Table 4. Regions of overlap between whole genome scans in multiple sclerosis

US	UK	Canada	Finland
	1p36-p33	1p36-p33	
2p23	2p23-p21	2p23-21	
	3p14-p13	3p14-p13	
3q22-q24		3q22-q24	
4q31-qter	4q31-qter		
		5p14-p12	5p14-22
5q13-q23	5q12-q13	5q12-q13	
6p21	6p21		6p21
6q27	6q22-27		
7q11-q22		7q21-q22	
	17q22		17q22-24
18p11		18p11	
19q13	19q12-13	19q13	
	Xq	Xq	

Table 5. Model of genetic contributions to MS

1. Multiple genes of moderate effect
2. No major MS gene with the exception of the MHC
3. Susceptibility genes vs. disease modifiers
4. Complex gene-gene and gene-environment interactions
5. Genetic heterogeneity may result in clinical isoforms

Thus, MS is most likely a polygenic disorder. It is also possible that genetic heterogeneity exists. Results from our familial MS dataset confirm the genetic importance of the MHC region in conferring susceptibility to MS. Susceptibility may be mediated by the class II genes themselves (DR, DQ or both) related to the known function of these molecules in the normal immune response, e.g. antigen binding and presentation and T-cell repertoire determination. The possibility that other genes in the MHC or the telomeric region of the MHC are responsible for the observed genetic effect cannot be excluded. The data also show that although the MHC region plays a significant role in MS susceptibility, much of the genetic effect in MS remains to be explained. In comparison with emerging data on the genetic basis of animal models for autoimmune demyelination, it will be of particular interest to identify whether some loci are involved in the initial pathogenic events, while others influence the development and progression of the disease. Due to the complex heterogeneous nature of MS, large studies of patients using multi-analytical approaches that incorporate gender and reproductive history, genetic polymorphic profiles, as well as detailed clinical, demographic, environmental and serological data, are needed to uncover the pathogenesis of MS and operating genetic risk factors. Their characterization will help to define the basic aetiology of the disease, improve risk assessment and significantly influence the development of novel therapeutic strategies.

Patient stratification: new directions for complex diseases

Because of the likely role of an undefined environmental exposure, our partial knowledge of the full set of genes involved in conferring susceptibility, and the clinical heterogeneity of the disease, it has been difficult to formulate a unifying mechanism that explains the pathogenesis of MS. The all-genome screens certainly represent the most important foray into the genetics of MS published in recent years, and propose a new experimental view to elucidate the pathogenic mechanisms of this disease. The analysis of the MS genome with larger DNA collections and more dense and informative genetic markers will continue. Disease heterogeneity provides an opportunity to determine the relative efficacy of different strategies. Some of that heterogeneity is reflected in age- and ethnicity-related differences in disease symptomatology, pathology and severity. Genetic analysis of responders and nonresponders in therapeutic trial may prove extremely informative as well. Studies such as these will be necessarily linked to the development of novel mathematical formulations designed to identify modest genetic effects, as well as epistatic interactions between multiple genes, and interactions between genes, environmental factors and clinical variables. Whether the genotype dictates different forms of MS in response to a common causative agent or trigger, or whether the genotype reflects different diseases with different environmental causes is not known. In all likelihood, the use of phenotypic and demographic variables will assume increasing importance as stratifying elements for future genetic studies of MS. Paediatric MS cases may prove to be a useful clinical subset for analysis. The relative prevalence of the condition lies in contradiction to the old dogma that MS pathogenesis required a 15-year latency from environmental exposure to disease onset. Regardless of whether the differences between paediatric MS and adult MS are dictated by genetic factors or different environmental agents, paediatric cases should prove to be a subject worthy of further study. The true significance of MS in children remains to be elucidated.

Acknowledgements: Ari J. Green is a fellow of the Howard Hughes Medical Institute.

References

Adams, A.B., Tyor, W.R. & Holden, K.R. (1999): Interferon beta-1b and childhood multiple sclerosis. *Pediatr. Neurol.* **21**, 481–483.

Baoxun, Z., Dosan, L., Weiming, H., Xiugin, L., Shihe, L., Yinchang, Y., Sinmei, J. & Huifen, H. (1982): MS in China: a clinical study of 256 cases. In: *Multiple Sclerosis East and West*, eds. Y. Kuroiwa & L.T. Kurland, pp. 71–81. Fukuoka: Kyushu University Press.

Bauer, H.J., Hanefeld, F. & Christen, H.J. (1990): Multiple sclerosis in early childhood: letter. *Lancet* **336**, 1190.

Becker, K.G., Mattson, D.H., Powers, J.M., Gado, A.M., Biddison, W.E., McFarland, H.F. & Trent, J.M. (1998): Clustering of non-major histocompatibility complex susceptibility candidate loci in human autoimmune diseases. *Proc. Natl. Acad. Sci. USA* **95**, 9979–9984.

Bo, L., Mark, S., Kong, P., Nyland, H., Pardo, C. & Trapp, B.D. (1994): Detection of MHC class II antigens on macrophages and microglia, but not astrocytes and endothelia in active MS lesions. *J. Neuroimmunol.* **51**, 135–146.

Bonetti, B. & Raine, C.S. (1997): Multiple sclerosis: oligodendrocytes display cell-death related molecules *in situ* but do not undergo apoptosis. *Ann. Neurol.* **42**, 74–84.

Boutin, B., Esquivel, E., Mayer, M., Chaumet, S., Ponsot, G. & Arthuis, M. (1988): Multiple sclerosis in children: report of clinical and paraclinical features of 19 cases. *Neuropediatr.* **19**, 118–123.

Brandt, S., Glydenstad, C., Offner, H. & Melchior, J.C. (1981): Multiple sclerosis with onset in a two year old boy. *Neuropediatr.* **12**, 75–82.

Bye, M.E., Kendall, B. & Wilson, J. (1985): Multiple sclerosis in childhood: a new look. *Dev. Med. Child Neurol.* **27**, 215–222.

Chataway, J., Feakes, R., Coraddu, F., Gray, J., Deans, J., Fraser, M., Robertson, N., Broadley, S., Jones, H., Clayton, D., Goodfellow, P., Sawcer, S. & Compston, A. (1998): The genetics of multiple sclerosis: principles, background and updated results of the United Kingdom systemic genome screen. *Brain* **121**, 1869–1887.

Cole, G.F. & Stuart, C.A. (1995): A long perspective on childhood MS. *Dev. Med. Child Neurol.* **37**, 661–666.

Cole, G.F., Auchterlonie, L.A. & Best, P.V. (1995): Very early onset multiple sclerosis. *Dev. Med. Child Neurol.* **37**, 667–672.

Compston, A. (1997): Genetic epidemiology of multiple sclerosis. *J. Neurol. Neurosurg. Psych.* **62**, 553–561.

De Stefano, N., Matthews, P.M., Fu, L., Narayanan, S., Stanley, J., Francis, G.S., Antel, J.P. & Arnold, D.L. (1998): Axonal damage correlates with disability in patients with relapsing-remitting multiple sclerosis: results of a longitudinal magnetic resonance spectroscopy study. *Brain* **121**, 1469–1477.

Duquette, P., Murray, T.G., Pleines, J., Ebers, G.C., Sadovnick, D., Weldon, P., Warren, S., Paty, D.W., Upton, A. & Hader, W. (1987): MS in childhood: clinical profile in 125 patients. *J. Pediatr.* **111**, 359–363.

Ebers, G.C. & Sadovnick, A.D. (1994): The role of genetic factors in multiple sclerosis susceptibility. *J. Neuroimmunol.* **54**, 1–17.

Ebers, G.C., Kukay, K., Bulman, D.E., Sadovnick, A.D., Rice, G., Anderson, C., Armstrong, H., Cousin, K., Bell, R.B., Hader, W., Paty, D.W., Hashimoto, S., Oger, J., Duquette, P., Warren, S., Gray, T., O'Connor, P., Nath, A., Auty, A., Metz, L., Francis, G., Paulseth, J.E., Murray, T.J., Pryse-Phillips, W., Risch, N. *et al.* (1996): A full genome search in multiple sclerosis. *Nature Genet.* **13**, 472–476.

Ebers, G.C., Sadovnick, A.D. & Risch, N.J., The Canadian Collaborative Study Group (1995): A genetic basis for familial aggregation in MS. *Nature* **377**, 150–151.

Elian, M. & Dean, G. (1987): MS among the UK-born children of immigrants from the West Indies. *J. Neurol. Neurosurg. Psych.* **50**, 327–332.

Eraksoy, M., Demir, G.A. & Yapycy, Z. (1998): Multiple sclerosis in childhood (abstract). *Brain. Dev.* **20**, 427.

Ghezzi, A., Deplano, V., Faroni, J., Grasso, M.G., Liguori, M., Marrosu, G., Pozzilli, C., Simone, I.L. & Zaffaroni, M. (1997): Multiple sclerosis in childhood: clinical features of 149 cases. *Mult. Scler.* **3**, 43–46.

Glasier, C.M., Robbins, M.B., Davis, P.C., Ceballo, E. & Bates, S.R. (1995): Clinical, neurodiagnostic, and MR findings in children with spinal and brainstem MS. *Am. J. Neuroradiol.* **16**, 87–95.

Gourie-Devi, M. & Nagaraja, D. (1982): Multiple scelrosis in South India. In: *Multiple Sclerosis East and West*, eds. Y. Kuroiwa & L.T. Kurland, pp. 135–148. Fukuoka: Kyushu University Press.

Haas, G., Scroth, G., Krageloh-Mann, I. & Buchwald-Saal, M. (1987): MRI of the brain of children with multiple sclerosis. *Dev. Med. Child Neurol.* **29**, 586–591.

Hanefeld, F., Bauer, H.J., Christen, H.J., Kruse, B., Bruhn, H. & Frahm, J. (1991): MS in childhood: report of 15 cases. *Brain. Dev.* **13,** 410–416.

Hauser, S.L. & Goodkin, D.E. (1998): Multiple sclerosis and other demyelinating diseases. In: *Harrison's Principles of Internal Medicine* (14th edn.), eds. A.D. Fauci, E. Braunwald, J.D. Isselbacher, J.B. Martin, D.L. Kasper, S.L. Hauser & D.L. Longo, pp. 2419–2418. New York: McGraw Hill.

Hauser, S.L., Bhan, A.K., Gilles, F., Kemp, M., Kerr, C. & Weiner, H.L. (1986): Immunocytochemical analysis of the cellular infiltrates in multiple sclerosis lesions. *Ann. Neurol.* **19,** 578–587.

Hauser, S.L., Bresnan, M.J., Reinherz, E.L. & Weiner H.L. (1982): Childhood multiple sclerosis: clinical features and demonstration of changes in T-cell subsets with disease activity. *Ann. Neurol.* **11,** 463–468.

Higa, H., Toyonaga, K., Nishihara, T., Sakugawa, H., Ikuta, F. (1982): Multiple Sclerosis in Okinawa. In: *Multiple Sclerosis East and West*, eds. Y. Kuroiwa & L.T. Kurland, pp. 49–56. Fukuoka: Kyushu University Press.

Hung, T.P. (1982): Multiple Sclerosis in Taiwan: a reappraisal. In: *Multiple Sclerosis East and West*, eds. Y. Kuroiwa & L.T. Kurland, pp. 83–96. Fukuoka: Kyushu University Press.

Izquierdo, G., Lyon-Caen, O., Marteau, R., Martinez-Parra, Lhermitte, F., Castaigne, P. & Hauw, J.J. (1986): Early onset MS. Clinical study of 12 pathologically proven cases. *Acta. Neurol. Scand.* **73,** 493–497.

Kalman, B., Lublin, F.D. & Alder, H. (1996): Characterization of the mitochondrial DNA in patients with multiple sclerosis. *J. Neurol. Sci.* **140,** 75–84.

Kellar-Wood, H., Robertson, N., Govan, G.G., and Compston, D.A. (1994): Leber's hereditary optic neuropathy mitochondrial DNA mutations in multiple sclerosis. *Ann. Neurol.* **36,** 109–112.

Kermode, A.G. (1990): Breakdown of the blood-brain barrier precedes symptoms and other MRI signs of new lesions in multiple sclerosis. *Brain* **113,** 1477–1489.

Kim, S.W. & Kim, S.K. (1982): Multiple Sclerosis in Busan, Korea: clinical features and prevalence. In: *Multiple Sclerosis East and West*, eds. Y. Kuroiwa & L.T. Kurland, pp. 57–70. Fukuoka: Kyushu University Press.

Kira, J., Kanai, T., Nishimura, Y., Yamasaki, K., Matsushita, S., Kawano, Y., Hasuo, K., Tobimatsu, S. & Kobayashi, T. (1996): Western versus Asian types of multiple sclerosis: two immunogenetically and clinically distinct patient groups. *Ann. Neurol.* **40,** 569–574.

Kumar, K., Toth, C. & Jay, V. (1998): Focal plaque of demyelination mimicking cerebral tumor in a pediatric patient. *Pediatr. Neurosurg.* **29,** 60–63.

Kuokkanen, S., Gschwend, M., Rioux, J.D., Daly, M.J., Terwilliger, J.D., Tienari, P.J., Wikstrom, J., Palo, J., Stein, L.D., Hudson, T.J., Lander, E.S. & Peltonen, L. (1997): Genomewide scan of multiple sclerosis in Finnish multiplex families. *Am. J. Hum. Genet.* **61,** 1379–1387.

Lassman, H., Suchanek, G. & Ozawa, K. (1994): Histopathology and the blood-cerebrospinal fluid barrier in multiple sclerosis. *Ann. Neurol.* **36,** S42–S46.

Lewis, C.M., Wise, L.H. & Lanchburry, J.S. (1998): Meta-analysis of genome search results. *Am. J. Hum. Genet.* **63,** A1351.

Lucchinetti, C.F., Brueck, W., Rodriguez, M. & Lassmann, H. (1998): Multiple sclerosis: lessons from neuropathology. *Sem. Neurol.* **18,** 337–349.

Lucchinetti, C.F., Kiers, L., O'Duffy, A., Gomez, M.R., Cross, S., Leavitt, J.A., O'Brien, P. & Rodriguez, M. (1997): Risk factors for developing MS after childhood ON. *Neurology* **49,** 1413–1418.

McAlpine, D. (1973): MS: a review. *Br. Med. J.* **2,** 292–295.

McDonald, W.I. (1994): The pathological and clinical dynamics of multiple sclerosis. *J. Neuropathol. Exp. Neurol.* **53,** 338–343.

Milanov, I., Topalov, N. & Kmetski, T. (1999): Prevalence of multiple sclerosis in Gypsies and Bulgarians. *Epidemiology* **18,** 218–222.

Muller, R. (1949): Studies on disseminated sclerosis, with special reference to symptomatology, course, and prognosis. *Acta Medica Scandinav.* Suppl 222, 5–214.

Mumford, C.J., Wood, N.W., Kellar-Wood, H., Thorpe, J., Miller, D. & Compston, D.A.S. (1994): The British Isles survey of multiple sclerosis in twins. *Neurology* **44**, 11–15.

Navarro, J.C., Sobrevega, E.E., Gamez, G.L. & Cuanang, J.R. (1982): The clinical manifestations of 51 cases of MS in the Philippines. In: *Multiple Sclerosis East and West*, eds. Y. Kuroiwa & L.T. Kurland, pp. 97–104. Fukuoka: Kyushu University Press.

Ohlenbusch, A., Wilichowski, E. & Hanefeld, F. (1998): Characterization of the mitochondrial genome in childhood MS: I. Optic neuritis and LHON mutations. *Neuropediatr.* **29**, 175–179.

Oksenberg, J.R. & Hauser, S.L. (1999): Emerging concepts of pathogenesis: relationship to MS therapeutics. In: *Multiple sclerosis: experimental and applied therapeutics*, eds. R.A. Rudick & D.E. Goodkin, pp. 115–142. London: Martin Dunitz.

Oksenberg, J.R., Seboun, E. & Hauser, S.L. (1996): Genetics of demyelinating diseases. *Brain Pathol.* **6**, 289–302.

Olerup, O. & Hillert, J. (1991): HLA class II-associated genetic susceptibility in multiple sclerosis: a critical evaluation. *Tissue Antigens* **38**, 1–15.

Ozawa, K. Suchanek, G. Breitschopf, H., Bruck, W., Budka, H., Jellinger, K. & Lassman, H. (1994): Patterns of oligodendroglia pathology in multiple sclerosis. *Brain* **117**, 1311–1322.

Pinhas-Hamiel, O., Barak, Y., Siev-Ner, I. & Achiron, A. (1998): Juvenile multiple sclerosis: clinical features and prognostic characteristics. *J. Pediatr.* **132**, 735–737.

Poser, C.M. (1995): Viking voyages: the origin of multiple sclerosis? An essay in medical history. *Acta Neurol. Scand.* **161** (Suppl), 11–22.

Poser, S., Raun, N.E. & Poser, W. (1982): Age at onset, initial symptomatology and the course of multiple sclerosis. *Acta Neurol. Scandinav.* **66**, 355–362.

Prineas, J.W., Barnard, R.O., Kwon, E.E., Sharer, L.R. & Cho, E.S. (1993): Multiple sclerosis. Remyelination of nascent lesions. *Ann. Neurol.* **33**, 137–151.

Raine C.S. (1994): The Dale E. McFarlin memorial lecture: the immunology of the multiple sclerosis lesion. *Ann. Neurol.* **36**, S61–S72.

Risch, N. (1992): Corrections to linkage strategies for genetically complex traits. III. The effect of marker polymorphism on analysis of affected relative pairs. *Am. J. Hum. Genet.* **51**, 673–675.

Riser, M., Geraud, J., Rascol, A., Benazet, A.M. & Segria, M.G. (1971): The course of MS, study of 203 cases followed up for more than 10 years (French). *Rev. Neurol. (Paris)* **124** (6), 479–486.

Rodriguez, M., Scheithauer, B.W., Forbes, G. & Kelly, P.J. (1993): Oligodendrocyte injury is an early event in lesions of multiple sclerosis. *Mayo Clin. Proc.* **68**, 627–636.

Ruggieri, M., Polizzi, A., Pavone, L. & Grimaldi, L.M. (1999): Multiple sclerosis in children under 6 years of age. *Neurology* **53**, 478–484.

Sadovnick, A.D., Armstrong, H., Rice, G.P.A., Bulman, D., Hashimoto, L., Paty, D.W., Hashimoto, S.A., Warren, S., Hader, W. & Murray, T.J. (1993): A population-based study of multiple sclerosis in twins: update. *Ann. Neurol.* **33**, 281–285

Sadovnick, A.D., Ebers, G.C., Dyment, D.A., Risch, N.J. & the Canadian Collaborative Study Group (1996): Evidence for genetic basis of multiple sclerosis. *Lancet* **347**, 1728–1730.

Sanders, V., Conrad, A.J. & Tourtellote, W.W. (1993): On classification of post-mortem multiple sclerosis plaques for neuroscientists. *J. Neuroimmunol.* **46**, 207–216.

Sawcer, S., Jones, H.B., Feakes, R., Gray, J., Smaldon, N., Chataway, J., Robertson, N., Clayton, D., Goodfellow, P.N. & Compston A. (1996): A genome screen in multiple sclerosis reveals susceptibility loci on chromosome 6p21 and 17q22. *Nature Genet.* **13**, 464–468.

Scaioli, V., Rumi, V., Cimino, C. & Angelini, L. (1991): Childhood MS: multimodal evoked potentials and magnetic resonance imaging comparative study. *Neuropediatr.* **22,** 15–23.

Seboun, E., Oksenberg, J.R. & Hauser, S.L. (1997): Molecular genetics of multiple sclerosis. In: *The molecular and genetic basis of neurological disease* (2nd edn.), eds. R.N. Rosenberg, S.B. Prusiner, S. DiMauro, R.L. Barchi & L.M. Kunkel, pp. 631–662. Boston: Butterworth-Heinemann.

Sheremata, W., Brown, S.B. & Curless, R.R. (1981): Childhood MS: a report of 12 cases, abstract. *Ann Neurol.* **10,** 304.

Sindern, E., Haas, J., Stark, E. & Wurster, U. (1992): Early onset MS under the age of 16: clinical and paraclinical features. *Acta. Neurol. Scand.* **86,** 280–284.

Sorensen, T.L. & Ransohoff, R. (1998): Etiology and pathogenesis of multiple sclerosis. *Sem. Neurol.* **18,** 287–294.

Stein, M.C., Ebb, D.H., Zalneritas, E.L., Schaeffer, P.W., Louis, D.N. & Vonsattel, J.P. (1998): Case records of the Massachusetts General Hospital. Weekly clinicopathological exercises. Case 26-1998. A 15-year-old girl with hemiparesis, slurred speech, and an intracranial lesion. *N. Engl. J. Med.* **339** (8), 542–549.

The Multiple Sclerosis Genetics Group (1996): A complete genomic screen for multiple sclerosis underscores a role for the major histocompatibility complex. *Nature Genet.* **13,** 469–471.

The Multiple Sclerosis Genetics Group (1998): Linkage of the MHC to familial multiple sclerosis suggests genetic heterogeneity. *Hum. Molec. Genet.* **7,** 1229–1234.

Trapp, B.D., Peterson, J., Ranshoff, R.M., Rudick, R., Mork, S. & Bo, L. (1998): Axonal transection in the lesions of multiple sclerosis. *N. Engl. J. Med.* **338,** 278–285.

Traugott, U. (1987): Relevance of class I and class II MHC-expressing cells to lesion development. *J. Neuroimmunol.* **15,** 283.

Vejjajiva, A. (1982): Some clinical aspects of MS in Thai patients. In: *Multiple Sclerosis East and West*, eds. Y. Kuroiwa & L.T. Kurland, pp. 117–122. Fukuoka: Kyushu University Press.

Wu, E. & Raine, C.S. (1992): Multiple sclerosis: interactions between oligodendrocytes and hypertrophic astrocytes and their occurrence in other, non-demyelinating conditions. *Lab. Invest.* **67,** 88–99.

Zelnik, N., Gale, A.D. & Shelburne, S.A. (1991): MS in black children. *J. Child. Neurol.* **6,** 53–57.

Chapter 5

Multiple sclerosis in childhood: clinical aspects

Nicoletta Milani, Alex Gravante and Federica Zibordi

Department of Child Neurology, Istituto Nazionale Neurologico 'C. Besta', via Celoria 11, 20133 Milan, Italy

Summary

Multiple sclerosis is a very well known disease in adults, but is still poorly studied in children, in which it is rare and probably still misdiagnosed. Literature on the topic is reviewed: studies are very heterogeneous, hardly comparable and mostly dealing with small samples of patients, if not single case reports. The existence of peculiar clinical pictures typical of MS in children is still under debate. We studied a group of 20 patients with clinically defined MS, eight females and 12 males, aged 8 years 2 months to 14 years 2 months at onset, selected from patients admitted to our child neurology department from 1985 to 1998. Symptoms at onset were due to brainstem, sensitive, motor and cerebellar dysfunction in decreasing order. Clinical course was relapsing-remitting in 75 per cent, relapsing-progressive in 25 per cent, with no case of progressive disease from the beginning. Patients relapsed within the first year in 85 per cent. In the seven patients with a disease duration more than 8 years long-term outcome was relatively favourable, with 42 per cent showing only mild disability (EDSS < 4).

Historical review

The first reports about relapsing-remitting neurological diseases resembling multiple sclerosis (MS) date back to the fourteenth century, the most ancient of which being the case of St. Lidwina of Schiedam (1380–1433), but only in the early nineteenth century was the disease described in terms of clinical and pathological manifestations. In 1868 a description of the disease in its classical form was finally provided by Charcot in his lecture on 'sclérose en plaques'. Still child onset was not taken into consideration and it was only in 1912 that Schilder (1912) reported the case of a 14-year-old girl with periaxial encephalomyelitis which can be considered the first description of MS onset in the very young, even if the relationship between MS and Schilder disease is still under debate.

With time passing, the occurrence of MS in childhood was well established: 129 patients with onset before the age of 18 had already been reported by 1980 and 176 more were added in the ten years following (Hanefeld *et al.*, 1991). In the same period more and more reports on very young affected children (i.e. with onset under the age of 5) were published, but the younger the child, the more doubtful the diagnosis. At least some of the reported cases with onset at age 2 or less, with fever, headache and paraparesis as main neurological signs and rapidly worsening course, were probably acute diffuse encephalomyelitis (ADEM) misdiagnosed as MS.

Even not taking into account single reports of very young children, juvenile MS is still poorly defined: most studies, if not case reports, are about small groups of patients, retrospectively studied, and only in a very few cases collected from a definite geographic area and compared to the adult MS population from the same area. This is of great relevance since MS in adults seems to differ not only in incidence but also in clinical aspects, such as symptoms at onset, according to different geographic areas. Besides, symptoms such as visual or sensitive impairment can be very difficult to detect in a child. This makes it very hard to date the onset of the disease (mostly if the child was not directly observed from the beginning), and even to follow up patients afterwards.

Reviewing literature on the topic of the last 14 years we found only eight studies on reasonably large groups of patients (Table 1). Only four of them (Duquette *et al.*, 1987; Sindern *et al.*, 1992; Cole & Stuart, 1995; Ghezzi *et al.*, 1997) reported a comparative study of the adult and child population in their series.

Table 1. Multiple sclerosis paediatric series (from 1985)

Izquierdo *et al.*	1986	12 patients
Duquette *et al.*	1987	125 patients
Boutin *et al.*	1988	19 patients
Hanefeld *et al.*	1991	18 patients
Sindern *et al.*	1992	31 patients
Guilhoto *et al.*	1994	15 patients
Cole & Stuart	1995	28 patients
Ghezzi *et al.*	1997	149 patients

In these series (Table 2), the percentage of child MS compared to the total MS population varied from 1.8 to 5 per cent. The preponderance of females reported in adults, with a sex ratio of 1.5–1.9 in different series, was even more striking in children, with a sex ratio exceeding 2 in three series and up to 3 in Duquette *et al.* (1987). Children with onset under the age of 11 varied from 6 per cent in Duquette *et al.* to 25 per cent in Cole & Stuart, who also reported the younger patient (1 year at onset), while in the remaining three series the younger patients were older than 5 years. Family history was positive in 21 per cent of patients in Duquette's series, but was not reported in the others.

Table 2. Paediatric series compared: sample features

	Child MS/ Total MS	Youngest age at onset	% < 11 years	Sex ratio (f/m)	Family history
Duquette	2.7%	5 years	6%	3	21%
Sindern	5.0%	9 years	10.5%	2.4	na
Cole	1.8%	1 year	25%	1.5	na
Ghezzi	4.4%	6 years	12.5%	2.2	na

Symptoms at onset were different in the four groups (Table 3): afferent structures of CNS were involved both in Duquette's and in Sindern's series, with sensitive dysfunctions being more frequent in the first case and visual dysfunctions in the second one. Pure motor symptoms were by far the more frequent presenting complaint in Cole & Stuart, while visual, motor, sensitive and brainstem dysfunctions were reported by Ghezzi et al., with slight prevalence of the latter. Cerebellar symptoms were unfrequent in all groups; other complaints, such as sphincteric disturbances or transverse myelitis, rare.

In the two series of Ghezzi and of Sindern, in which presenting symptoms in children were compared to presenting symptoms in adults, no significant difference was reported. So, discrepancies among the series, and not between children and adults, may be related to geographical differences or even to differences in collecting and analysing clinical and instrumental data.

Table 3. Paediatric series compared: symptoms at onset

	Motor	Motor-sensitive	Sensitive	Visual	Brainstem	Cerebellar
Duquette	1%	5%	26%	14%	12%	5%
Sindern	6%	–	16%	52%	6%	6%
Cole	46%	–	–	28%	21%	10%
Ghezzi	17.5%	–	18.3%	16.5%	20.3%	9.1%

Clinical course was relapsing-remitting (RR) in more than 50 per cent of patients in all series (varying from 56 per cent in Duquette to 78 per cent in Cole), relapsing progressive (RP) in 8 to 32 per cent, and primary progressive (PP) in 5.5 to 22 per cent, respectively in Duquette and Ghezzi (Table 4).

Data on patients relapsing during the first year from onset were available only in Cole (60 per cent) and Ghezzi (34.9 per cent).

Table 4. Paediatric series compared: clinical course

	RR	RP	PP	Patients relapsed within 1 year	Follow-up
Duquette	56%	22%	22%	na	15 years
Sindern	61%	32%	7%	na	11.4 ± 7.7 years
Cole	78%	8%	14%	60%	3–47 years
Ghezzi	65%	29.5%	5.5%	34.9%	14.2 ± 9.1 years

RR = relapsing-remitting; RP = relapsing-progressive; PP = primary-progressive.

Long-term outcome was better than in adults in Sindern and Cole, with more than 50 per cent of patients scoring < 3 at Kurtzke disability scale after at least 10 years from onset, while Duquette and Ghezzi did not report significant differences between child and adult MS populations, apart from an early onset group of patients in Ghezzi's series, with disease duration less than 8 years, in which an Expanded Disability Status Scale (EDSS) score of > 6 was slightly more frequent than in the adult population from the same study (Table 5).

Table 5. Paediatric series compared: long-term outcome

Duquette	EDSS < 3	60 per cent of patients with disease duration > 8 years
Sindern	EDSS =1	50 per cent of patients (mean duration 15 years)
Cole		No significant difference in disease progression between children and adults
Ghezzi (I)	EDSS < 4	72.7 per cent of patients with duration < 8years 40 per cent of patients with duration > 8 years
Ghezzi (II)	EDSS > 6	20.8 per cent of patients with duration < 8 years (9.2 per cent in adults) 28.7 per cent of patients with duration > 8 years (25.75 per cent in adults)

Subjects and methods

Twenty patients with child or juvenile MS (with onset before 15 years) were collected from the general population admitted to our department of child neurology between 1985 and 1998 and retrospectively studied (1985 being the first year in which MR was routinely performed in our institute).

Five patients were admitted within one month from onset, seven within 6 months and eight at more than 6 months from onset, with a maximum of 44 months. Patients who were not observed from the beginning of the disease were selected only when medical records which confirmed anamnestic information were available.

Only 50 per cent of patients were from Milan or Lombardia, while the others came from other Italian regions, mostly from the South. Disease duration was longer than 8 years only in seven patients (35 per cent), while in four (20 per cent) it was less than 1 year (minimum 5 months). Only 10 patients were still followed up when this sample was collected: lost cases were almost all from other regions.

All the patients were diagnosed as 'clinically defined' MS, according to Poser's criteria. MR was performed in all patients (within the first year in 80 per cent, within one month in 35 per cent): radiological findings fitted in with the diagnosis of MS in 100 per cent.

CSF examination was performed in 19/20 patients: oligoclonal banding was present in 18/19 (94.7 per cent). Visual, auditory and somatosensory evoked potentials were performed respectively in 16, 17 and 12 patients, being pathological respectively in 62 per cent, 47 per cent and 41 per cent.

For each patient the following data were obtained: sex, age at onset, family history, symptoms at onset, clinical course, disease duration, EDSS after the first episode and at the last clinical control. For the seven patients with disease duration longer than 8 years also the following were recorded: time interval between onset and first relapse, total number of *poussées*, mean number of *poussées* per year, EDSS at 1 year from onset.

Results

Age at onset ranged from 8 years 2 months to 14 years 2 months, with a mean age of 12 years for females and of 10 years 8 months for males. The youngest boy was 8 years 2 months, the youngest girl 9 years 2 months. Eight patients (40 per cent) were younger than 11 years.

Sex ratio (female/male ratio) was 0.75:1 on the whole sample, but strikingly varied with age at onset, being 0.14:1 in children younger than 11 at onset and 1.4:1 in older children.

Table 6. Clinical features (total sample)

Patient	Sex	Age at onset	Symptoms at onset	Disease duration	EDSS at onset	EDSS at last control	Clinical course
1	M	8.2	B	5.9	0	3.5	RR
2	M	8.8	S	3.4	0	3.0	RR
3	M	8.11	B	11	1.5	4.0	RP
4	M	8.11	CB	0.5	1.5	1.0	RR
5	F	9.2	B	7.2	3.0	5.5	RP
6	M	9.10	V	1	0	1.0	RR
7	M	10.6	V	13.7	0	1.5	RR
8	M	10.10	PS	13.5	0	2.5	RR
9	F	11.0	BPS	7.4	0	4.0	RP
10	M	11.9	B	3.5	2.0	2.5	RR
11	F	12	P	0.6	0	3.5	RR
12	M	12.1	BCP	8.3	1.0	2.5	RR
13	F	12.2	PC	13.10	3.5	7.5	RP
14	F	12.2	S	0.6	1.0	1.0	RR
15	F	12.6	S	9.6	2.0	6.0	RP
16	F	13.2	SPB	2.2	2.5	2.0	RR
17	M	13.4	C	5.3	1.0	2.0	RR
18	M	13.6	VCP	5.2	2.5	2.5	RR
19	M	13.7	S	1.11	0	2.5	RR
20	F	14.2	SBC	2.1	1.5	1.5	RR

B = brainstem; C = cerebellar; P = pyramidal; S = sensory; V = visual.

Family history was positive only in one case: the patient's twin became affected later (no other information on this family was available since the twins were adopted).

Onset was monosymptomatic in only 9/20 patients, the others showing dysfunction of two or even three functional systems. Forty-five per cent of patients showed symptoms from brainstem dysfunction, 40 per cent sensitive, 35 per cent pyramidal, 30 per cent cerebellar and only 15 per cent pure visual symptoms (the total exceeds 100 per cent because of cases in which onset was polysymptomatic). Only 15 per cent presented with malaise, fever, headache, nausea or vomiting, suggesting diffuse CNS involvement, which was previously reported as being relatively frequent in children at onset. Epilepsy was reported in only one case, and not as a presenting complaint.

As many as 17/20 patients (85 per cent) relapsed within the first year. The interval between the first and second episode ranged from 2 to 26 months. Clinical course was relapsing-remitting in 75 per cent, relapsing-progressive in the remaining 25 per cent. No one showed a progressive course from the beginning. Patients with disease duration > 8 years had a relapsing progressive course in a higher percentage (57.1 per cent).

EDSS after the first episode ranged from 0 to 3.5. 14 patients scored < 2, of which seven out of eight patients with onset before 11 years, but only seven out of 12 in the older group.

Considering the seven patients (four males and three females) with a disease duration > 8 years, long-term impairment was mild (EDDS < 4) in three (42.8 per cent), severe (EDSS > 4) in four (57.2 per cent). Only two patients lost deambulation, scoring respectively 6.0 and 7.0. Both patients were female.

Results are summarized in Table 6 (total sample) and in Tables 7a and 7b (patients with disease duration > 8 years).

Table 7a. Clinical features (patients with disease duration > 8 years)

Patient	Sex	Age at onset	Symptoms at onset	Interval 1st–2nd episode	Mean number of relapses/year	Total number of relapses
3	M	8.11	B	26	0.6	7
7	M	10.6	V	12	0.7	10
8	M	10.10	PS	11	1.3	18
9	F	11	BPS	10	0.5	4
12	M	12.1	BCP	8	1.5	13
13	F	12.2	PC	5	2.4	34
15	F	12.6	S	2	2.10	20

Table 7b. Clinical features (patients with disease duration > 8 years)

Patient	Sex	Disease duration	EDSS at onset	EDSS after 1 year	EDSS at last control	Clinical course
3	M	11	1.5	0	4.0	RP
7	M	13.7	0	0	1.5	RR
8	M	13.5	0	0	2.5	RR
9	F	8	0	3.5	4	RP
12	M	8.3	1.0	2.0	2.5	RR
13	F	13.10	3.5	2.5	7.5	RP
15	F	9.6	2.0	2.5	6.0	RP

Comments

The most peculiar aspect in our study is the unusual male preponderance, particularly when compared to other paediatric series in which the female preponderance generally observed in adults with MS was even more marked. This male preponderance, mostly evident in children with onset before age 11, decreases with age at onset raising. This has already been reported by Ghezzi et al. and suggests the possibility that changes in sexual hormones in the puberal period may play a role in triggering disease onset. Obviously, since our sample is small and collected from a large geographic area, selection bias is possible.

Symptoms at onset were most frequently due to brainstem dysfunction, followed by sensitive and pyramidal symptoms. The published literature shows great variability on this point, but Ghezzi *et al.* (1997) reported the same distribution, even if in a far larger sample.

Patients relapsing within the first year were 85 per cent, a very high percentage compared with other series. The fact that ours is a tertiary referral centre could have played a role in selecting a sample with a particularly active disease, at least at the very beginning.

On the other hand, clinical course was never progressive from the beginning, compared to other series in which progressive cases ranged from 5.5 per cent (Ghezzi) to 22 per cent (Duquette).

Long-term outcome was relatively favourable, with only 28.5 per cent patients scoring > 6 after a minimum disease duration of 8 years, compared to the estimated 50 per cent scoring > 6 after 10 years of the total adult MS population (Bradley *et al.*, 1996).

Even if in a very small sample, the correlation reported in adults between time elapsed between onset and first relapse and long-term outcome was confirmed in our series, the two patients with shortest interval being the most severely affected at the last control.

In conclusion, both from literature review and our sample results, clinical features typical for childhood or juvenile MS do not clearly emerge, even if a relatively favourable long-term outcome is suggested at least by some series, ours included. MS is still a rare disease in childhood, even now that it is surely less underestimated than in the past. More data are needed on the topic, from large multicentric prospective studies, according to strict diagnostic and follow-up protocols.

Acknowledgements: The authors wish to thank Dr. Elvio Maccagnano for neuroradiological consulting. The topic of this paper was the subject of the dissertation for MD degree of Alex Gravante, University of Milan.

References

Bradley, W.G., Daroff, R.B., Fenichel, G.B. & Marsden, C.D. (1996): *Neurology in clinical practice*. Boston: Butterworth-Heinemann.

Boutin, B., Esquivel, E., Mayer, M., Chaumet, S., Ponsot, G. & Arthuis, M. (1988): Multiple sclerosis in children: report of clinical and paraclinical features of 19 cases. *Neuropediatrics* **19**, 118–123.

Cole, G.F. & Stuart, C.A. (1995): A long perspective on childhood multiple sclerosis. *Dev. Med. Child Neurol.* **37**, 661–666.

Duquette, P., Murray, T.J., Pleines, J., Ebers, G.C., Sadovnik, D., Weldon, P., Warren, S., Paty, W., Upton, A., Hader, W., Nelson, R., Auty A., Neufeld, B. & Meltzer, C. (1987). Multiple sclerosis in childhood. clinical profile in 125 patients. *J. Pediatr.* **111**, 359–363.

Ghezzi, A., Deplano, V., Faroni, J., Grasso, M.G., Liguori, M., Marrosu, G., Pozzilli, C., Simone, I.L. & Zaffaroni, M. (1997): Multiple sclerosis in childhood: clinical features of 149 cases. *Multiple Sclerosis* **3**, 43–46.

Guilhoto, L.M. de F.F., Osorio, C.A.M. & Machado L.R. (1994): Pediatric multiple sclerosis report of 14 cases. *Brain Dev.* **17**, 9–12.

Hanefeld, F., Bauer, H.J., Christen, H., Kruse, B., Bruhn, H. & Frahm, J. (1991): Multiple sclerosis in childhood: report of 15 cases. *Brain Dev.* **13**, 410–416.

Izquierdo, G., Lyon-Caen, O., Marteau, R., Martinez-Parra, Lhermitte, F., Castaigne, P. & Hauw, J.J. (1986): Early onset multiple sclerosis. Clinical study of 12 pathologically proven cases. *Acta Neurol. Scand.* **73,** 493–497.

Poser, C.M., Paty, D.W., Scheiberg, L., McDonald, I., Davis, F.A., Ebers, G.C., Johnson, K.P., Sibley, W.A., Silberger, D.H. & Tourtellotte, W.W. (1983): New diagnostic criteria for multiple sclerosis: guidelines for research protocols. *Ann. Neurol.* **13,** 227–231.

Schilder, P. (1912): Zur Kenntnis der sogenannten diffusen Sklerose. *Z. Ges. Neurol. Psychiatr.* **10,** 1–60.

Sindern, E., Haas, J., Stark, E. & Wurster, U. (1992): Early onset MS under the age of 16: clinical and paraclinical features. *Acta Neurol. Scand.* **87,** 280–284.

Chapter 6

Acute disseminated encephalomyelitis

Marianna Bugiani, Chiara Conti, Elio Maccagnano* and Lucia Angelini

*Departments of Child Neurology and *Neuroradiology, Istituto Nazionale Neurologico 'C. Besta', via Celoria 11, 20133 Milan, Italy*

Summary

Acute disseminated encephalomyelitis (ADEM) is an immune-mediated demyelinating disease of the central nervous system (CNS) which seldom complicates systemic viral and mycoplasma pneumoniae infections or vaccinations. Following the evidence of diffuse brain involvement (sensitized T-lymphocytes reach CNS myelin through the venous system), focal signs develop reflecting the occurrence of multiple large perivenous demyelinating areas easily detectable by MRI. Gravity rests on the degree of parenchimal oedema and, on rare occasions, of vessel wall necrosis leading to blood extravasation. Clinical presentation may reflect selective vulnerability responsible for site-restricted forms (optic neuritis, cerebellitis, brinstem encephalitis or myelitis). Combined forms involving the peripheral nervous system are also known. The disease is usually monophasic and sensitive to high-dose steroid treatment, plasma exchange or intravenous immunoglobulins administration. Recurrent and multiphase forms often require immunosuppression.

The results of a retrospective analysis carried out on 16 patients are reported, focusing on the clinical and radiological features suggestive for diagnosis and prognosis.

Introduction

Acute disseminated encephalomyelitis (ADEM) is a demyelinating disease which follows a viral infection or a vaccination. Mostly, ADEM complicates measles, mumps, chickenpox and rubella (either infection or vaccination), and upper respiratory tract infections due to influenza, parainfluenza, Epstein-Barr, herpes simplex, adenovirus and *Mycoplasma pneumoniae* (Miller *et al.*, 1956; Kaji *et al.*, 1996; Pellegrini *et al.*, 1996; Kumada *et al.*, 1997; Nagai & Mori, 1999). Incidence ranges 1:200,000 to 1:1,000 depending on age and vaccination policy. ADEM is characterized pathologically by multiple perivenous demyelinating areas in the white matter, which often cluster into larger lesions, while axons are remarkably preserved. Inflammatory reaction is characterized by microglial cells and macrophages, which are superimposed to demyelination, and by lymphocytes and mononuclear cells which cuff intraparenchimal veins, often extending into the cerebral cortex and subcortical gray structures (Prineas & McDonald, 1997; Olivero *et al.*, 1999). Dispersed inflammatory infiltrates are detectable in the meninges. Following demyelination and inflammatory reaction localized around intraparenchimal veins and the absence of virus in CSF and brain tissue, ADEM is regarded as induced by polyclonal antibodies secreted by B-lymphocytes cross-reacting with myelin proteins. T-lymphocytes favour inflammation by releasing lymphokynes. A disease closely resembling ADEM can be experimentally produced by inoculating laboratory animals with myelin proteins. Thus, experimental allergic encephalomyelitis and ADEM share the same lesions. Moreover, in both diseases the myelin basic protein can be isolated from CFS, while this protein also induces T-lymphocyte proliferation *in vitro* (Prineas & McDonald, 1997; Pohl-Koppe *et al.*, 1998).

The clinical features of ADEM reflect a diffuse involvement of the brain. Fever, fatigue, malaise and shooting pains in the limbs are rapidly followed by neck stiffness, headache, drowsiness, fits, and a rostrocaudal deterioration syndrome with stupour and coma in the most severe cases. Subsequently, focal signs develop due to focal demyelination in the white matter. Rarely, onset is characterized by focal signs or acute psychotic syndromes (Johnsen *et al.*, 1989; Moscovich *et al.*, 1995). Based on clinical features, several forms have been identified ranging from silent forms incidentally found by MRI, to lethal forms (Table 1). Most commonly, ADEM is characterized by a single episode. Multiple episodes are uncommon, increasingly recurrent (the first episode is followed by recovery and recurrences are clinically stereotyped), pseudorecurrent (patients are affected by a steroid-dependent disease), and multiphase (two or more acute episodes differing in clinical presentation) forms (Kamio *et al.*, 1982; Gutowski *et al.*, 1993; Khan *et al.*, 1995). Since demyelination can be restricted to selected structures, ADEM seldom presents as optic neuritis, cranial nerve neuritis, brainstem or cerebellar encephalitis, and transverse myelitis (Al Deeb *et al.*, 1997; Sakakibara *et al.*, 1996; Smith & Traquina, 1998; Asenbauer *et al.*, 1997). Combined forms involving the central and peripheral nervous system are known (Kinoshita *et al.*, 1996).

Table 1. ADEM and related demyelinating disorders

- ADEM (uniphasic form)
- Acute haemorrhagic form (Hurst's disease)
- Site-restricted forms:
  - Optic neuritis
  - Other cranial nerve neuritis
  - Cerebellitis
  - Brainstem encephalitis
  - Transverse myelitis
- Chronic-recurrent forms:
  - Recurrent
  - Pseudorecurrent
  - Multiphasic
- Combined CNS-PNS form

Increased white blood cell counts and erythrocyte sedimentation rate can be demonstrated at onset, while disappearing within a few days. In most cases, CSF examination reveals a moderately increased number of lymphocytes (20–50 cell/ml, rarely more) and protein content (usually less than 100 mg/dl), while transient endogenous IgG oligoclonal bands have been found in a few patients only (Khan *et al.*, 1995; Francis *et al.*, 1996). EEG abnormalities are a

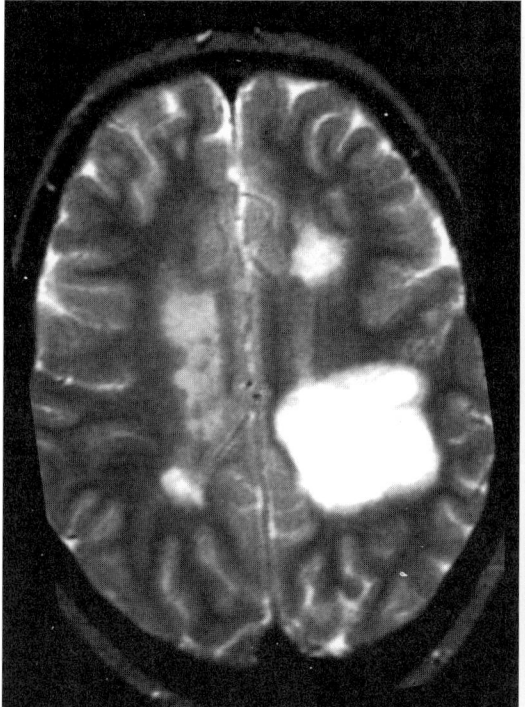

Fig. 1. Case 3, seven months after onset. Axial T2-weighted image (TR/TE = 2350/90) demonstrates a large area of marked hyperintensity involving posteriorly the white matter of the centrum semiovale, with no significant mass effect. Multiple diffuse smaller hyperintense areas are present within the white matter on both sides.

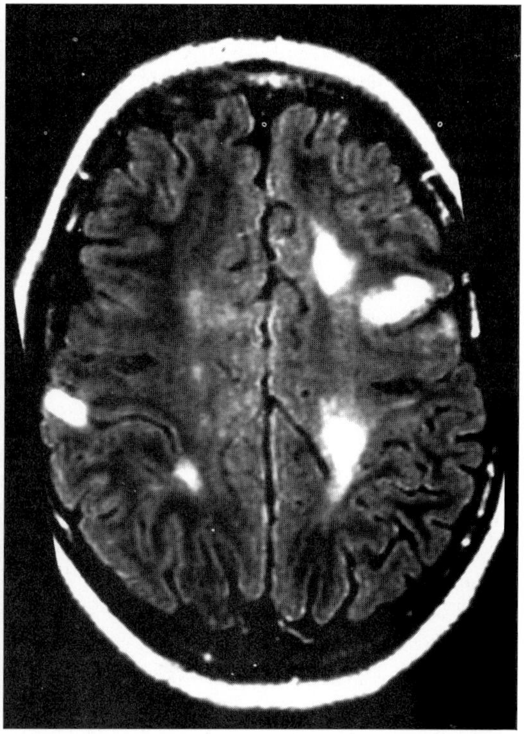

Fig. 2. Case 3, 12 months after onset. Axial FLAIR image (TR/TE = 11000/140; TI = 2500) demonstrates a considerable reduction in size of the left centrum semiovale white matter lesion, while remaining smaller lesions are only slightly reduced. Two new lesions with no mass effect have appeared in the left frontal and right parietal subcortical white matter respectively, partly involving the cortex.

frequent, however unspecific finding. On the contrary, MRI investigation is diagnostic, since it shows multifocal, symmetric, often large T2 prolongation abnormalities in the white matter, possibly extending into the gray structures, which appear in a 4-week time span from the onset. Sequential MRIs often demonstrate oedema in the white matter leading sometimes to herniations at the beginning of the disease, while demyelinating lesions can be detected within 3–4 weeks from onset. In most cases, focal abnormalities disappear or change into glial scars within 12–24 months (Kesselring *et al.*, 1990; Triulzi & Scotti, 1998; Perdue *et al.*, 1985, Dagher & Smirniotopoulos, 1996). Additional lesions can be found along with recurrence (Fig. 1), or may develop without new symptoms.

In most cases, ADEM has a good prognosis due to high efficacy of steroid therapy (methylprednisolone, 15–20 mg/kg iv) which is related to both anti-inflammatory and anti-oedematous actions (Straub *et al.*, 1997). Alternative drugs (immune suppressants such as azathioprine, intravenous immunoglobulins and plasma exchange) have been employed against relapses and treatment failure following steroid treatment (Kleiman, 1995; Kanter *et al.*, 1995; Hahn *et al.*, 1996; Apak *et al.*, 1999; Pradhan *et al.*, 1999). Mortality rate ranging 10–30 per cent is mostly

Table 2. Clinical, CSF and MRI features at onset and follow-up

N	Sex	Age	Infection	Interval after infection	Prodromal illness	Clinical syndrome at onset	CSF	Initial MRI	Course	Interval	Clinical outcome	MRI
1	F	3.6 y	Mycopl	1 wk	+	Encephalopathy ataxia	prot	Multiple pv and sc lesions	Monoph	8 m	Complete recovery	Marked but incomplete resolution
2	F	5.1 y	NURT	1 wk	–	Myelopathy	prot cells	Swelling and high signal in lumbar cord	Monoph	11 m	Partial recovery	Unchanged
3	F	9 y	Mycopl	6 wks	–	Encephalopathy spasticity, 7 cn palsy	Normal	Multiple pv, dc and sc lesions, basal nuclei	Multiph	4 m (II) 7 m (III) 1 y	Frontal sy Unchanged Partial recovery	New lesions New lesions New lesions
4	F	1 y	?	?	–	Encephalopathy psychomotor regression	Np	Np	Monoph	1.6 y	Partial recovery (hypotonia, ataxia, mental deter)	Multiple pv and dc
5	M	2.9 y	Measles	3 wks	+	Encephalopathy seizures	Normal	Multiple confluent dc	Monoph	2 m	Partial recovery (ataxia, spasticity)	Unchanged, atrophy
6	F	6 y	Measles	4 wks	–	Encephalopathy	prot cells	Multiple pv and dc	Monoph	12 y	Partial recovery (mental deterioration)	Unchanged, atrophy
7	F	4 m	NGI	6 wks	–	Encephalopathy psychomotor regression, dystonia	Normal	Dc (temporal, occipital)	Monoph	11 m	Partial recovery (mental deterioration, dystonia)	Diffuse extensive cerebral lesions, atrophy
8	F	8 y	?	?	+	Encephalopathy seizures	cells	Basal nuclei lesions	Pseudorec	1 m	Complete recovery	New lesions (multiple dc)
9	M	6.3 y	NURT	4 wks	+	Encephalopathy ataxia	Np	Multiple dc	Monoph	4 m	Partial recovery (hyperreflexia)	Complete resolution, no new lesions
10	F	1.3 y	NURT	2 wks	–	Encephalopathy	Np	Multiple pv and dc	Monoph	3.6 y	Complete recovery	Unchanged

Table 2. (contd).

#	Sex	Age	Prodrome	Interval	OB	Clinical	CSF prot/cells	MRI	Mono/Multi	Follow-up	Clinical outcome	MRI outcome
11	M	6.9 y	NURT	3 wks	+	Encephalopathy seizures	Normal		Multiph	2 m (II)	Encephalopathy (flaccid paraparesis)	Cerebellar hemispheric, bulbar, cervical cord
										5 m (III)	Encephalopathy (spastic tetraparesis)	New lesions (pv, dorsal cord)
										7 m (IV)	Encephalopathy (ataxia, spasticity, visual impairment)	Unchanged
										1 y	Partial recovery (spasticity, dystonia)	Complete resolution of cerebral lesions, partial recovery of cord lesions
12	M	10.7 y ?	?	?	+	Encephalopathy ataxia, spasticity	Np	Multiple pv and dc	Monoph	1.2 y	Complete recovery	Unchanged
13	M	1.5 y	NURT	1 wk	+	Encephalopathy spasticity	cells	Multiple confluent pv and dc, middle cerebellar peduncle, bulbar	Multiph	3 m (II)	Encephalopathy (brainstem dysf)	New lesion (basal nuclei)
										8 m (III)	Encephalopathy (spasticity)	Unchanged
										11 m	Severe spasticity, exophoria	Unchanged
14	F	4 y	NURT	2 wks	–	Ataxia, intention tremor	OB	Multiple pv and dc, pons	Monoph	6.6 y	Partial recovery (hypotonia, intention tremor)	Unchanged
15	M	8 y	NURT	1 wk	–	Bilateral visual failure, spastic paraparesis	Normal	Multiple, confluent pv and dc	Monoph	6 y	Unchanged	Unchanged
16	F	13.6 y	NURT	1 wk	+	Encephalopathy seizures, spasticity	prot	Multiple confluent dc, middle cerebellar peduncle, pons	Monoph	6 m	Complete recovery	Marked but incomplete resolution

NURT: nonspecific upper respiratory tract infection. NGI: nonspecific gastrointestinal infection. Prodromal illness: fever, malaise, myalgia. Encephalopathy: headache, vomiting, altered sensorium. OB: transient oligoclonal IgG bands. Prot: increased protein content. Cells: increased cell count. MRI pv: periventricular lesions; sc: subcortical lesions; dc: discrete cerebral lesions. Np: not performed.

related to the severity of oedema and the occurrence of a necrotic vasculitis responsible for haemorrhagic softenings in the white matter (this form is referred to as acute haemorrhagic leukoencephalitis, Hurst type, and usually follows a *Mycoplasma* infection; Prineas & McDonald, 1997; Francis *et al.*, 1996; Watson *et al.*, 1984; Huang *et al.*, 1988). Fifty per cent of survivors present a full recovery within 6 to 8 months, while others have permanent sequelae.

Results and discussion

We have observed 16 patients (six males, 10 females, age at onset 4 months to 13 years), who underwent a follow-up study ranging 5 months to 12 years (Table 2). A trivial infection anticipating onset could be assessed in all but three patients. Measles and *Mycoplasma* were demonstrated in four patients. Symptoms at onset reflected diffuse brain involvement in 13 out of 16 patients, and focal involvement in three patients. The disease was monophasic in 12 patients, pseudorecurrent in one, and multiphase in three. Full recovery could be assessed in five out of 16 patients, while focal signs and/or cognitive deterioration and behavioural troubles persistent in nine and four patients respectively. CSF abnormalities were observed in 10 patients (seven out of 10 at onset, three out of four after recurring), while transient IgG oligoclonal bands were found only in one. MRI showed diagnostic signal abnormalities in all patients, with involvement of grey structures in one third of them.

Ten patients out of 16 received a 2 months to 12 years follow up because of persisting focal signs and cognitive impairment associated with MRI abnormalities. In five more patients, the clinical recovery was completed in 1 month to 3.6 years despite persisting MRI abnormalities. The opposite occurred in one patient within 4 months. At the end of the follow-up, none of the patients had attained either clinical or full neuroradiological recovery. This observation suggests the need for a longer follow-up in ADEM patients. Based on these data and in comparison with the experience of other authors, we have devised a diagnostic work-up to be applied prospectively at onset of symptoms and during follow-up (Table 3).

Table 3. Diagnostic work-up

At onset/after recurrence
• Routine blood analysis

• CSF analysis:
    Glucose and protein content, cell count
    IgG isoelectrofocusing
    Antibodies against measles, mumps, HSV-1 and HSV-2, VZV, influenza, EBV, coxsackie, Borrelia, mycoplasma, leptospira

• Contrasted MRI of the brain and spinal cord (to be repeated after 1 month)
• Multimodal evoked potentials (VEP, ABR, SSEP)
During follow-up (6 months, 12 months, 24 months)
• CSF analysis, in case of previous detection of positive oligoclonal bands
• Contrasted MRI of the brain and spinal cord
• Multimodal evoked potentials (VEP, ABR, SSEP), if already altered at a previous examination

The course of the disease is difficult to predict on purely clinical and radiological grounds. Moreover, it is still to be established if such features may help distinguish disease recovery in asymptomatic patients or in the case of permanent sequelae from eventually recurrent forms, in order to guide surveillance and therapeutic decisions.

References

Al Deeb, S.M., Yaqub, B.A., Bruyn, G.W. & Biary, N.M. (1997): Acute transverse myelitis: a localized form of postinfectious encephalomyelitis. *Brain* **120**, 1115–1122.

Apak, R.A., Anlar, B. & Saatci I. (1999): A case of relapsing acute disseminated encephalomyelitis with high-dose corticosteroid treatment. *Brain Dev.* **21**, 279–282.

Asenbauer, B., McConachie, N.S., Allcutt, D., Farrell, M.A. & King, M.D. (1997): Acute near-fatal parainfectious cerebellar swelling with favourable outcome. *Neuropediatrics* **28**, 122–125.

Dagher, A.P. & Smirniotopoulos, J. (1996): Tumefactive demyelinating lesions. *Neuroradiology* **38**, 560–565.

Francis, G.S., Duquette, P. & Antel, J.P. (1996): Inflammatory demyelinating diseases of the central nervous system. In: *Neurology in clinical practice*, eds. W.G. Bradley, R.B. Daroff, G.M. Fenichel & C.D. Marsden, pp. 1307–1343. Newton: Butterworth-Heinemann.

Gutowski, N.J., Davenport, R.J., Heron, J.R. & Miller, D.M. (1993): Benign relapsing meningo-encephalomyelitis. *J. Neurol. Neurosurg. Psychiatry* **56**, 568–569.

Hahn, J.S., Siegler, D.J. & Enzmann, D. (1996): Intravenous gammaglobulin therapy in recurrent acute disseminated encephalomyelitis. *Neurology* **46**, 1173–1174.

Huang, C.C., Chu, N.S. & Chen, T.J. (1988): Acute haemorrhagic encephalitis with a prolonged clinical course. *J. Neurol. Neurosurg. Psychiatry* **51**, 870–874.

Johnsen, S.D., Sidel, A.D & Bird, R. (1989): Subtle encephalomyelitis in children: a variant of acute disseminated encephalomyelitis. *J. Child Neurol.* **4**, 214–217.

Kaji, M., Kusuhara, T., Hino, H., Shoji, H. & Nagao, T. (1996): Survey of herpes simplex virus infections of the central nervous system, including acute disseminated encephalomyelitis, in the Kyushu and Okinawa regions of Japan. *Multiple Sclerosis* **2**, 83–87.

Kamio, M., Tahira, K., Ono, J. & Ikehara, C. (1982): Acute relapsing disseminated encephalomyelitis: case report and study of 24 patients in previous reports. *J. Japan. Pediat. Soc.* **86**, 559–566.

Kanter, D.S., Horensky, D., Sperling, R.A., Kaplan, J.D., Malachowski, M.E. & Churchill, W.H. Jr. (1995): Plasmapheresis in fulminant acute disseminated encephalomyelitis. *Neurology* **45**, 824–827.

Kesselring, J., Miller, D.H., Robb, S.A., Kendall, B.E., Moseley, I.F., Kingsley, D., Du Boulay, G.H. & McDonald, W.I. (1990): Acute disseminated encephalomyelitis: MRI findings and the distinction from multiple sclerosis. *Brain* **113**, 291–302.

Khan, S., Yaqub, B.A., Poser, C.M., Al Deeb, S.M. & Bohlega, S. (1995): Multiphasic disseminated encephalomyelitis presenting as alterning hemiplegia. *J. Neurol. Neurosurg. Psychiatry* **58**, 467–470.

Kleiman, M. (1995): Acute disseminated encephalomyelitis: response to intravenous immunoglobulin. *J. Child Neurol.* **10**, 481–483.

Kinoshita, A., Hayashi, M., Miyamoto, K., Oda, M., & Tanabe, H (1996): Inflammatory demylinating polyradiculitis in a patient with acute disseminated encephalomyelitis (ADEM). *J. Neurol. Neurosurg. Psychiatry* **60**, 87–90.

Kumada, S., Kusaka, H., Okaniwa, M., Kobayashi, O. & Kusunoki, S. (1997): Encephalomyelitis subsequent to mycoplasma infection with elevated serum anti-Gal C antibody. *Pediatr. Neurol.* **16**, 241–244.

Miller, H. G., Stanton, J. B. & Gibbons, J.L. (1956): Para-infectious encephalomyelitis and related syndromes. *Quarterly J. Med.* **25**, 427–505.

Moscovich, D.G., Singh, M.B., Eva, F.J. & Puri, B.K. (1995): Acute disseminated encephalomyelitis presenting as an acute psychotic state. *J. Nerv. Ment. Dis.* **183**, 116–117.

Nagai, K. & Mori, T. (1999): Acute disseminated encephalomyelitis with probable measles vaccine failure. *Pediatr. Neurol.* **20,** 399–402.

Olivero, W.C., Deshmukh, P. & Gujrati, M. (1999): Bilateral enhancing thalamic lesions in a 10 year old boy: case report. *J. Neurol. Neurosurg. Psychiatry* **66,** 633–635.

Pellegrini, M., O'Brien, T.J., Hoy, J. & Seidal, L. (1996): *Mycoplasma pneumoniae* infection associated with an acute brainstem syndrome. *Acta Neurol. Scand.* **93,** 203–206.

Perdue, Z., Bale, J.F. Jr, Dunn, V.D. & Bell, W.E. (1985): Magnetic resonance imaging in childhood disseminated encephalomyelitis. *Pediatr. Neurol.* **1,** 370–374.

Pohl-Koppe, A., Burchett, S.K., Thiele, E.A. & Hafler, D.A. (1998): Myelin basic protein reactive Th2 T-cells are found in acute disseminated encephalomyelitis. *J. Neuroimmunol.* **91,** 19–27.

Pradhan, S., Gupta, R.P., Shashank, S. & Pandey, N. (1999): Intravenous immunoglobulin therapy in acute disseminated encephalomyelitis. *J. Neurol. Sci.* **165,** 56–61.

Prineas, J.W. & McDonald, W.I. (1997): Demyelinating diseases. In: *Grienfield's neuropathology*, eds. D.I. Graham & P.L. Lantas, pp. 813–896. London: Arnold.

Sakakibara, R., Hattori, T., Yasuda, K. & Yamanishi, T. (1996): Micturitional disturbance in acute disseminated encephalomyelitis (ADEM). *J. Auton. Nerv. Syst.* **60,**, 200–205.

Smith, V. & Traquina, D.N. (1998): Pediatric bilateral facial palsy. *Laryngoscope* **108,** 519–523.

Straub, J., Chofflon, M. & Delavelle, J. (1997): Early high-dose intravenous methylprednisolone in acute disseminated encephalomyelitis: a successful recovery. *Neurology* **49,** 1145–1147.

Triulzi, F. & Scotti, G. (1998): Differential diagnosis of multiple sclerosis: contribution of magnetic resonance techniques. *J. Neurol. Neurosurg. Psychiatry* **64,** S6–S14.

Watson, R.T., Ballinger, W.E. & Quisling, R.G. (1984): Acute haemorrhagic leukoencephalitis: diagnosis by computed tomography. *Ann. Neurol.* **15,** 611–612.

Chapter 7

Opsoclonus-myoclonus syndrome in children

Giovanna Zorzi, Nardo Nardocci, Anna Erba and Giovanni Lanzi*

Department of Child Neurology, Istituto Nazionale Neurologico 'C. Besta', via Celoria 11, 20133 Milan; *Dept of Developmental Neurology and Psychiatry, Fondazione 'C. Mondino', via Palestro 3, 27100 Pavia, Italy

Summary

The opsoclonus-myoclonus syndrome (OMS) is a neurological disorder of children and adults consisting of opsoclonus, myoclonus, cerebellar signs and mental and emotional features. The disease has an acute onset and treatment with corticosteroids is dramatically effective. The clinical course is characterized by frequent recurrence of symptoms coincident with infectious disorders or reduction of dose therapy. It can be the consequence of a viral infection (parainfectious OMS) or can be associated with neuroblastoma (paraneoplastic OMS). In both conditions, immunological mechanisms play an essential role. The analysis of our series of patients demonstrates that OMS is a chronic disease, which implies disabling cognitive and neurological deficits.

Introduction

In 1962 Kinsbourne described six cases affected by a unique form of myoclonic encephalopathy with acute onset following a non-specific respiratory or gastrointestinal infection (Kinsbourne, 1962). A few years later, a similar clinical picture was reported in two children with neuroblastoma, in which the myoclonic status was the first sign of the disease (Solomon & Chutorian, 1968).

Since the original report, more than 100 infantile cases have been reported in the literature under several names including 'infantile polymyoclonia', 'dancing eyes, dancing feet syndrome', 'Kinsbourne syndrome'. The opsoclonus-myoclonus syndrome (OMS) is now recognized as a neurological syndrome, presenting also in adulthood, that can be the manifestation of remote cancer, toxic, metabolic, and infectious disorders (Pranzatelli, 1992).

Clinical aspects

With the accumulation of additional cases, the symptomatology originally reported has been confirmed. The age at onset is almost invariably in the second year of life, but exceptional cases with an earlier or later onset have been reported (Rivner *et al.*, 1982; Shawkat *et al.*, 1993). The clinical picture consists of opsoclonus, myoclonus, cerebellar signs and mental and emotional features; the disorder has usually an acute or subacute onset, reaching its peak within 2 days to one week from onset.

Opsoclonus refers to conjugate or semiconjugate, chaotic, rapid, randomly directed eye movements. It is increased by saccadic movements or fixation and may persist in sleep, but diminished. Electro-oculographic recordings have shown bursts of saccades without saccadic intervals in horizontal and vertical planes (Vignaendra & Lim, 1977; Shawkat *et al.*, 1993).

Myoclonus consists of shock-like muscular contractions, involving any region of the body; it is present at rest and exacerbated by action, excitement or stress, and it is usually irregular in duration, amplitude and distribution. The functional disability due to abnormal movements is, in most cases, severe and the sitting or standing position is excluded or compromised. Electrophysiological studies do not demonstrate spikes or complex wave forms on EEG coincident with the EMG discharges (Pampiglione & Maria, 1972; Lott & Kinsbourne, 1986).

Cerebellar signs are mainly represented by ataxia, tremor, hypotonia, and dysarthria. Another striking feature of the disease, almost invariably present, is a variety of *behavioural disturbances*, ranging from emotional lability to a marked irritability; vomiting frequently accompanies the onset of the disease.

There is no temporal association of opsoclonus with the other symptoms that may follow or precede its appearance, but all the symptoms are usually present in the conclamate disease, making the clinical picture distinctive and unlike that seen in any other condition.

Corticosteroid treatment is dramatically effective, determining an almost total remission of symptoms expecially during the first phases of the disease (Kinsbourne, 1962; Pranzatelli, 1992).

The clinical course is characterized by recurrences precipitated by intercurrent infections or decrease in the dose therapy. After this initial phase, during which most patients require steroid treatment, the disease course becomes stable, myoclonus and opsoclonus eventually disappear, but motor and mental deficits are observed in more than half the cases (Koh *et al.*, 1994; Hammer *et al.*, 1995; Rodriguez-Barrionuevo *et al.*, 1998).

The prognosis of the disease does not seem to be correlated with the age at onset, treatment, frequency and duration of the recurrences, or aetiology (Hammer *et al.*, 1995).

Aetiology

Approximately half of the cases of opsoclonus-myoclonus syndrome in children are associated with neuroblastoma. The tumour is more frequently located in the mediastinal region (49–61 per cent), but may also originates from retroperitoneal, adrenal, sacrococcigeal or superior cervical ganglion locations (Pranzatelli, 1992).

Opsoclonus-myoclonus syndrome can follow an infectious illness, in most cases due to a viral infection. In some patients the aetiological agent has been identified: EBV (Sheth *et al.*, 1995), coxsackie B3 (Kuban *et al.*, 1983), mumps (Ichiba *et al.*, 1988), poliovirus (Vieira & Rosa, 1985), rubella (Christoff, 1969); more often the infectious aetiology can only be suspected.

The recognition of a viral agent does not rule out the presence of neuroblastoma.

The neurological symptoms can precede up to several years the finding of the tumour, that can remain occult and the spontaneous regression of which has been sometimes demonstrated (Engle *et al.*, 1995). Moreover, it has been shown that the viral infection of the neural crest cells can be a carcinogenic event, so that brain damage and tumour induction can be independent but simultaneous events. Each patient presenting with opsoclonus-myoclonus syndrome should therefore be extensively investigated for neuroblastoma, even years after the onset of neurological symptoms. The most sensitive investigations in the detection of the neuroblastoma are the MRI and the metaiodobenzylguanidine radionuclide scans; increased urinary catecholamine excretion is found in only 60 per cent of the cases (Mitchell & Snodgrass, 1990).

Anatomical bases

The anatomical localization of the abnormalities underlying OMS is still uncertain and several structures of the CNS, including the cerebellum and the brainstem, are thought to play a role.

Neuroradiological investigations (brain CT and/or MRI) are normal in the majority of patients with opsoclonus-myoclonus syndrome; only two infantile cases are reported in the literature, in which it was possible to demonstrate lesions of the cerebellum (Willis *et al.*, 1983; Tuchman *et al.*, 1989). In one of these patients, follow-up radiological studies have revealed cerebellar atrophy (Willis *et al.*, 1983). In adults OMS has been observed also in association with brainstem abnormalities (Hattori *et al.*, 1988; Luque *et al.*, 1991). Electrophysiological studies by mean of electro-oculographic recordings to assess the eye movements in five children have indicated the cerebellum, and in particular the fastigial nuclei, as the structure mainly involved (Shawkat *et al.*, 1993).

Very few data are reported regarding the anatomical findings in autopsied cases, both in adults and children, with controversial results (Shawkat *et al.*, 1993).

Immunological aspects

Several findings support the concept that immunological mechanisms are involved in the pathogenesis of paraneoplastic or parainfectious opsoclonus-myoclonus syndrome (Pranzatelli, 1992):

1. Spontaneous regression of neuroblastoma;
2. CSF abnormalities (pleocytosis, increased IgG and/or protein);
3. Better prognosis for survival in patients with neuroblastoma and OMS compared to those with no paraneoplastic manifestations;
4. Presence of specific anti-CNS antibodies.

While in adulthood paraneoplastic syndromes the association of certain autoantibodies with specific tumours is well established, very few data are available for the childhood population (Liblau *et al.*, 1998).

Circulating anti-neurofilament antibodies were found in the serum of three children with OMS and no neuroblastoma, but these antibodies are thought to be less specific and have also been found in other diseases as well as in healthy subjects (Noetzel *et al.*, 1987; Stefansson *et al.*, 1985). More interestingly, in six children with OMS specific anti-Purkinje cell antibodies were detectable, and in all cases these antibodies were no longer measurable after corticosteroid treatment (Plioplys *et al.*, 1989). The frequency and the role of such autoantibodies in the pathogenesis of this neurological syndrome is yet to be established (Pranzatelli, 1992; Liblau *et al.*, 1998).

Case studies

Table 1. Neurological and cognitive outcome of the 16 patients with opsoclonus-myoclonus syndrome

Patient no.	Age at onset	Follow-up	Duration of treatment	Neurological outcome (age)	Cognitive and psychological outcome (age)
1	18 m	1 m	1 m	Normal	Irritable (19 m)
2	20 m	1 m	1 m	Normal	Irritable (21 m)
3	2 yrs	6 m	2 m	Normal	Normal (2.6 yrs)
4	17 m	6 m	6 m	Normal (2 yrs)	Speech delay (23 m)
5	19 m	8 m	8 m	Normal (2.5 yrs)	Speech delay, irritable (2.5 yrs)
6	1.9 yrs	8 m	7 m	Normal (2.5 yrs)	IQ: 76 (2 yrs) Severely irritable (2.5 yrs)
7	15 m	2 yrs	2 yrs	Normal	Speech delay, irritable
8	13 m	2.9 yrs	2.9 yrs	Normal (3.1 yrs)	Speech delay, irritable (3.10 yrs)
9	18 m	3.2 yrs	3.2 yrs	Normal (4.1 yrs)	IQ: 78 (3.2 yrs) IQ: 87 (4.10 yrs)
10	14 m	5 yrs	5 yrs	Clumsy, mild ataxia (6.3 yrs)	IQ: 77 (2 yrs) Special education (6.3 yrs)
11	18 m	6.4 yrs	6.4 yrs	Clumsy, tremor (7.9 yrs)	IQ: 74 (5.5 yrs) IQ: 78 (7.9 yrs)
12	17 m	8.7 yrs	8.7 yrs	Clumsy, tremor (10 yrs)	IQ: 80 (6 yrs) Special education (10 yrs)
13	2.10 yrs	9 yrs	9 yrs	Ataxia, dysmetria, tremor (12 yrs)	IQ: 60 (6 yrs) IQ: 50 (12 yrs)
14	2.4 yrs	9.7 yrs	9.7 yrs	Severly clumsy, tremor (10.6 yrs)	Developmental age: 4 yrs and psychosis (10 yrs)
15	16 m	10.7 yrs	10.7 yrs	Ataxia (12 yrs)	IQ: 64 (5.4 yrs) IQ: 31 (10 yrs)
16	18 m	18.3 yrs	18.3 yrs	Clumsy, dysmetria (19 yrs)	

We retrospectively evaluated the medical records of 16 patients (10 females and six males) affected by opsoclonus-myoclonus syndrome. The children have been evaluated during the last 15 years at the Department of Child Neuropsychiatry of the Neurological Institute 'Carlo Besta' in Milan and at the Department of Child Neuropsychiatry of the Institute 'C. Mondino' in Pavia.

All the patients were extensively investigated during a mean follow-up of 6 years (range: 1 month – 18.4 years).

Pregnancy and delivery were uneventful and early psychomotor development was normal in all patients. In one child (patient no. 4) diabetes mellitus was diagnosed 6 months before the onset of neurological symptoms.

The age at onset of the disease ranged between 14 months and 3 years (mean 19 months). The symptoms reached their peak within 2 days to 3 weeks from the onset, and all patients presented opsoclonus, myoclonus, ataxia, and marked irritability.

Prior to the onset of the disease nine patients suffered an infectious disease of presumed viral aetiology with upper respiratory or gastrointestinal symptoms; two other patients presented a defined viral illness, and two patients underwent immunization.

In none of the patients was it possible to demonstrate a neuroblastoma during follow-up. In four patients the investigations pointed out a viral infection of established origin: Coxsackie B3 (patient no. 11), Coxsackie A (patient no. 10), Poliovirus in two (patients nos. 6 and 14).

All patients were initially treated with corticosteroids (ACTH in nine patients and dexamethasone in seven patients), with a complete regression of the neurological symptoms. At the end of the follow-up 12 patients were still on corticosteroid therapy at the lowest possible dosage. In the remaining four patients treatment was withdrawn after 4–7 years, and in none of them did exacerbation of symptoms occur after 1–11 years.

In all patients the initial course of the disease was characterized by exacerbations of symptoms due to an intercurrent infectious illness or reduction of dose therapy. Subsequently, fixed neurological signs, mainly characterized by severe clumsiness, cerebellar signs, moderate to severe cognitive deficits, and behavioural disturbances, were observed in all cases with a duration of the disease longer than 3 years. The long-term outcome of the 16 patients is summarized in Table 1.

Conclusions

Our results allow us to conclude, in accordance with the literature, that OMS is a chronic disease: in all patients with a follow-up longer than 4 years, disabling cognitive and neurological sequels are present (Papero *et al.*, 1995). We could not find any differences of outcome in respect of age at onset, frequency of exacerbation, or aetiology, but further studies are needed in order to identify prognostic factors.

To conclude, we would like to recommend a diagnostic protocol for each patient with OMS, which should include:

- Extensive virological investigations, both on serum and CSF;
- Repeated investigations for the detection of neuroblastoma (MRI of thorax and abdomen);
- Immunological investigations with the detection of specific circulating autoantibodies (anti-Purkinje cells, anti-Ri, anti-Hu, anti-Yo).

Acknowledgements: We thank Dr. Pierangelo Veggiotti, Istituto 'C. Mondino', Pavia, for referring patients nos. 4 and 7.

References

Christoff, N. (1969): Myoclonic encephalopathy of infants. A report of two cases and observation of related disorders. *Arch. Neurol.* **21,** 229–234.

Engle, E.C., Schaefer, P.W. & Hedley-White, E.T. (1995): A 29 month-old girl with worsening ataxia, nystagmus, and subsequent opsoclonus and myoclonus (Case Record of the Massachusetts General Hospital). *N. Eng. J. Med.* **339,** 579–586.

Hammer, M.S., Larsen, M.B. & Stack, C.V. (1995): Outcome of children with opsoclonus-myoclonus regardless of etiology. *Pediatr. Neurol.* **13,** 21–24.

Hattori, T., Hirayama, K., Imai, T., Yamada, T. & Kojima, S. (1988): Pontine lesion in opsoclonus-myoclonus syndrome shown by MRI. *J. Neurol. Neurosurg. Psychiatry* **51,** 1572–1575.

Ichiba, N., Miyake, Y., Sato, K., Oda, N. & Kimoto, H. (1988): Mumps-induced opsoclonus-myoclonus and ataxia. *Ped. Neurol.* **4,** 224–227.

Kinsbourne, M. (1962): Myoclonic encephalopathy of infants. *J. Neurol. Neurosurg. Psychiatry.* **25**, 271–276.

Koh, P.S., Raffensperger, J.G., Berry, S., Larsen, M.B., Johnstone, H.S., Chou, P., Luck, S.R., Hammer, M. & Cohn, S.L. (1994): Long-term outcome in children with opsoclonus-myoclonus and ataxia and coincident neuroblastoma. *J. Pediatr.* **125**, 712–716.

Kuban, K.C., Ephros, M.A., Freeman, R.L., Laffell, L.B. & Bresnan, M.J. (1983): Syndrome of opsoclonus-myoclonus caused by Coxsackie B3 infection. *Ann. Neurol.* **13**, 69–71.

Liblau, R., Benyahia, B. & Delattre, J.Y. (1998): The pathophysiology of paraneoplastic neurological syndromes. *Ann. Med. Interne (Paris)* **8**, 512–520.

Lott, I. & Kinsbourne, M. (1986): Myoclonic encephalopathy of infants. *Adv. Neurol.* **43**, 127–136.

Luque, F.A., Furneaux, H.M., Ferziget, R., Rosenblum, M.K., Wray, S.H., Schold, C., Glantz, M.J., Jaeckle, K.A., Biran, H., Lesser, M., Paulsen, W.A., River, M.E. & Posner, J.B. (1991): Anti-Ri: an antibody associated with paraneoplastic opsoclonus and breast cancer. *Ann. Neurol.* **29**, 241–251.

Mitchell, W.G. & Snodgrass, S.R. (1990): Opsoclonus and ataxia due to childhood neural crest tumors: a chronic neurologic syndrome. *J. Child. Neurol* **5**, 153–155.

Noetzel, M., Cawley, L.P., James, V.L., Minard, B.J. & Agrawal, H.C. (1987): Anti-neurofilament protein antibodies in opsoclonus-myoclonus. *J. Neuroimmunol.* **15**, 137–145.

Pampiglione, G. & Maria, M. (1972): Syndrome of rapid irregular movements of eyes and limbs in childhood. *Br. Med. J. (Clin. Res.)* **1**, 469–473.

Papero, P.H., Pranzatelli, M.R., Margolis, L.J., Tate, E., Wilson, L.A. & Glass, P. (1995): Neurobehavioral and psychosocial functioning of children with opsoclonus-myoclonus syndrome. *Dev. Med. Child Neurol.* **10**, 915–932.

Plioplys, A.V., Greaves, A. & Yoshida, W. (1989): Anti-CNS antibodies in childhood neurological diseases. *Neuropediatrics* **20**, 93–102.

Pranzatelli, M.R. (1992): The neurobiology of the opsoclonus-myoclonus syndrome. *Clin. Neuropharmacol.* **15**, 186–228.

Rivner, M.H., Jay, W.M., Green, J.B. & Dyken, P.R. (1982): Opsoclonus in *Haemophilus influenzae* meningitis. *Neurology* **32**, 661–663.

Rodriguez-Barrionuevo, A.C., Caballero-Morales, M.A., Delgado-Marques, M.P., Mora-Ramirez, M.D. & Martinez-Anton, J. (1998): Kinsbourne syndrome: review of our cases. *Rev. Neurol.* **26**, 956–959.

Shawkat, F.S., Harris, M.Ch., Wilson, J. & Taylor, D.S.I. (1993): Eye movements in children with opsoclonus-polymyoclonus. *Neuropediatrics* **24**, 218–223.

Sheth, R.D., Horwitz, S.J., Aronoff, S., Gingold, M. & Bodensteiner, J.B. (1995): Opsoclonus-myoclonus syndrome secondary to Epstein-Barr virus infection. *J. Child. Neurol.* **10**, 297–299.

Solomon, G.E. & Chutorian, A.M. (1968): Opsoclonus and occult neuroblastoma. *N. Eng. J. Med.* **279**, 475–477.

Stefansson, K., Marton, L.S., Dieperinik, M.E., Molnar, G.K., Schlaepfer, W.W. & Helgason, C.M. (1985): Circulating autoantibodies to the 20,000 Dalton proteins of neurofilaments in the serum of healthy individuals. *Science* **228**, 1117–1119.

Tuchman, R.F., Alvarez, L.A., Kantrowitz, A.B., Moser, F.G., Llena, J. & Moshe, S.L. (1989): Opsoclonus-myoclonus syndrome: correlation of radiographic and pathological observation. *Neuroradiology* **31**, 250–252.

Vieira, J.B.A. & Rosa, E.D. (1985): Polymyoclonia-opsoclonus. Kinsbourne's syndrome. A case report. *Arq. Neuropsiquiatr.* **43**, 194–197.

Vignaendra, V. & Lim, C.L. (1977): Electro-oculographic analysis of opsoclonus: its relation to saccadic and nonsaccadic eye movements. *Neurology* **27**, 1129–1133.

Willis, J., Collada, M. & Robertson, H.J. (1983): Cerebellar lesion in myoclonic encephalopathy of infants. *Arch. Neurol.* **40**, 818–819.

Chapter 8

Rasmussen's syndrome

Tiziana Granata^, Elena Freri^, Carlo Antozzi•, Renato Mantegazza•,
Marina Casazza*, Flavio Villani*, Federica Zibordi^, Lucia Angelini^,
Francesca Ragona^, Luisa Chiapparini§ and Roberto Spreafico*

^Department of Child Neurology; *Department of Neurophysiology; •Department of Neuromuscular Research;
§Department of Neuroradiology, Istituto Nazionale Neurologico 'C. Besta', via Celoria 11, 20133 Milan, Italy

Summary

Rasmussen's encephalitis (RE) is a rare syndrome characterized by childhood onset of partial and secondarily generalized seizures, often with epilepsia partialis continua (EPC) and recurrent status epilepticus, progressive dysfunction of one cerebral hemisphere and cognitive decline. Neuroimaging shows progressive atrophy of the affected hemisphere. Neuropathology of affected brain tissue is characterized by inflammatory changes such as perivascular lymphocytic cuffing and microglial nodules composed of T-cells and macrophages or microglia; neuronal loss, laminar necrosis and variable degrees of glial scarring are also prominent features. The aetiology of RE is still unknown. A viral pathogenesis has long been suspected on the basis of histopathological findings. However, serological studies have been inconclusive, and positive findings from polymerase chain reaction or *in situ* hybridization analyses of brain samples could not be associated specifically to the disease. The recent observation that rabbits immunized with a fusion protein containing a portion of the extracellular domain of glutamate receptor 3 (GluR3) developed seizures and histopathological features similar to those of RE suggested a role for anti-GluR3 antibodies in the pathogenesis of the animal model, and of the human disease. Indeed, evidence of immunoreactivity to GluR3 was found by immunoblot analysis of sera from three patients with pathologically proven RE. Moreover, rabbit and human sera, as well as purified IgG, were able to activate currents in kainate-responsive neurons in culture.

Introduction

Rasmussen's encephalitis (RE) is a rare childhood disease clinically characterized by the association of intractable partial seizures and symptoms of progressive hemispheric dysfunction. Neuroimaging shows progressive atrophy of the affected hemisphere; neuropathologic studies reveal chronic encephalitis with perivascular lymphocytic cuffing, glial nodules, laminar necrosis and eventually spongy degeneration.

The aetiopathogenesis of the disease is still unknown and the role of viral infections and immunomediated disorders remains under study.

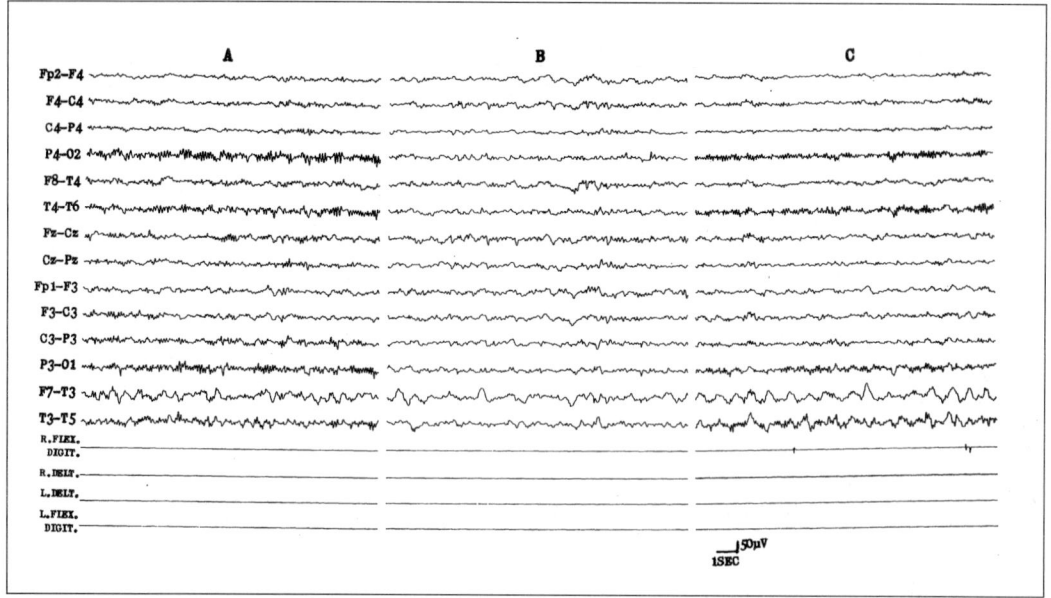

Fig.1. Intermittent polymorphic delta activity is evident in the left temporal area (A and C), the slow activity decreases during sleep (B). [From Capovilla et al., 1997, with permission.]

Clinical features

The disease is sporadic and affects males and females in childhood or early adolescence (mean age 6.8 ± 5.1 years; range 1–15 years); only a few adult-onset cases have been reported (Gray et al., 1987; McLachlan et al., 1993; Hart et al., 1997). The previous personal history is uneventful, although the occurrence of febrile illness (usually minor viral illness such as influenza, tonsillitis or gastrointestinal upset) in the months preceding the first seizure is frequently reported.

The onset is typically marked by epileptic seizures, either simple motor partial, complex partial, or generalized convulsive. In a number of cases (20 per cent in the Montreal Neurologic Institute series of 51 cases, Rasmussen & Andermann, 1991) the initial event consisted of generalized or focal status epilepticus. The epilepsy course is characterized by recurrence of different types of seizures at increasing frequency, and refractory to antiepileptic drugs (Piatt et al., 1988; Vining et al., 1993; Andrews et al., 1997). Partial motor seizures are frequently followed by transient hemiparesis. Epilepsia partialis continua (EPC) develops in about half of the patients and partial status epilepticus may recur. The EEG recordings reveal slowing of background activity, with early evidence of focal slow abnormalities (Capovilla et al., 1997; Fig.1) and multifocal interictal epileptic discharges, all confined, in the early stages, to the affected hemisphere. As the illness progresses, bilateral abnormalities become evident and in some cases asynchronous epileptic abnormalities over the unaffected hemisphere may be recorded. During the course of the disease progressive neurological deficits appear, consisting of hemiparesis and hemianopia as well as cortical sensory loss and speech deficits (aphasia and dysarthria) depending on which hemisphere is affected. Progressive intellectual deterioration is also a constant feature. In most although not all cases, the progression of neurologic and mental impairment seems to be related to the malignancy of epilepsy. The natural course of the disease

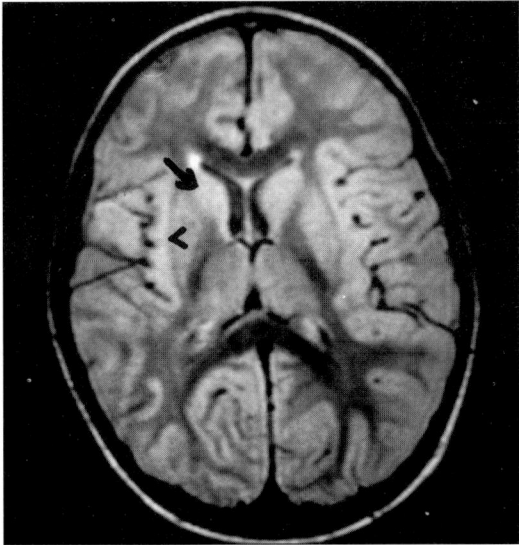
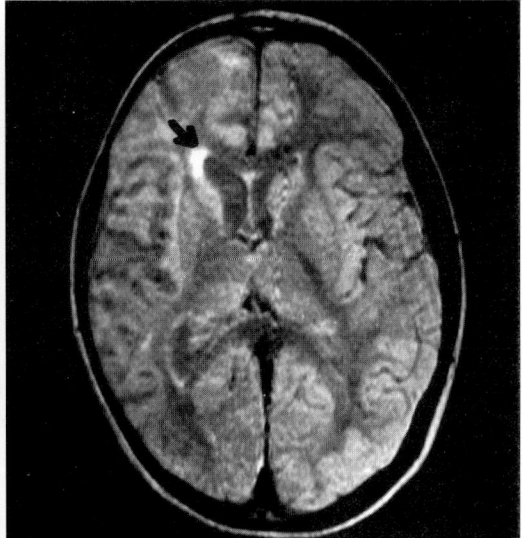
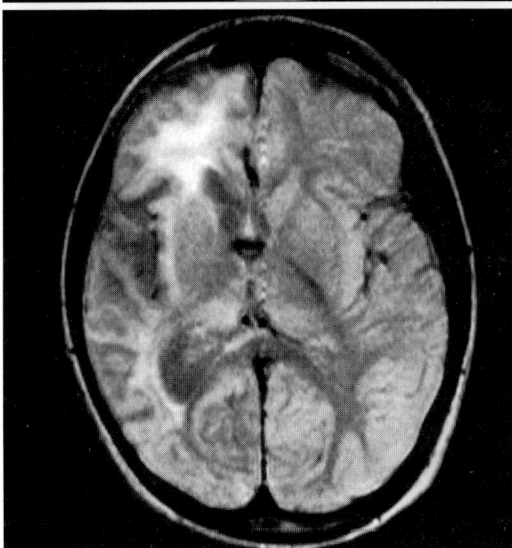

Fig.2. MR axial proton density image at the onset of the disease shows atrophy of the right caudate nucleus head (arrow), associated with a mild enlargement of the frontal horn on the same side. Note the mild signal hyperintensity in the right insula (arrowhead) (A, top left). One year later, MR axial proton-density image shows the progression of the atrophy of the right caudate nucleus head, the progressive atrophy of the right frontal lobe and the enlargement of the sylvian fissure; slight enlargement of the right ventricle is also present. Note the signal hyperintensity in the deep white matter around the frontal horn (arrow) (B, top right). In the following years, axial proton density MR image shows atrophic right hemisphere. Right frontal horn is dilated owing to caudate nucleus atrophy. Right putamen and insula are extremely atrophic. Note the progression of the hyperintensity in the white matter of the frontal and parietal lobes (C, bottom left).

is generally characterized by a relentless progression for many years, usually reaching a stable condition characterized by a moderate to severe hemiparesis, visual field defect, intellective and language impairment.

Neuroradiologic findings

The neuroimaging correlate of RE is a progressive hemispheric damage well documented by CT, MRI and functional neuroimaging.

On CT and MRI the prominent feature is the progressive unilateral atrophy that usually first affects the temporoinsular region and progresses over a few years to involve the large part of the hemisphere, particularly the frontal lobe (Tien *et al.*, 1992; Bhatjiwale *et al.*, 1998). In the last few years the extensive use of MRI has allowed a better definition of the pathologic changes from the early stages of the disease. Beside the hemispheric atrophy, common features include focal white matter hyperintensity, and atrophy of basal ganglia, particularly centred on the head of the caudate nucleus (Fig. 2). Data on magnetic resonance spectroscopy (MRS) have been sporadically reported: a decrease in the N-acetylaspartate peak in the affected hemisphere, involving both grey and white matter, is a constant finding (Cendes *et al.*, 1995; Sundgren *et al.*, 1999). This finding confirms the original observation of low N-acetylaspartate and glutamate levels detected by MRS in tissues from surgically treated RE cases (Peeling & Sutherland, 1993).

Laboratory findings

Blood tests are usually unrevealing; antibodies titre of HSV 1 and 2, EBV, and CMV may be elevated in sera and cerebrospinal fluid (CSF). CSF may be normal or show non-specific abnormalities such as a mild increase in the white cell count and proteins. In a number of cases, oligoclonal bands have been found.

Neuropathologic findings

The histopathological picture is characterized by the typical microscopic features of active encephalitis, with many large and small vessels showing perivascular cuffs of lymphocytes and monocytes and glial nodules scattered throughout the grey and white matters (Rasmussen, 1978); the microglial nodules, often exhibiting neuronophagia, are mainly represented in the medium-sized pyramidal cells of the external pyramidal layer. Spongy degeneration following coalescence of multifocal neuronal loss is the final aspect. Different inflammatory stages may coexist in the same specimen.

Diagnostic clues

Hart *et al.* (1994) suggested the following diagnostic criteria:

(a) Children with epilepsia partialis continua and at least one of the following: (1) progressive neurologic deficit at the beginning or after the onset of EPC; (2) progressive hemispheric atrophy on CT and/or MRI; (3) presence of oligoclonal banding on CSF examination; (4) biopsy evidence of chronic encephalitis.

(b) Children who do not have EPC but do have focal epilepsy and biopsy evidence of chronic encephalitis, and meet criteria 1, 2 or 3.

Biological basis and pathogenesis

The aetiopathogenesis of the disease is still unknown and the role of viral infections and immunomediated disorders is still under study.

Since the original Rasmussen's description, a possible viral aetiology has been postulated based on the clinical course and the histological findings similar to those seen in other encephalitis, but despite several epidemiological and virologic studies aimed at detecting viral particles or genetic evidence of viral material in brain tissue taken by patients with RE, the role of viral infection is still questionable. Moreover, the viral hypothesis is challenged by the lack of geographic, seasonal or clustering effects.

Serologic and cerebrospinal fluid searching for antecedent viral infection or inflammatory response has given inconsistent results, as well as direct search for virus on resected brain tissues. Positive *in situ* hybridization for CMV and Epstein-Barr viral genome (Walter & Renella, 1989; Power *et al.*, 1990), and detection of CMV and HSV1 by polymerase chain reaction (Jay *et al.*, 1995) have been reported, but these data were not confirmed by other studies (Farrell *et al.*, 1991; Vinters *et al.*, 1993; Atkins *et al.*, 1995). Atkins *et al.* (1995) systematically studied 34 tissue blocks from seven patients with RE using biotinylated double-stranded DNA probes to CMV, HSV, and EBV; two cases were also evaluated by electron microscopy and one case by immunoperoxidase techniques. The authors failed to identify any evidence of viral material, challenged the role of viruses as the sole factor in the development of RE and suggested that more complex mechanisms involving immune response to viral infection could underlay the disease. The role of immunopathogenetic mechanisms was also suggested by Andrews *et al.* (1990) who found, on an hemispherectomy specimen from a child with RE, widespread vasculitis with immunofluorescence staining for IgG, IgM, IgA, C3 and C1q; in this patient, ultrastructural studies disclosed signs of vascular injury, beside severe cortical atrophy with marked neuronal loss. The role of the immunologic system was further supported by the presence of elevated serum antinuclear body titres and of cerebrospinal fluid oligoclonal bands.

A new interest in the pathogenesis of RE as an autoimmune disorder was raised by the report of Rogers and colleagues who induced clinical and pathologic changes mimicking RE in two out of four rabbits immunized with the putative extracellular fragment of the AMPA receptor subunits GluR3 (Rogers *et al.*, 1994). The two rabbits developed high titres of GluR3 antibodies, anorexia and behavioural abnormalities consistent with seizures (unresponsiveness, clonic movements). Microscopic examination disclosed inflammatory changes characterized by microglial nodules, perivascular lymphocytic infiltration mainly located in the cerebral cortex, and lymphocyte infiltration of the meninges. Neither behavioural abnormalities nor pathologic changes were seen in rabbits injected with fusion proteins containing GluR1, 2, 5, 6. These observations suggested the hypothesis that antibodies directed at a GluR3 subunit regulate neuronal excitability by binding and modulating glutamate receptors. The authors also detected immunoreactivity to GluR3 fusion protein in sera samples from two patients affected by RE with high frequency seizures, but not in one more RE patient who was seizure-free since the hemispherectomy performed some years before. The authors thus suggested that GluR immunoreactivity is correlated with disease activity. The same group later proposed that glutamate receptor antibodies activate a subset of receptors and reveal an agonist binding site and suggested that excessive activation of GluR3 might directly trigger seizures (Twyman *et al.*, 1995). In a more recent paper the same authors challenged their original hypothesis and suggested that neuronal cell death might result from activation of the complement system by anti-GluR3 antibodies more than from the direct excitotoxic effect of overstimulated glutamate receptors (He *et al.*, 1998).

Treatment

It is common experience that conventional antiepileptic drugs have only partial, if any, effect on seizure control in RE. Furthermore the question whether the progressive neurologic disorder could be explained by the effect of the high seizure frequency or by the underlaying encephalitis process is still unsolved. Clinicians have therefore tried, in addition to antiepileptic drugs, a number of medical treatments, mainly antiviral or immunosuppressant agents, on the basis of the different proposed aetiologies.

The rarity of the condition and the variability in the rate of progression of the disease make clinical trials and evaluation of treatment efficacy difficult. Most treatments have been tried on an empirical basis and information about their efficacy is mostly derived from retrospective studies of single case reports and of few case series.

Zidovudine at the dose of 800 mg/die was employed by De Toledo & Smith (1994) in a 18-year-old girl with a 4-year history of RE. Zidovudine was given for 2 months and then withdrawn because of granulocytopenia. Within 6 weeks of treatment, seizures stopped and neurologic deterioration was in remission for 21 months, then seizures relapsed involving the previously unaffected hemisphere and a new trial with zidovudine was precluded by severe side effects.

Ganciclovir was administered by McLachlan *et al.* (1996) in four patients with a clinical picture suggestive of RE. In a young girl treated early in the course of the disease, ganciclovir (given intravenously at 10 mg/kg/day for 10 days) was dramatically effective, leading to disappearance of seizures and neurological deficits and to EEG normalization. A less striking effect was observed in two more patients who had a reduction in seizure frequency, whereas the treatment was ineffective in the fourth case. According to the authors, these findings support the viral role in the pathogenesis of RE and suggest that any patient suspected of having chronic encephalitis should be given a trial of ganciclovir early in the course of the disease.

Intraventricular recombinant alpha interferon (rIFNA) has also been tried (Maria *et al.*, 1993; Dabbagh *et al.*, 1997) on the basis of its immunomodulatory and antiviral effect: rIFNA enhances phagocytic activity of macrophages, cytotoxicity of lymphocytes for target cells, and inhibits virus replication in virus infected cells. The two reported patients had a significant improvement in seizure frequency and neurologic conditions during the rIFNA chronic treatment.

Corticosteroids (dexamethasone, prednisone, methylprednisolone and ACTH) have been used by many authors at different dosages and treatment schedules (Gupta *et al.*, 1984; Piatt *et al.*, 1988; Dulac *et al.*, 1992; Hart *et al.*, 1994; Kraus *et al.*, 1996). Repeated bolus of IV methylprednisolone 400 mg/m^2 associated with chronic administration of oral prednisolone have been proposed by Dulac and coworkers; in the authors' experience the treatment was effective both in seizure control (with cessation of epilepsia partialis continua in three out of the five cases) and in contrasting the progression of motor and cognitive deterioration. Promising results with long term immunomodulatory treatment with human IV immunoglobulin have been reported (Hart *et al.*, 1994; Leach *et al.*, 1999); this treatment seems to be particularly effective in adult onset RE (Leach *et al.*, 1999; Villani *et al.*, 2001).

The use of immunosuppressant agents, such as cyclophosphamide and azathioprine has been reported in very few cases (Krauss *et al.*, 1996; Andrews *et al.*, 1996). In our experience neither IV monthly administration (two patients) nor chronic oral treatment (one patient) with cyclophosphamyde produced any significant effect on seizure frequency and neurologic picture.

Based on the review of the medical treatment given to 19 patients in different centres, Hart and colleagues proposed a treatment protocol (Hart *et al.*, 1994): the treatment should start with intravenous immunoglobulin (IV IG) at the dose of 400 mg/kg/day on three consecutive days. Patients who benefit from the treatment should be maintained with a monthly single IV IG administration, whereas patients who do not show any improvement should be switched to high dose steroid treatment with an intermittent infusion of IV methylprednisolone 400 mg/m^2 associated with chronic administration of oral prednisolone.

The use of plasma exchange was first reported by Rogers and colleagues following their finding of GluR immunoreactivity in RE (Rogers *et al.*, 1994). The result of plasma exchange in a child severely affected was transient (lasting 4 weeks) with a decrease in seizure frequency and an improvement in the neurological status. The same team later reported the use of repeated plasmapheresis in four children, three of whom had a striking repeated, albeit transient reduction of seizure frequency, interruption of status epilepticus, and improvement of neurological functions (Andrews *et al.*, 1996). In the authors' view, given the transient response, risks (e.g. infections, anaemia, coagulopathy), and expense of plasma exchange (PEX), this treatment should be used as an adjunct to other therapies. The authors therefore suggested a protocol of sequential combination of PEX and IVIG or intermittent PEX combined with immunotheraphy to limit costs and prolong the improvement after each cycle of plasma exchange. Moreover, the authors underlined the specific potential applications of PEX, including treatment of status epilepticus, and the preoperative assessment of residual function of the affected cortex, that could be masked by the transient improvement induced by PEX.

We evaluated the efficacy of periodic IgG immunoadsorption with protein A in a patient with treatment-resistant RE (Antozzi *et al.*, 1998). Because antibodies to GluR3 are IgG, we assumed that the periodic, selective removal of IgG by protein A immunoadsorption could be a feasible alternative to plasmapheresis in a 15-year-old patient with RE, never submitted to surgery, and positive for antiGluR3 antibodies. In fact, selectivity, efficiency and tolerability make protein A immunoadsorption suitable for long-term treatment. We adopted a standardized protocol already applied to the treatment of severe immunosuppression-resistant myasthenia gravis patients in which periodic removal of IgG led to significant improvement of their neurological function (Antozzi *et al.*, 1994).

Our patient's conditions were markedly improved by protein A immunoadsorption. Seizure frequency was reduced and a dramatic improvement of her neuropsychological deficit was observed along the 3-year follow-up. AntiGluR3 antibodies were always significantly reduced by immunoadsorption. A worsening of the patient's neurological function and seizures was observed at the attempt of delaying treatment, notwithstanding cyclophosphamyde chronic administration.

Despite the several attempts to find rational medical therapies, none of the proposed treatments has shown a persistent effect on the course of the disease, and the surgical option still remain inevitable in most cases. Hemispherectomy, or functional hemispherectomy (Polkey 1990; Villemure & Mascott, 1995; Peacock *et al.*, 1996), is the only procedure that stops the progression of the disease. It is unanimously considered the treatment of choice in patients who have already developed hemiparesis and hemianopia and even, according to some authors (Vining *et al.*, 1993) in the early phases, given the inevitable progression of symptoms. Less destructive procedures such as subpial cortical resection are on the contrary preferred by others in earlier phases.

References

Andrews, J.M., Thompson, J.A., Pysher, T.J., Walker, M.L. & Hammond, M.E. (1990): Chronic encephalitis, epilepsy, and cerebrovascular immune complex deposits. *Ann. Neurol.* **28**, 88–90.

Andrews, P.I., Dichter, M.A., Berkovic, S.F., Newton, M.R. & McNamara, J.O. (1996): Plasmapheresis in Rasmussen's encephalitis. I. **46**, 242–246.

Andrews, P.I., McNamara, J.O. & Lewis, D.V. (1997): Clinical and electroencephalographic correlates in Rasmussen's encephalitis. *Epilepsia* **38**, 189–194.

Antozzi, C., Berta, E., Confalonieri, P., Zuffi, M., Cornelio, F. & Mantegazza, R. (1994): Protein-A immunoadsorption in immunosuppression-resistant myasthenia gravis. *Lancet* **343**, 124.

Antozzi, C., Granata, T., Aurisano, N., Zardini, G., Confalonieri, P., Airaghi, G., Mantegazza, R. & Spreafico, R. (1998): Long-term selective IgG immunoadsorption improves Rasmussen's encephalitis. *Neurology* **51**, 302–305.

Atkins, M.R., Terrell, W. & Hulette, C.M. (1995): Rasmussen's syndrome: a study of potential viral etiology. *Clin. Neuropathol.* **14**, 7–12.

Bhatjiwale, M.G., Polkey, C., Cox, T.C.S., Dean, A. & Deasy, N. (1998): Rasmussen's encephalitis: neuroimaging findings in 21 patients with a closer look at the basal ganglia. *Pediatr. Neurosurg.* **29**, 142–148.

Capovilla, G., Paladin, F. & Dalla Bernardina, B. (1997): Rasmussen's syndrome: longitudinal EEG study from the first seizure to epilepsia partialis continua. *Epilepsia* **38**, 483–488.

Cendes, F., Andermann, F., Silver, K. & Arnold, D.L. (1995): Imaging of axonal damage *in vivo* in Rasmussen's syndrome. *Brain* **118**, 753–758.

Dabbagh, O., Gascon, G., Crowell, J. & Bamoggadam, F. (1997): Intraventricular interferon-alpha stops seizures in Rasmussen's encephalitis: a case report. *Epilepsia* **38**, 1045–1049.

De Toledo, J.C. & Smith, D.B. (1994): Partially successful treatment of Rasmussen's encephalitis with zidovudine: symptomatic improvement followed by involvement of the contralateral hemisphere. *Epilepsia* **35**, 352–355.

Dulac, O., Chinchilla, D., Plouin, P., Pinel, J.F. & Robain, O. (1992): Follow-up of Rasmussen syndrome treated by high-dose steroids. *Epilepsia* **33** (S3), 128.

Farrell, M., Cheng, L., Cornford, M.E., Grody, W.W. & Vinters, H.V. (1991): Cytomegalovirus and Rasmussen's encephalitis. *Lancet* **337**, 1551–1552.

Gray, F., Serdau, M., Baron, H., Daumas-Duport, C., Loron, P., Sauron, B. & Poirier, J. (1987): Chronic localised encephalitis (Rasmussen's) in an adult with epilepsia partialis continua. *J. Neurol. Neurosurg. Psych.* **50**, 747–751.

Gupta, P.C., Rapin, I., Houroupian, D.S., Roy, S., Liena, J.F. & Tandon, P.N. (1984): Smouldering encephalitis in children. *Neuropediatrics* **15**, 191–197.

Hart, Y.M., Cortez, M., Andermann, F., Hwang, P., Fish, D.R., Dulac, O., Silver, K., Fejerman, N., Cross, H., Sherwin, A. & Caraballo, R. (1994): Medical treatment of Rasmussen's syndrome (chronic encephalitis and epilepsy): effect of high-dose steroids or immunoglobulins in 19 patients. *Neurology* **44**, 1030–1036.

Hart, Y.M., Andermann, F., Fish, D.R., Dubeau, F., Robitaille, Y., Rasmussen, T., Berkovic, S., Marino, R., Yakoubian, E.M., Spillane, K. & Scaravilli, F. (1997): Chronic encephalitis and epilepsy in adults and adolescents: a variant of Rasmussen's syndrome? *Neurology* **48,**, 418–424.

He, X.P., Patel, M., Whitney, K.D., Janumpalli, S., Tenner, A. & McNamara, J.O. (1998): Glutamate receptor GluR3 antibodies and death of cortical cells. *Neuron* **20**, 153–163.

Jay, V., Becker, L.E., Otsubo, H., Cortez, M., Hwang, P., Hoffman, H.J. & Zielenska, M. (1995): Chronic encephalitis and epilepsy (Rasmussen's encephalitis): detection of cytomegalovirus and herpes simplex virus 1 by polymerase chain reaction and *in situ* hybridisation. *Neurology* **45**, 108–117.

Krauss, G.L., Campbell, M.L., Roche, K.W., Huganir, R.L. & Niedermeyer, E. (1996): Chronic steroid-responsive encephalitis without autoantibodies to glutamate receptor GluR3. *Neurology* **46**, 247–249.

Leach, J.P., Chadwick, D.W., Miles, J.B. & Hart, I.K. (1999): Improvement in adult-onset Rasmussen's encephalitis with long-term immunomodulatory therapy. *Neurology* **52**, 738–742.

Maria, B.L., Ringdahl, D.M., Mickle, J.P., Smith, L.J., Reuman, P.D., Gilmore, R.L., Drane, W.E. & Quisling, R.G. (1993): Intraventricular alpha interferon therapy for Rasmussen's syndrome. *Can. J. Neurol. Sci.* **20**, 333–336.

McLachlan, R.S., Girvin, J.P., Blume, W.T. & Reichman, H. (1993): Rasmussen's chronic encephalitis in adults. *Arch. Neurol.* **50**, 269–274.

McLachlan, R.S., Levin, S. & Blume, W.T. (1996): Treatment of Rasmussen's syndrome with ganciclovir. *Neurology* **47**, 925–928.

Peacock, W.J., Wehby-Grant, M.C., Shields, W.D., Shewmon, D.A., Chugani, H.T., Sankar, R. & Vinters, H.V. (1996): Hemispherectomy for intractable seizures in children: a report of 58 cases. *Child's Nerv. Syst.* **12**, 376–384.

Peeling, J. & Sutherland, G. (1993): 1H Magnetic resonance spectroscopy of extracts of human epileptic neocortex and hippocampus. *Neurology* **43**, 589–594.

Piatt, J.H., Hwang, P.A., Armstrong, D.C., Becker, L.E. & Hoffman, H.J. (1988): Chronic focal encephalitis (Rasmussen syndrome): six cases. *Epilepsia* **29**, 268–279.

Polkey, C.E. (1990): The place of hemispherectomy and major cortical resection in the control of drug-resistant epilepsy. *Acta Neurochirurgica* **50**, 131–133.

Power, C., Poland, S.D., Blume, W.T., Girvin, J.P. & Rice, G.P. (1990): Cytomegalovirus and Rasmussen's encephalitis. *Lancet* **336**, 1282–1284.

Rasmussen, T. (1978): Further observations on the syndrome of chronic encephalitis and epilepsy. *Appl. Neurophysiol.* **41**, 1–12.

Rasmussen, T. & Andermann, F. (1991): Rasmussen's syndrome: symptomatology of the syndrome of chronic encephalitis and seizures: 35-year experience with 51 cases. In: *Epilepsy surgery*, ed. H. Lüders, pp. 173–178. New York: Raven Press.

Rogers, S.W., Andrews, P.I., Gahring, L.C., Whisenand, T., Cauley, K., Crain, B., Hughes, T.E., Heinemann, S.F. & McNamara, J.O. (1994): Autoantibodies to glutamate receptor GluR3 in Rasmussen's encephalitis. *Science* **265**, 648–651.

Sundgren, P.C., Burtscher, I.M., Lundgren, J., Geijer, B. & Holtas, S. (1999): MRI and proton spectroscopy in a child with Rasmussen's encephalitis. Case report. *Neuroradiology* **41**, 935–940.

Tien, R.D., Ashdown, B.C., Lewis, D.V., Atkins, M.R. & Burger, P.C. (1992): Rasmussen's encephalitis: neuroimaging findings in four patients. *Am. J. Radiol.* **158**, 1329–1332.

Twyman, R.E., Gahring, L.C., Spless, C. & Rogers, S.W. (1995): Glutamate receptor antibodies activate a subset of receptors and reveal an agonist binding site. *Neuron* **14**, 755–762.

Villani, F., Spreafico, R., Farina, L., Giovagnoli, A.R., Bernasconi, P., Granata, T. & Avanzini, G. (2001): Positive response to immunomodulatory therapy in an adult patient with Rasmussen's encephalitis. *Neurology* **56**, 248–250.

Villemure, J.G. & Mascott, C.R. (1995): Peri-insular hemispherectomy: surgical principles and anatomy. *Neurosurgery* **37**, 975–981.

Vining, E.P., Freeman, J.M., Brandt, J., Carson, B.S. & Uematsu, S. (1993): Progressive unilateral encephalopathy of childhood (Rasmussen's syndrome): a reappraisal. *Epilepsia* **34**, 639–650.

Vinters, H.V., Wang, R. & Wiley, C.A. (1993): Herpes viruses in chronic encephalitis associated with intractable childhood epilepsy. *Hum. Pathol.* **24**, 871–879.

Walter, G.F. & Renella, R.R. (1989): Epstein-Barr virus in brain and Rasmussen's encephalitis. *Lancet* **i**, 279–280.

Chapter 9

Rheumatic fever and its neurologic features

Maria Bardare

Paediatric Rheumatology Centre, First Paediatric Clinic, University of Milan, via Commenda 9, 20122 Milan, Italy

Summary

Rheumatic fever (RF) is a multisystemic disease which follows an infection from group A ß-haemolitic streptococcus (GAS) and is characterized by major and minor signs and symptoms. Major criteria are carditis, arthritis, chorea and cutaneous involvement (erythema marginatum and subcutaneous nodules); minor criteria are fever, arthralgies, prolonged P-R interval, high phlogosis indexes and antistreptococcal antibodies. Rheumatic chorea (or Sydenham's chorea) is an extrapyramidal disorder characterized by fast, clonic, involuntary movements, especially of the face and limbs, muscular hypotonus, lability, irritability and bizarre behaviour. Recently, a relationship between rheumatic chorea and obsessive-compulsive disorders (OCD) has been claimed and, moreover, other investigations have demonstrated that OCD occur in over 70 per cent of children affected with rheumatic chorea.

There is much evidence that chorea is due to an autoimmune reaction: antineuronal antibodies which arise in response to GAS infection cross-react with unknown epitope on neurons within the basal ganglia. Rheumatic chorea is usually a late manifestation and can be the sole manifestation of rheumatic fever, but in 50 per cent of cases it is associated with valvular involvement. Resolution of symptoms can take few weeks, but not unfrequently many months. Laboratory tests usually assay normal except for antiDNAase B antibodies; D8/17 antigen is often present on B-lymphocytes. The differential diagnosis must be done principally with lupic chorea, which is generally associated with other systemic lupus erythematosus (SLE) signs and symptoms and is characterized by the presence of ANA and antiDNA antibodies and low levels of C4.

Many treatments have been tried with equivocal results; haloperidol is one of the most frequently used drugs and can induce marked improvements. There is no agreement on the employment of steroids, which have been used on the rationale of basal ganglia encephalitis. As in RF with full-blown features, even in chorea benzathine penicillin secondary prophylaxis is mandatory.

Introduction

Rheumatic fever (RF) is an inflammatory systemic disease aetiologically related to group A ß-haemolitic streptococcus (GAS), characterized by a wide spectrum of disorders of the humoral as well as of the cellular immunity.

Among the clinical presentations of GAS infection, RF and acute glomerulonephritis are non-suppurative sequelae, the others being noninvasive and invasive infections and toxic shock syndrome (see Table 1).

Table 1. Clinical presentations of group A streptococcal infection

Noninvasive infections
        Mucous membrane: pharingitis, tonsillitis, otitis media, sinusitis and vaginitis
        Cutaneous: impetigo

Scarlet fever

Invasive infections: defined as isolation of GAS from a normally sterile site in patients not meeting case definition
        of streptococcal toxic shock syndrome:
        Isolated bacteraemia
        Focal infections with or without bacteraemia
        – Meningitis, pneumonia, peritonitis
        – Necrotizing fasciitis, osteomyelitis, septic arthritis
        – Puerperal sepsis, surgical wound infection
        – Cellulitis, erysipelas

Streptococcal toxic-shock syndrome

Non-suppurative sequelae:
        Acute post-streptococcal glomerulonephritis
        Acute rheumatic fever

The first description of RF was made in 400 BC by Hippocrates, but only in 1944 did T.D. Jones establish the criteria for the diagnosis. The first documented epidemic of rheumatic chorea occurred in 1418, but as late as 1831 Richard Bright associated chorea with RF.

The incidence of RF has dramatically declined in the 1960s and the 1970s: in Taplow, Great Britain, for example, the yearly hospitalization of this disease decreased from 150 in 1952 to less than 20 in 1972 (Ansell, 1980). Anyway, in the mid-1980s a new outbreak occurred in the United States with somewhat different features (Veasy et al., 1987; Congeni et al., 1987; Hosier et al., 1987; Mason et al., 1991, Hefelfinger, 1992) and the incidence is still very high in developing countries: while in Great Britain and in Japan the incidence is 0.06/1000 people and 0.7 in USA, in Brazil it is 3.6 and in South Africa 19.2/1000 subjects (data reported by Da Silva et al., 1997). Estimates suggest there will be from 10 to 20 million new cases of RF a year in those countries where two thirds of the world's population live (Gibofsky et al., 1998).

The resurgence of RF could be due to a loss of surveillance, increased resistance of GAS to antibiotics or to a still unascertained increase in GAS virulence (mucoid phenotype associated with organisms rich in M proteins, like serotypes 1, 3, 5; 6, 18) (Stollerman, 1990; Kaplan et al., 1989; Bronze & Dale, 1996).

The pathogenesis of RF is still uncompletely understood: a cross-reactivity between GAS components and organic tissues such as skin, synovial membrane, cardiac valves and cardiac muscle has been widely documented, but in recent years the role of cell-mediated immunity has been recognized (reviewed by Carapetis et al., 1996a) and a superantigen mechanism for streptococcus has been suggested, the same as in toxic-shock syndrome. M protein could act as a superantigen, directly stimulating T-cells that bear specific TCR Vß repertoires (Bronze & Dale, 1996; Tomai et al., 1990).

As for chorea, beside the demonstration in the affected patients of antibodies cross-reacting with the cells of nucleus caudatus and the astrocytes and neutralized by streptococcal membrane antigens (Kingston & Glynn, 1971; Hosier *et al.*, 1987), Bronze and Dale (Bronze, 1993) found that synthetic peptides from different streptococcal M proteins could produce in rabbits antibodies cross-reacting with various brain proteins and that the same antibodies could inhibit in patients with chorea antibodies cross-reacting with cerebral proteins. Moreover, these antibodies can interfere with the transmission pathways of the basal ganglia, thus producing chorea or other behavioural disturbances (Gibofsky *et al.*, 1998; Swedo, 1994).

The resurgence of RF in developed countries and its persistence in developing countries make rapid diagnosis necessary in order to avoid life-threatening sequelae.

The revised Jones criteria (Special Writing Group of the Committee on Rheumatic Fever, 1993) are still invaluable guidelines to establish diagnosis (Table 2), but there are at least two exceptions which allow diagnosis in the absence of any other sign or symptom: indolent carditis and isolated chorea.

Table 2. 1992 modification of Jones criteria for first attacks of acute rheumatic fever*

1. Evidence of a preceding group A streptococcal infection plus:
2. Either two major manifestations or one major and two minor manifestations

Major manifestations:	**Minor manifestations:**
Carditis	Clinical findings
Polyarthritis	– Arthralgia
Chorea	– Fever (temperature of at least 39°)
Erythema marginatum (rare)	Laboratory findings
Subcutaneous nodules (rare)	– Elevated acute-phase reactants
	Erythrocyte sedimentation rate
	C-reactive protein
	– Prolonged PR interval

*Caveats and changes include the following: (1) the diagnosis of acute rheumatic fever should never be made on the basis of minor manifestations alone; (2) early administration of anti-inflammatory drugs may mask symptoms; and (3) some patients with rheumatic fever may present with indolent carditis or Sydenham's chorea alone, without other features of Jones criteria.

The presence of mitral – or aortic – regurgitation detected by both clinical evaluation and echocardiography is generally sufficient to diagnose RF, but echocardiographic findings should meet strict criteria to be reliable (Minich *et al.*, 1997). Anyway, echocardiographic signs of valvulitis without accompanying auscultatory findings are insufficient as the sole criteria of carditis (Da Silva & De Faria Pereira, 1997).

Chorea

Sydenham's chorea, or chorea minor, is a disorder of the central nervous system characterized by abrupt, purposeless, nonrhytmic involuntary movements, muscular weakness and emotional disturbances. They disappear during sleep, but may occur at rest and may interfere with voluntary activity. Initially, it may be possible to suppress these movements, which generally affect all the voluntary muscles, especially those of the face and hands. Grimaces and inappropriate smiles are common. Abnormalities of ocular movements, specifically hypometric saccades and oculogyric crises, are recognized in the majority of patients (probably due to damage to connections between basal ganglia and superior colliculuses) (De Carvalho Coelho Mota & Alves Meira, 1999); handwriting usually becomes clumsy and provides a convenient way of following the patient's course. Speech is often slurred. The movements are generalized, but commonly more marked on one side, and are occasionally completely unilateral (hemichorea).

The first documented outbreak of chorea was seen in 1418, but only in 1686 did Thomas Sydenham first provide a detailed description of the disease (hence Sydenham's chorea). Cheadle (1889) described the full rheumatic syndrome of carditis, polyarthritis and chorea, as well as the subcutaneous nodules and erythema marginatum (less frequent features).

Chorea may follow streptococcal infection after the usual latent period (15–20 days), but more often it appears months or years later. It may be isolated but in some cases follows arthritis and is associated with carditis in a percentage ranging from 40 to 50 per cent (Da Silva & De Faira Pereira, 1997; Al-Eissa, 1993; Carapetis et al., 1996b). Chorea affects almost 25 per cent of patients with RF, is more often seen in females and has an average duration of many months (9.9 ± 13.4) (Cardoso et al., 1997). Other authors report different durations: 5–40 days for Kulkarni & Anees (1996), 7 days–3 years for Al-Eissa (1993).

The average age of patients at onset of chorea is 9.2 ± 9.7 years (Cardoso et al., 1997).

Most often the laboratory tests, such as ESR and CRP, assay normal and so do the antistreptococcal antibodies, with the only exception of anti DNAse B. In more than 80 per cent of patients D8/17 antigen can be detected on B-lymphocyte surface (Feldman et al., 1993; Swedo et al., 1997). Brain CT and MRI are often normal and on the whole the diagnosis is clinical.

Rheumatic chorea must be distinguished from systemic lupus erythematosus (SLE) chorea, but in the latter there are always other signs and symptoms: C_4 is low and ANA and anti dsDNA antibodies are present in the serum, while in the former D8/17 antigen can be detected on B-lymphocytes.

As in RF, also chorea incidence has declined: in Israel, for instance, 27 cases were observed in the period ranging from the 1960s to the 1980s and only one case from the 1980s to the 1990s (Eshel et al., 1993). In our experience five cases of chorea out of 48 cases of RF were observed in the last eight years, and three of them were associated with valvulitis (Table 3).

Table 3. Experience of the rheumatology centre (First Paediatric Clinic, Milan University)

	1991–1994	1995–1998
RF (only with arthritis)	9	6
Arthritis + carditis	12	8
Carditis	2	2
Chorea	2	3
Isolated mitral regurgitation	0	4
Total	25	23

In recent years an interesting new chapter has unfolded, concerning the relationship between chorea and behavioural disorders such as tics or obsessive-compulsive disorders (OCD) (Moore, 1996; Ashbar et al., 1998; Abbas et al., 1996). In fact, OCD are seen in 17–20 per cent of cases with chorea, and during the acute phase of chorea the irritability and/or psycotic symptoms can be observed. OCD can also follow at a distance from the recovery. Moreover, in OCD as well as in chorea D8/17 Ag is present on B-cells in 85 per cent of cases (Swedo et al., 1997; Murphy et al., 1997). This relationship provides support for the hypothesis of the involvement of the corticostriatal loops in the pathophysiology of the disorder.

Treatment

The mainstay of treatment for RF is anti-inflammatory agents, most commonly acetil-salicilic acid (ASA), at the dosage of 70–80 mg/kg/day (to reach serum levels of 20–25 mg/dl). Duration of therapy can vary (but is not inferior to 4–6 weeks) and usually must be continued until symptoms are absent and laboratory tests are normal. Steroid therapy must be instituted if carditis is present, at a dosage of 1–2 mg/kg/day of prednisone for 2 weeks, tapered over the next two weeks, when ASA may be added. Whether or not signs of pharyngitis are present, antibiotic therapy with penicillin must be started and maintained for 10 days.

When chorea appears during the acute phase of RF, the treatment is the same, but these drugs are not required when chorea is an isolated manifestation. In this case, haloperidol can yield good results with an initial dose of 0.5–1 mg/day, adding 0.5 mg every 3 days, if necessary, until a maximum of 5 mg/day (Da Silva & De Faria Pereira, 1997; Miyakawa et al., 1995). Other drugs possibly effective are sodium valproate (15–20 mg/kg/day), reserpine and perphenazine (Da Silva & De Faria Pereira, 1997). There is no proven benefit from steroids, which have been used on the rationale of basal ganglia encephalitis. In resistant cases plasmapheresis and intravenous gammaglobulins can be used. Secondary prophylaxis with 1,200,000 U of benzathine penicillin G every 3 weeks is also mandatory for chorea, to avoid recurrences. There is no agreement on the end point of prophylaxis, but 10 years from the attack seems a reasonable period.

Until now there have been many difficulties to prepare a vaccine against GAS, due to potential cross-reactivity between T-cells stimulated by the chosen region of the M protein and the host cardiac myosin, but recently good results have been obtained immunizing mice with a conserved region of the M protein (residues 7-20 of the p 145 sequence): the antibodies produced were able to bind and opsonize the organism GAS (Hayman et al., 1997). Moreover, Bronze and Dale (1996) were able to construct hybrid genes that encoded defined aminoterminal regions of some M protein, which evoked protective antibodies against multiple serotypes of GAS, in the absence of potentially harmful tissue-cross-reactive antibodies.

A vaccine is anyway the hope for the future.

References

Abbas, S., Khanna, S. & Taly, A.B. (1996). Obsessive-compulsive disorders and rheumatic chorea: is there a connection? *Psychopathology* **29,** 193–197.

Al-Eissa, A. (1993): Sydenham's chorea: a new look at an old disease. *Brit. J. Clin. Pract.* **47,** 14–16.

Ansell, B.M. (1980): *Rheumatic fever. A changing scene in rheumatic disorders in childhood*, ed. J. Apley, pp. 152–166. London: Butterworth.

Asbahr, F.R., Negrao, A.B., Gentil, V., Zanetta, D.M., da Paz, J.A., Marques-Dias, M.J. & Kiss, M.H. (1998): Obsessive-compulsive and related symptoms in children and adolescents with rheumatic fever with and without chorea: a prospective 6-month study. *Amer. J. Psychiatry* **155,** 1122–1124.

Bronze, M.S. (1993): Epitopes of streptococcal M 6, 5, 19 proteins that evoke antibodies that cross-react with human brain. *J. Immunol.* **151,** 2820–2828.

Bronze, M.S. & Dale, J.B. (1996): The reemergence of serious group A streptococcal infections and acute rheumatic fever. *Am. J. Med. Sci.* **311,** 41–54.

Carapetis, J.R., Currie, B.J. & Good, M.F. (1996a): Towards understanding the pathogenesis of rheumatic fever. *Scand. J. Rheumatol.* **25,** 127–131.

Carapetis, J.R., Wolff, D.R. & Currie, B.J. (1996b): Acute rheumatic fever and rheumatic heart disease in the top end of Australia's Northern Territory. *Med. J. Australia* **164,** 146–149.

Cardoso, F., Eduardo, C., Silva, A.P & Mota, C.C. (1997): Chorea in fifty consecutive patients with rheumatic fever. *Movement Disorders* **12,** 701–713.

Cheadle, W.B. (1889): Various manifestations of the rheumatic state as exemplified in childhood and early life. *Lancet* **1,** 871–877, 921–927.

Congeni, B., Rizzo, C., Congeni, J. & Sreenivasan, V.V. (1987): Outbreak of acute rheumatic fever in Northeast Ohio. *J. Pediatr.* **111,** 176–179.

Da Silva, N.A. & De Faria Pereira, B.A. (1997): Acute rheumatic fever, still a challenge. *Rheum. Dis. Clin. North Am.* **23,** 545–568.

De Carvalho Coelho Mota, C. & Alves Meira, Z.M. (1999): Rheumatic fever. *Cardiol. Young* **9,** 239–248.

Eshel, G., Lahat, E., Azizi, E., Gross, B. & Aladjem, M. (1993): Chorea as a manifestation of rheumatic fever – a 30-year survey (1960–1990). *Eur. J. Paediatr.* **152,** 645–646.

Feldman, B.M., Zabriskie, J.B., Silverman, E.D. & Laxer, R.M. (1993): Diagnostic use of B-cell alloantigen D8/17 in rheumatic chorea. *J. Pediatric.* **123,** 84–86.

Gibofsky, A., Suresh Kerwar, J.D. & Zabriskie, J.B. (1998): Rheumatic fever: the relationship between host, microbe and genetics. *Rheumatic Disease Clinics of North America* **24,** 237–259.

Hayman, W.A., Brandt, E.R., Relf, W.A., Cooper, J., Saul, A. & Good, M.F. (1997): Mapping the minimal murine T-cell and B-cell epitopes within a peptide vaccine candidate from the conserved region of the M protein of group A streptococcus. *Intern. Immunol.* **9,** 1723–1733.

Hefelfinger, D.C. (1992): Resurgence of acute rheumatic fever in West Alabama. *South Med. J.* **85,** 761–765.

Hosier, D.M., Craenen, J.M., Teske, D.W. & Wheller, J.J. (1987): Resurgence of acute rheumatic fever. *Am. J. Dis. Child.* **141,** 730–733.

Husby, G., van de Rijn, I., Zabrieski, J.B. *et al.* (1976): Antibodies reacting with cytoplasm of subthalamic and caudate nuclei neurons in chorea and acute rheumatic fever. *J. Exp. Med.* **144,** 1094–1110.

Kaplan, E.L., Johnson, D.R. & Cleary, P.P. (1989): Group A streptococcal serotypes isolated from patients and sibling contacts during the resurgence of rheumatic fever in the United States in the mid-1980s. *J. Infect. Dis.* **159,** 101–103.

Kingston, D. & Glynn, L.E. (1971): A cross-reaction between *streptococcus pyogenes* and human fibroblasts, endothelial cells and astrocytes. *Immunology* **21,** 1003–1017.

Kulkarni, M.L. & Anees, S. (1996): Sydenham's chorea. *Indian Pediatrics* **33,** 112–115.

Mason, T., Fisher, M. & Kujala, G. (1991): Acute rheumatic fever in West Virginia. *Arch. Intern. Med.* **151,** 133–136.

Minich, L.L., Tani, L.Y., Pagotto, L.T., Shaddy, R.E. & Veasy, L.G. (1997): Doppler echocardiography distinguishes between physiologic and pathologic 'silent' mitral regurgitation in patients with rheumatic fever. *Clin. Cardiol.* **20,** 924–926.

Miyakawa, M., Ohkubo, O., Fuchigami, T., Fujita, Y., Poriuchi, R., Hiyoshi, K., Ejiri, K. & Harada, K. (1995): Effectiveness of haloperidol in the treatment of chorea minor. *Brain and Development* **27,** 191–196.

Moore, D.P. (1996): Neuropsychiatric aspects of Sydenham's chorea: a comprehensive review. *J. Clin. Psychiatry* **57,** 407–414.

Murphy, T.K., Goodman, W.K., Fudge, M.W., Williams, R.C. Jr., Ayoub, E.M., Dalal, M., Lewis, M.H. & Zabriskie, J.B. (1997): B-lymphocytes antigen D8/17: a peripheral marker for childhood-onset obsessive-compulsive disorder and Tourette syndrome? *Am. J. Psychiatry* **153,** 402–407.

Special Writing Group of the Committee on Rheumatic Fever, Endocarditis, and Kawasaki Disease of the Council on Cardiovascular Disease in the Young of the American Heart Association. Guidelines for the diagnosis of rheumatic fever: Jones criteria, 1992 update. *Jama* 268, 2069–2073. Correction 1993: *Jama* 269, 476.

Stollerman, G.H. (1990): Rheumatogenic group A streptococci and the return of rheumatic fever. *Adv. Intern. Med.* **35,** 1–25.

Swedo, S.E. (1994): Sydenham's chorea: a model for childhood autoimmune neuropsychiatric disorders. *JAMA* **272,** 1788-

Swedo, S.E., Leonard, H.L., Mittleman, B.B., Allen, A.J., Rapoport, J.L., Dow, S.P., Kanter, M.E., Chapman, F. & Zabriskie, J. (1997): Identification of children with pediatric autoimmune neuropsychiatric disorders associated with streptococcal infections by a marker associated with rheumatic fever. *Am. J. Psychiatry* **154,** 110–112.

Tomai, M., Kotb, M., Majumdar, G. & Beachey, E.H. (1990): Superantigenicity of streptococcal M protein. *J. Exp. Med.* **172,** 359–362.

The Working Group on Severe Streptococcal Infections (1993). *JAMA* **269,** 390–391.

Veasy, V., Wiedmeier, S.E., Orsmond, G.S., Ruttenberg, H.D., Boucek, M.M., Roth, S.J. *et al.* (1987): Resurgence of acute rheumatic fever in the intermountain area of the United States. *N. Engl. J. Med.* **316,** 421–427.

Chapter 10

Neurological manifestations of rheumatic fever

Nardo Nardocci and Anna Erba

Istituto Nazionale Neurologico 'C. Besta', via Celoria 11, 20133 Milan, Italy

Summary

Sydenham's chorea (SC), one of the major neurological manifestations of rheumatic fever (RF), is thought to be determined by an autoimmune attack of the central nervous system triggered by group A ß-haemolitic streptococcal infection. It usually appears in childhood and is characterized by the subacute appearance of abnormal movements associated with behavioural disturbances. Recently a correlation between tics and/or obsessive-compulsive disorders and streptococcal infection was evidenced leading to the identification of a new entity called PANDAS (Paediatric Autoimmune Neuropsychiatric Disorders Associated with Streptococcal infection).

A delineation of the clinical spectrum of SC as reported in the literature and as observed in a series of patients observed at the Neurological Institute 'C. Besta' of Milan will be presented.

Introduction

Sydenham's chorea (SC) is one of the major neurological manifestations of rheumatic fever and is the most common acquired chorea in childhood. It was described by Thomas Sydenham in 1686 (Sydenham, reprinted in 1939), while the association with rheumatic fever (RF) was suggested by Bright in 1831.

In developed countries, where the overall incidence of rheumatic fever has been declining due to prompt treatment of *Streptococcal pharyngitis*, the frequency of SC has declined; however epidemics of RF have occurred in the United States since 1985 despite penicillin therapy and SC is reported in 32 per cent of RF cases (Ayoub, 1992). A recent study conducted in Brazil reports the occurrence of SC in 26 per cent of RF cases (Cardoso *et al.*, 1997).

Pathophysiology

The pathophysiology of SC is still unclear. Chorea seems to result from a diminished activity of the indirect pathway involving, as demonstrated by most neural circuitry models, the external component of the globus pallidus and the subthalamic nucleus. The underactivity of the indirect pathway, due to dysfunction either of the striatum or of the subthalamic nucleus, results in the inappropriate disinhibition of thalamic projections to the premotor and motor cortex (Albin, 1995).

Basal ganglia involvement in SC is supported by *post mortem* studies and functional and structural brain imaging.

Neuropathological studies have shown inflammatory vascular changes in the acute phases with dense perivascular lymphocytic infiltration, thrombosis, occlusion of smaller vessels and capillaries by emboli, fibrinoid vessel necrosis and small haemorrhages. In more advanced cases the anomalies are of subacute degenerative character without inflammatory or vascular components. These alterations are pronounced in the basal ganglia, but also involve the cerebral cortex and the brainstem (Moore, 1996).

Recent studies using positron emission tomography (PET) and single photon emission computed tomography (SPECT) revealed variable imaging features. SPECT showed no abnormalities or hypo or hyperperfusion, PET disclosed striatal hypermetabolism with normal or increased thalamic metabolism (Hill *et al.*, 1994; Heye *et al.*, 1993; Weindle *et al.*, 1993; Lee *et al.*, 1999).

A quantitative MRI study performed in 24 patients with SC and compared with matched controls demonstrated a slight but significant increase in size of the caudate, putamen and globus pallidus (Giedd *et al.*, 1995).

Studies of the metabolites of serotonine and dopamine in CSF have generally been unrewarding. CSF 5-hydroxy-indolacetic acid (5-HIAA) and homovanillic acid (HVA) levels in CSF were found either increased, decreased or not significantly different from controls (Moore, 1996).

SC is presumed to be determined by an autoimmune-mediated inflammatory process incited by the streptococcal infection. Specific cross-reactivity of IgG antibodies towards neuronal cytoplasmic antigens of the caudate and subthalamic nuclei was demonstrated using immunofluorescent staining. Serological antibodies directed against the human central nervous system are found in about 46 per cent of children with Sydenham chorea (Husby *et al.*, 1976). A recent survey has demonstrated that streptococcal M proteins contain brain cross-reactive epitopes that could be potentially involved in the pathogenesis of chorea (Bronze & Dale, 1993). Other authors suggest that the cross-reactive antigen-antibody reaction releases circulating cellular products such as interleukin-1 or -6 that may act on neuronal receptors (Swedo *et al.*, 1997). Circulating streptococcal-antistreptococcal immune complexes are likely to initiate an immunologic reaction against neuronal tissue resulting in vasculitis, perivasculitis and exudation. The basal ganglia inflammation with focal blood-brain barrier disruption and oedema is also suggested by neuroimaging studies. A recent study reports basal ganglia proton MR spectroscopy findings suggestive of inflammation and cell breakdown, without ischaemia (Castillo *et al.*, 1999).

Several studies suggest that susceptibility to SC is linked to HLA-linked antigen expression. A marker found on a subset of B-cells recognized by a monoclonal antibody designated as D8/17 seems to be highly specific and sensitive to identify individuals with rheumatic fever (Swedo *et al.*, 1997).

Clinical features

Chorea usually appears insidiously, weeks to months after group A ß-haemolytic streptococcal infection (GABHS), usually of the pharynx. It is more common in females; age at onset ranges usually from 5 to 15 years but later onset may be observed.

Despite the fact that chorea is the most frequent symptom at onset, it may be preceded by a decrease in school performance or by mood disturbances. Rarely is the onset acute and characterized by signs of encephalopathy like headache, vomiting and disturbances of consciousness (Swedo et al., 1997). The following onset has been observed in two of a series of 25 patients observed at the Neurological Institute 'C. Besta' in Milano, in the last ten years. Predominance of the abnormal movements on one side or true hemichorea is not infrequent. In our series nine patients showed unilateral chorea. Oral facial involvement may be prominent with dysarthria, explosive speech and disturbances of chewing and swallowing. Chorea usually subsides during sleep and as other movement disorders is exaggerated by emotions. In severe cases the continuous abnormal motions during wakefulness impair coordination and can make writing, feeding or dressing difficult or impossible.

In the fully expressed syndrome chorea is associated with other movement disorders: in our series 13 patients presented athetosis, three patients dystonia, three patients tics. The clinical syndrome also includes hypotonia and motor impersistence. Disturbances of ocular movements as hypometria or saccades have been recently reported in a small proportion of cases (Cardoso et al., 1997) and also observed in four patients of our series. Behavioural disturbances such as irritability, depression, attention deficit disorder and obsessive-compulsive disorders have also been reported (Moore, 1996). In our series depression was frequent, occurring in about 50 per cent of the patients, while attention deficit and obsessive compulsive disorders were very rare (10 per cent).

Most patients recover completely in a period ranging from 2 to 3 months but a longer course is possible and recurrences may occur. Some emotional lability may persist for years. In our patients the duration ranged from 1 month to 3.3 years and six patients presented recurrences.

Persistent SC lasting more than 2 years has been reported to correlate with female gender, probably related to endocrine factors, and carditis (Cardoso et al., 1999). No definite risk factors for recurrences have been detected; however, these may occur during pregnancy or during treatment with oral contraceptives (Nausieda, 1986).

As chorea is usually a late feature of rheumatic disease, serological evidence of streptococcal infection may be absent and therefore diagnosis is made on a clinical basis.

Several laboratory tests may be useful to prove prior streptococcal infection: throat culture is occasionally positive. Antistreptolysin appears early and decrease rapidly (in 65 per cent of patients); anti DNAse B may be present for longer periods.

CT does not usually show abnormalities and MRI either fails to show signal alterations or discloses transient increased signal intensity on T2-weighted images and enlargement of the caudate and putamen bilaterally (Moore, 1996). A case of permanent MRI abnormalities after resolution of SC has been reported in one patient (Emery & Vieco, 1997). In our series of patients MRI was performed in 14 cases and no basal ganglia alterations were disclosed.

EEG may show generalized slowing with posterior prominence and occasionally high voltage slow waves (Moore, 1996).

Differential diagnosis of SC includes a long list of genetic and acquired conditions.

In a series of 52 patients affected by chorea observed at the Neurological Institute in the last 10 years, acquired chorea accounted for 77 per cent of cases. SC was the most frequent cause (65 per cent) followed by other immune-mediated diseases (primary antiphospholipid syndrome 11 per cent, systemic lupus erythematosus 3 per cent, post-infectious 6 per cent); other causes were toxic (8 per cent), brain tumours (5 per cent) and post-pump chorea (2 per cent).

Paediatric Autoimmune Neuropsychiatric Disorders Associated with Streptococcal infection (PANDAS)

The first mention of a bacterial infection as a possible direct aetiologic cause for tic disorder was in 1929 with the description of three children with tics presenting onset and exacerbation in association with acute sinusitis. Several reports of patients with clearly postinfectious disease followed.

More observation demonstrated that some children with obsessive-compulsive disorder manifested a fluctuating course.

In recent years a correlation among tics and OCD and streptococcal infection was highlighted and lead to the identification of a new entity called PANDAS (Paediatric Autoimmune Neuropsychiatric Disorders Associated with Streptococcal infection).

The acronym PANDAS describes a novel group of patients who develop and undergo repeated exacerbations of tic disorders, obsessive-compulsive disorders (OCD), and attention-deficit hyperactivity disorder (ADHD) following GABHS. The pathophysiology is considered similar to that proposed for Sydenham's chorea in which group A ß-haemolytic streptococcal antibodies cross-react with basal ganglia, resulting in abnormal behaviour and involuntary movements.

The diagnostic criteria established in a series of 50 patients are: presence of OCD or tic disorder or both; onset before puberty; episodic clinical course with 'explosive' onset or sudden exacerbations and remissions or both; a temporal relation between symptoms and group A ß-haemolytic streptococcal infection; presence of 'adventitious' movements such as motor hyperactivity and choreiform movements (Swedo et al., 1998).

The concept of infection-triggered OCD and tic disorder has raised discussion and the existence of PANDAS is not free from controversy (Kurlan, 1998; Giuliano et al., 1998). Diagnostic criteria established for PANDAS can be blurred by the variability commonly associated with tic disorders which normally show fluctuations in the frequency and severity of symptoms and by the absence of a precise definition of choreiform movements. Further studies on the epidemiology and natural history of paediatric OCD and tic disorders are needed to determine the role of GABHS infections in the aetiology of these group of disorders.

References

Albin, R.L. (1995): The pathophysiology of chorea/ballism and Parkinsonism. *Parkinsonism & Related Disorders* **1**, 3–11.

Ayoub, E.M. (1992): Resurgence of rheumatic fever in the United States. The changing picture of a preventable illness. *Postgrad. Med.* **92**, 133–142.

Bronze, M.S. & Dale, J.B. (1993): Epitopes of streptococcal M proteins evoke antibodies that cross-react with human brain. *J. Immunol.* **151**, 2820–2828.

Castillo, M., Kwock, L. & Arbelaez, A. (1999): Sydenham's chorea: MRI and proton spectroscopy. *Neuroradiology* **41**, 943–945.

Cardoso, F., Eduardo, C., Silva, A.P. & Mota C.C. (1997): Chorea in 50 consecutive patients with rheumatic fever. *Mov. Disord.* **12,** 701–703.

Cardoso, F., Vargas, A.P., Oliveira, L.D., Guerra, A.A. & Amaral, S.V. (1999): Persistent Sydenham's chorea. *Mov. Disord.* **14,** 805–807.

Emery, E.S. & Vieco, P.T. (1997): Sydenham's chorea: magnetic resonance imaging reveals permanent basal ganglia injury. *Neurology* **48,** 531–533.

Giedd, J.N., Rapaport, J.N., Kruesi, M.J.P., Parker, C., Shapiro, M.B., Allen, A.J., Leonard, H.L., Kaysen, B.S., Dickstein, B.S., Marsh, W.L., Kozuch P.L., Vaituzis, A.C., Hamburger, S.D. & Swedo, S.E. (1995): Sydenham's chorea: magnetic resonance imaging of the basal ganglia. *Neurology* **45,** 2199–2202.

Giuliano, J.D., Zimmerman, A., Walktup, J.T. & Singer, H.S. (1998): Prevalence of pediatric autoimmune neuropsychiatric disorders associated with streptococcal infection by history in a consecutive series of community-referred children evaluated for tics. *Ann. Neurol.* **44,** 556

Heye, N., Jergas, M., Hotzinger, H., Farahati, J., Pöhlau, D. & Przuntek, H. (1993): Sydenham chorea: clinical, EEG, MRI and SPECT findings in the early stage of the disease. *J. Neurol.* **240,** 121–123.

Hill, A., Herkes G.K. & Roche, P. (1994): SPECT and MRI findings in Sydenham's chorea. *J. Neurol. Neurosurg. Psychiatry* **57,** 763.

Husby, G., Van De Rijn I., Zabriskie, J.B., Abdin, Z.H. & Willims, R.C. (1976): Antibodies reacting with cytoplasm of subthalamic and caudate nuclei neurons in chorea and acute rheumatic fever. *J. Exp. Med.* **144,** 1094–1110.

Kurlan, R. (1998): Tourette syndrome and 'PANDAS': will the relationship bear out? *Neurology* **50,** 1530–1534.

Lee, P.H., Nam, H.S., Lee, K.Y., Lee, B.I. & Lee, J.D. (1999): Serial brain SPECT images in a case of Sydenham's chorea. *Arch. Neurol.* **56,** 237–240.

Moore, D.P. (1996): Neuropsychiatric aspects of Sydenham's chorea: a comprehensive review. *J. Clin. Psychiatry* **57,** 407–414.

Nausieda, P.A. (1986): Sydenham's chorea, chorea gravidarum and contraceptive-induced chorea. In: *Handbook of clinical neurology*, eds. P.J. Vinken, G.W. Bruyn & H.L. Klawans, pp. 359–367. Amsterdam: Elsevier.

Swedo, S.E., Leonard, H.L., Mittleman, B.B., Allen, A.J., Rapoport, J.L., Dow, S.P., Kanter, M.E., Chapman, F. & Zabriskie, J. (1997): Identification of children with pediatric autoimmune neuropsychiatric disorders associated with streptococcal infection by a marker associated with rheumatic fever. *Am. J. Psychiat.* **154,** 110–112.

Swedo, S.E., Leonard, H.L., Garvey, M., Mittleman, B., Allen, A.J., Perlmutter, S., Dow, S., Zamkoff, J., Dubbert, B.K. & Lougee, L. (1998): Pediatric Autoimmune Neuropsychiatric Disorders Associated with Streptococcal infections: clinical description of the first 50 cases. *Am. J. Psychiatry* **155,** 264–271.

Sydenham, T. (1939): An essay on the rise of a new fever. *Medical Classics* **4,** 327–355.

Weindle, A., Kuwert, R. & Leenders, K.L. (1993): Increased striatal glucose consumption in Sydenham's chorea. *Mov. Disord.* **8,** 437–444.

Chapter 11

Systemic lupus erythematosus

Nicolino Ruperto and Alberto Martini*

*Laboratory of Medical Computer Science; *University Department of Paediatric Sciences, IRCCS San Matteo, Piazzale Golgi 19, 27100 Pavia, Italy*

Summary

Systemic lupus erythematosus (SLE) can be considered the prototype of human autoimmune diseases. It is an episodic, multisystem disease characterized by the presence, at high titre, of various autoantibodies and in particular antibodies directed towards nuclear components. The main pathological event is a widespread inflammation of small blood vessels that can involve many organs and lead to heterogenous clinical manifestations.

This chapter describes the main clinical manifestations, alterations in laboratory tests, criteria for diagnosis, current therapeutic modalities, and prognosis of the disease.

Introduction

Systemic lupus erythematosus (SLE) can be considered the prototype of human autoimmune diseases (Jacobs, 1992; Wallace & Hahn, 1993; Cassidy & Petty, 2001). It is an episodic, multisystem disease characterized by the presence, at high titre, of various autoantibodies and in particular antibodies directed towards nuclear components.

The main pathological event is a widespread inflammation of small blood vessels that can involve many organs and lead to heterogenous clinical manifestations. The presence of a spectrum of different clinical manifestations, ranging from benign to more rapidly progressive, and data obtained from experimental models of SLE raised the hypothesis that this disease should be considered as a syndrome, the final clinical expression of different pathogenetic processes all causing an abnormal and persistent autoimmune response. Alternatively SLE might be considered one disease with different clinical expressions according to the genetic background of the patient (Lippman et al., 1982).

About 15 per cent of patients develop the first symptoms at paediatric age (Siegel & Lee, 1973; Hochberg, 1985; Kaufman et al., 1986; Lehman et al., 1989). The disease, which is rare before the age of 10, is more common in adolescents (King et al., 1977). Like in adults, there is a large prevalence among females (80–90 per cent) (Celermajer et al., 1984) even if this difference is less evident in the first 10 years of life.

Clinical manifestations

The clinical manifestations are very heterogenous (see Table 1). Some organs or apparatus are involved more frequently than others and this aspect can considerably influence prognosis. Among the general symptoms we can list fever, as well as asthenia, anorexia and weight loss (Kornreich & Hanson, 1974).

Table 1. Clinical features of SLE

Constitutional	Fever, malaise, weight loss
Cutaneous	Butterfly rash, discoid lupus, periungual erythema, photosensitivity, mucocutaneous ulcerations, alopecia
Musculoskeletal	Polyarthritis and arthralgia, tenosynovitis, myopathy, aseptic necrosis
Vascular	Lupus crisis, Raynaud's phenomenon, erythromelalgia, thrombophlebitis, livedo reticularis, lupus profundus
Cardiovascular	Pericarditis and effusion, myocarditis, Libman-Sacks endocarditis
Pulmonary	Pleuritis, basilar pneumonitis, atelectasis, haemorrhage
Gastrointestinal	Abdominal crisis, esophageal motor dysfunction, colitis
Liver, spleen, and nodes	Hepatomegaly, splenomegaly, lymphadenopathy
Neurological	Organic brain syndrome, convulsions, psychosis, chorea, cerebrovascular accident, polyneuritis and peripheral neuropathy, cranial nerve palsies, pseudotumour cerebri
Ocular	Cotton-wool spots, papilloedema, retinopathy
Renal	Glomerulonephritis, nephrotic syndrome, uraemia, hypertension

Arthritis is frequent, usually migrant, short in duration but only occasionally erosive. Very rarely, articular deformities can be observed without bony erosions due to soft tissue contractures (Jaccoud's arthritis) (Martini *et al.*, 1987; Reilly *et al.*, 1990). *Myalgia* is also very common, but rarely associated with an increase of muscular enzymes (Foote *et al.*, 1982).

Cutaneous manifestations are present in most of the patients. The most classic manifestation is the *malar rash* (so called butterfly rash), that even if not pathognomonic is certainly suggestive of SLE; it is a maculopapular slightly squamous or simply erythematosus lesion, over the bridge of the nose and on both malar eminences. The lesion can be photosensitive with exacerbation during exposure to sunlight; sunlight can also exacerbate the overall disease activity. *Maculopapular rashes* are common particularly on the soles of the feet and palms of the hands. Frequently it is possible to find erythematosus and ulcerative lesions of the mucous membranes especially of the hard palate. Hair loss can be observed in almost every patient with active disease and sometimes may lead to patchy *alopecia*. The other two peculiar SLE skin lesions, very rare in children, are *subacute cutaneous lupus erythematosus* and *discoid lupus erythematosus*.

Ischaemic necrosis of bone (Smith *et al.*, 1976) due to the activity of the disease or, more frequently, to steroid treatment, can be observed usually some years after the onset of SLE.

The most frequent cardiovascular manifestation (Englund & Lucas-RV, 1983) is *pericarditis*. It can be observed in one-third of the patients and may rarely lead to cardiac tamponade. Heart failure can be the presenting sign of *myocarditis*. The classic lesion of the endocardium during SLE is the *Libman-Sacks verrucous endocarditis* (Galve *et al.*, 1988), usually at the mitral valve; it is characterized by small nodules of fibrinoid necrosis and has been associated with antiphospholipid antibodies; it rarely can lead to haemodynamic complications. Involvement of the coronary arteries can lead to *myocardial infarction* (Ishikawa et al., 1978; Spiera & Rothenberg, 1983). Accelerated atherosclerosis has been observed after long term administration of glucocorticoid drugs (Bulkley & Roberts, 1975).

Hypertension, usually associated with renal involvement, can be dangerous, leading to rapid kidney failure. *Raynaud's phenomenon* is rare in children.

Lupus crisis is the sudden development of overwhelming, often fatal, systemic disease from widespread vasculitis.

SLE is characterized by an increase in the frequency of venous or arterial *thrombosis*, often associated with the presence of antiphospholipid antibodies.

Lupus pneumonitis (Schaller, 1982; Emery, 1986; de-Jongste et al., 1986; Delgado et al., 1990) can be the consequence of vasculitis of the alveolar capillaries. Before making the diagnosis of lupus pneumonitis it is however necessary to exclude an *infective pneumonitis*, a frequent event in patients with SLE. Vasculitis of the pulmonary vessels may also be responsible of *acute pulmonary haemorrhage* (Miller et al., 1986). *Pulmonary hypertension*, either primary or secondary to parenchymal involvement, is another manifestation of SLE. *Pleuritis* is also frequent but usually not clinically relevant. Pulmonary function tests are altered also in children (Cerveri et al., 1992; Cerveri et al., 1996).

Episodes of *abdominal pain* are also frequent and vasculitis of the mesenteric arteries can lead to *perforation* or *infarction of the intestine* (Nadorra et al., 1987; Eberhard et al., 1991a). Another rare but dangerous complication is *pancreatitis* (Reynolds et al., 1982; Martini et al., 1983) consequent to either the disease or to glucocorticoid therapy. *Hepatomegaly* of mild degree is present in up to two-thirds of children (Meislin & Rothfield, 1968). *Splenomegaly* and *lymphadenopathy* can also be observed.

All the structures of the *eye* can be involved as a consequence of retinal vasculitis.

Central nervous system involvement is very heterogenous and can play an important role in the prognosis of the disease. It ranks second only to nephritis as a cause of morbidity and mortality (Dietze & Voegele, 1966; Yancey et al., 1981). *Headache* is very common in the active phases of the disease while *seizures* and *pseudotumour cerebri* are rare (DelGiudice et al., 1986). *Chorea* (Bruyn & Padberg, 1984; Arisaka et al., 1984) is also rare and can present in the early phase of the disease like *transverse myelitis* that is a severe complication requiring immediate and intensive treatment. *Aseptic meningitis* has also been reported. Less rare are *peripheral neuritides* that usually respond slowly to treatment. *Eye hallucination* or *sight loss* can be either of central origin or secondary to small vessel vasculitis; they are usually associated with other neurologic manifestations but sometimes appear isolated. *Behavioural change* (Silber et al., 1984), may range from minor conditions like *depression* to *psychoses* usually secondary to lupus vasculitis. The presence of small, repeated and multiple *cerebral infarctions* can lead to a progressive deterioration of cerebral functions; the possibility of a single massive haemorrhagic infarction is rare.

Renal involvement is present clinically in 50–80 per cent (Meislin & Rothfield, 1968) of the patients and is determinant for prognosis. Usually it is one of the presenting signs, or else it appears in the first 2 years of the disease (Garin et al., 1976). The glomerular lesions are variable. Since there is a good correlation between histology, clinical evolution and response to treatment (Rush et al., 1986), the different types of lupus glomerulonephritis can be classified according to histopathologic criteria (see Table 2) (Magil *et al.*, 1982; Golbus & McCune, 1994).

Table 2. Lupus nephritis. Histopathologic classification of the World Health Organization (Magil *et al.*, 1982; Golbus & McCune, 1994)

CLASS I	**Normal glomeruli**
CLASS II	**Mesangial glomerulitis** The deposits are limited to the mesangium. There are two types: (a) *minimal alteration* (absence of mesangial proliferation) (b) *mesangial glomerulitis* (presence of mesangial proliferation)
CLASS III	**Focal and segmental proliferative glomerulonephritis** Immunocomplex deposits are important, extended over the mesangium and associated with a marked cellular proliferation. The involvement is segmental (that is only some portion of the glomeruli are interested) and limited to less that 50 per cent of the glomeruli.
CLASS IV	**Diffuse proliferative glomerulonephritis** This is similar to class 3 but lesions are more important and widespread, and affect over 50 per cent of the glomeruli.
CLASS V	**Membranous glomerulonephritis** The typical lesion is a diffuse thickening of the basal membrane of the glomeruli with deposits on the epithelial site, and often also on the epithelial side. Frequently there is also a moderate degree of mesangial hypercellularity.
CLASS VI	**Glomerular sclerosis** Segmental or extensive sclerosis of glomeruli with frequent fibrous crescents.

Autoimmune endocrinopathy (Eberhard *et al.*, 1991b) and diabetes mellitus (Fruman, 1977) can also occur.

Laboratory tests

Table 3. Main laboratory test abnormalities in SLE

Laboratory tests	Abnormalities
Erythrocyte sedimentation rate (ESR)	Elevated
C-reactive protein (CRP)	Usually normal or slightly elevated
Haemoglobin	Reduced
Leukopenia	Frequent (in particular lymphopenia)
Thrombocytopenia	Sometimes
Hypergammaglobulinaemia	Often present
Coombs test	Often positive
Antinuclear antibodies (ANA)	Positive
Antibodies against native DNA (nDNA)	Positive in most patients
Antibodies against-Sm	Sometimes positive
Antiphospholipid antibodies	Sometimes positive
C3, C4	Often reduced

The main alterations of laboratory tests in SLE are reported in Table 3 (Rothfield, 1977; Hochberg *et al.*, 1985). Their abnormal values should always be considered in association with the clinical picture of the patient.

Since *C-reactive protein* is often normal, an important elevation of this test should be seen with suspicion as a possible index of an overlapping infection (Pepys *et al.*, 1982). A mild *inflammatory anaemia* is quite frequent. The *Coombs* test can be positive even without presence of haemolysis since a true haemolytic anaemia with positive Coombs is rare.

Table 4. Main ANA specificities and clinical correlation observed in the connective tissue diseases. (Modified from Burgio & Martini, 1990)

Antigen		Disorder	Clinical association
Original designation	Molecular definition		
Denatured DNA	Single-strand DNA	SLE, MCTD, RA, SS, drug induced LE	
Native DNA*	Double-strand DNA	SLE	Nephropathy
Histones	Histones	SLE, RA, JCA, drug induced LE	
Sm*	Protein complexed with U-rich RNAs	SLE	Central nervous system involvement (?)
Nuclear RNP	Protein complexed with U1 RNA	SLE, MCTD, SS	Raynaud's phenomenon
SSA/Ro	Protein complexed with RNAs	SLE, SS, PSS, RA	Neonatal LE, CHB, cutaneous SLE vasculitis
SSB/La	Phosphoprotein complexed with nascent RNA-polymerase transcripts	SLE, SS	Xerostomia and xerophthalmia in SS
Ku	Proteins	SLE, PSS/PM	
PCNA	Auxiliary protein of DNA polymerase 6	SLE	
Ribosomal RNP	Phosphoproteins associated with ribosomes	SLE	Psychotic syndromes in SLE (?)
Jo-1*	Histidyl tRNA synthetase	PM/DM	
PL-7*	Threonyl tRNA synthetase	PM/DM	
PL-12*	Alanyl tRNA synthetase	PM/DM	
PM-Scl (PM-1)	Complex of various proteins	PM/PSS, JDM	
Scl-70*	DBA topoisomerase I	PSS	
RNA Pol I*	RNA polimerase I complex of subunit proteins	PSS	High prevalence of internal organ involvement
Fibrillarin*	Protein, component of U3 RNP particle	PSS	
Centromere*	Proteins localized at inner and outer kinetochores plates	CREST syndrome	

*Disease specific.
CHB: congenital heart block; **CREST**: calcinosis, Raynaud's phenomenon, esophageal dysmotility, sclerodactyly, and teleangiectases; **DM**: dermatomyositis; **JCA**: juvenile chronic arthritis; **JDM**: juvenile dermatomyositis; **MCTD**: mixed connective tissue disease; **PM**: polymyositis; **PSS**: progressive systemic sclerosis; **RA**: rheumatoid arthritis; **SLE**: systemic lupus erythematosus; **SS**: Sjögren syndrome.

Antinuclear antibodies (ANA) are useful as a clue to the disease but are not specific of SLE (Petty *et al.*, 1977; Gillespie *et al.*, 1981), since they can be observed in many other connective tissue diseases, and at lower titre, in other inflammatory or infective diseases and also in a small percentage of normal children (Martini *et al.*, 1989). The ANA are a heterogenous group of antibodies and their specificities are reported in Table 4 (Burgio & Martini, 1990). The presence of *anti-native DNA antibodies* (n-DNA) (Lehman *et al.*, 1980) or *anti-Sm nuclear antigen antibodies* are specific of SLE, but are not present in all patients. Both the titre of anti n-DNA and the level of hypocomplementaemia are well correlated with the grade of disease activity and the presence of nephropathy (Singsen *et al.*, 1976). The so called *LE phenomenon* is suggestive but not specific of SLE and has now been substituted, in routine practice, by the different specificities of ANA. Also the search of Ig deposits and complement at the dermo-epidermis junction through a skin biopsy (*lupus band test*) is rarely used in routine practice since even if frequently positive it is not specific to SLE (Wertheimer & Barland, 1976). For *antiphospholipid antibodies* and the related *thrombotic events* see Chapters 13 and 14 of this book.

Diagnosis

The diagnosis of SLE is mainly clinical, even though some laboratory exams are useful. The American College of Rheumatology (ACR) criteria for diagnosis of SLE are reported in Table 5 (Tan *et al.*, 1982). These criteria (with the exception of discoid rash which is rare in childhood), may be useful for the clinical studies of SLE in children (Norris *et al.*, 1977; Passas *et al.*, 1985). Indeed, these criteria are very restricted and have been developed mainly for inclusion of patients in clinical studies and not for diagnosis in everyday clinical practice. A physician with expertise in SLE can therefore make the diagnosis of SLE even if the patient does not fulfil all the criteria set up by the ACR.

Therapy

Corticosteroids are the drugs of choice for the therapy of SLE (Norris *et al.*, 1977; Jacobs, 1977; Urman & Rothfield, 1977). The dosage and duration of treatment are mainly related to the severity of the clinical expression of the disease and to the organ(s) involved.

The renal involvement (in particular the diffuse proliferative glomerulonephritis or Class IV) and the CNS involvement are the most harmful events and require an aggressive therapy with dosage of prednisone up to 2 mg/kg/day (Hagge *et al.*, 1967). Prednisone must be slowly and progressively tapered until the minimum dosage for the maintenance of disease control has been reached.

In children with skin and/or articular manifestation, hydroxychloroquine can be useful: initial dosage 6–7 mg/kg/day and then maintenance 5 mg/kg/day (Laaksonen *et al.*, 1974).

If corticosteroid therapy is able to control the disease but is associated with substantial side effects, it is useful to combine the therapy with an immunosuppressant like azathioprine at a dosage of 2 mg/kg/day. In the event of a patient refractory to this standard treatment the infusion of intravenously methylprednisolone pulse therapy at the dosage of 30 mg/kg/day over 3 days may be advisable (Cathcart *et al.*, 1976; Kimberly *et al.*, 1981; Barron *et al.*, 1982).

In patients with serious renal involvement (Donadio-JV *et al.*, 1978, 1982; Austin *et al.*, 1986) or with important general involvement, the combination of corticosteroid therapy with monthly intravenous cyclophosphamide pulse therapy should be considered (Steinberg & Decker, 1974;

Steinberg & Steinberg, 1991) at the dosage of 500–1000 mg/m^2 followed by considerable oral and intravenous hydration. This combination must be administered monthly for the first 6 months and then every 3 months for 18 months.

Table 5. American College of Rheumatology criteria for the diagnosis of SLE (Tan *et al.*, 1982)

Criterion	Definition
(1) Malar rash	Fixed erythema, flat or raised, over the malar eminences, tending to spare the nasolabial folds
(2) Discoid lupus	Erythematous raised patches with adherent keratotic scaling and follicular plugging: atrophic scarring may occur in older lesions
(3) Photosensitivity	Skin rash as a result of unusual reaction to sunlight by patient history or physician observation
(4) Oral/nasal ulcerations	Oral or nasopharyngeal ulceration, usually painless, observed by a physician
(5) Non-erosive arthritis	Non-erosive arthritis involving two or more peripheral joints, characterized by tenderness, swelling, or effusion
(6) Serositis	(a) Pleuritis: convincing history of pleuritic pain or rub heard by a physician or evidence of pleural effusion, or (b) Pericarditis: documented by ECG or rub or evidence of pericardial effusion
(7) Nephritis	(a) Persistent proteinuria greater than 0.5 gm/d or greater than 3+ if quantitation not performed, or (b) Cellular casts, may be red cell, haemoglobins, granular, tubular, or mixed
(8) Neurologic disorder	(a) Seizures, in the absence of offending drugs or known metabolic derangements; i.e. uraemia, ketoacidosis, or electrolyte imbalance; (b) Psychosis, in the absence of offending drugs or known metabolic derangements, i.e. uraemia, ketoacidosis, or electrolyte imbalance
(9) Haematologic disorder	(a) Haemolytic anaemia with reticulocytosis, or (b) Leukopenia: less than 4,000/mm^3; (c) Lymphopenia: less than 1.500/mm^3 on two or more occasions; (d) Thrombocytopenia: less than 100,000/mm^3 in the absence of offending drugs
(10) Immunologic disorder	(a) Positive LE cell preparation, or (b) Anti-DNA antibody to native DNA in abnormal titre, or (c) Anti-MS: presence of antibody to MS nuclear antigen, or (d) False positive serologic test for syphilis known to be positive for at least 6 months and confirmed by *Treponema pallidum* immobilization or fluorescent treponemal antibody absorption test
(11) Antinuclear antibody	An abnormal titre of antinuclear antibody by immunofluorescence or an equivalent assay at any point in time and in the absence of drugs known to be associated with 'drug-induced lupus' syndrome

For the purpose of identifying patients in clinical studies, a patient shall be said to have SLE if any four or more of the 11 criteria are present, serially or simultaneously, during any interval of observation.

In the event of autoimmune haemolytic anaemia or thrombocytopenia, nonresponsive to steroid treatment, some patients may benefit from the combination of steroids and intravenous immunoglobulin at the dosage of 400 mg/kg/day for 5 days or 2000 mg/kg in a single infusion (Berkman *et al.*, 1988; Akashi *et al.*, 1990).

The efficacy and modality of administration of plasmapheresis are still under debate (Johannessen *et al.*, 1982; Wei *et al.*, 1983; Lewis *et al.*, 1992); it is reserved only for the most severely affected patients, usually in combination with steroids and cyclophosphamide.

Methotrexate (Abud-Mendoza *et al.*, 1993; Ravelli *et al.*, 1998) and cyclosporine-A (Feutren *et al.*, 1987) have also been advocated for refractory SLE.

During the entire course of the disease, particular attention must be given to the control of infection. Some patients with SLE, probably because of functional asplenia (Malleson *et al.*, 1988), are particularly prone to pneumococcus infections and therefore may benefit from vaccination against this bacteria.

Dialysis and renal transplantation are an efficacious treatment for severe renal failure (Jarrett *et al.*, 1983; Cheigh *et al.*, 1990).

Attention must be also shown to symptomatic control of possible complications (like hypertension), to protection from sunlight, and to general support care.

Prognosis

The disease is characterized by periodic remissions and relapses. Without treatment SLE can be rapidly progressive and often fatal. Renal and central nervous system involvement can significantly alter the prognosis (Walravens & Chase, 1976; Cassidy *et al.*, 1977). However, in the last decades, the introduction of corticosteroids first (Urman & Rothfield, 1977) and then immunosuppressive therapy, more effective antibiotics, and more precise immunologic monitoring has greatly improved prognosis (Meislin & Rothfield, 1968; King *et al.*, 1977). Survival at 5 and 10 years is now 100 per cent in children without renal involvement, and 80–90 per cent at 5 years and 70–80 per cent at 10 years in children with nephropathy (Wedgwood, 1977; Abeles *et al.*, 1980; Glidden *et al.*, 1983; Lacks & White, 1990; McCurdy *et al.*, 1992). This data are continuously improving. The most frequent causes of death are infections, malignant hypertension, and pulmonary or gastrointestinal acute haemorrhage.

Among the patients with nephropathy, those with diffuse proliferative glomerulonephritis (Class IV) have the worst prognosis and may require dialyses and renal transplantation for kidney failure.

With the reduction of mortality clinicians are now faced with new problems that should be addressed and solved during the course of the disease, such as stunted growth, aseptic necrosis of bones, cataract, neuropsychiatric involvement, specific organ damage, atherosclerosis.

Neonatal lupus

The incidence of abortion in pregnant women with SLE is increased (Mintz *et al.*, 1986). Most of the children born to women with SLE are premature and small for gestational age but otherwise normal. In some newborn children transplacental exchange of autoantibodies may lead to onset of neonatal lupus (Watson *et al.*, 1984), or congenital heart block (CHB) (Scott *et al.*, 1983).

Usually clinical manifestations of neonatal lupus are limited to the skin with a rash similar to discoid lupus and erythematosquamous papulae expanding outside, with an area of atrophy in the middle (annular erythema). The systemic manifestation like a Coomb's positive haemolytic anaemia, thrombocytopenia etc. are rare. These clinical manifestations are evident in the first weeks of life and then subside spontaneously with the disappearance of maternal immunoglobulin.

The most frequent clinical manifestation, more frequent than neonatal lupus, is CHB (Hardy *et al.*, 1979) isolated or associated with myocarditis with or without fibroelastosis. Neonatal lupus is considered the cause of one-third of CHB.

Neonatal lupus can also be evident in newborn babies from mothers with other connective tissue diseases or in asymptomatic mothers. A pathogenetic role has been attributed to the autoantibodies anti-Ro (Petri *et al.*, 1989; Alexander *et al.*, 1989). The persistence of this antibody in the serum of a mother is associated with an elevated risk of having another baby with neonatal lupus in a subsequent pregnancy.

Drug-induced lupus

More than 50 drugs have been associated with the occurrence of lupus (Table 6) (Jacobs, 1972; Beernink & Miller, 1973; Miller, 1977; Hess, 1982). Drug-induced lupus presents with the same clinical manifestations of idiopathic lupus but it is usually less severe; in particular, central nervous system and renal involvement are rare. Diagnosis can be advocated when SLE appears after a prolonged administration of a drug suspected to induce SLE. All the patients are ANA positive and more than 95 per cent present with anti-histone antibodies. On the contrary anti n-DNA and anti-Sm antibodies are negative and complement is normal. Therefore the presence of these more restricted ANA specificities can be useful in discriminating drug-induced lupus from idiopathic lupus. The disease most of the time disappears spontaneously with the discontinuation of the suspected drug while the serologic abnormalities can persist for a long time. In the most severe cases, treatment similar to the one for idiopathic lupus may be necessary.

Table 6. List of the main drugs suspected of inducing lupus

Hydralazine	Methyldopa	Phenytoin
Procainamide	D-penicillamine	Ethosuximide
Isoniazid	Captopril	Methimazole
Chlorpromazine	Carbamazepine	Propylthiouracil

The same drugs may also induce the formation of ANA more frequently then the drug-induced lupus itself; anyway the positivity of ANA is not an indication to discontinue drug treatment.

References

Abeles, M., Urman, J.D., Weinstein, A., Lowenstein, M. & Rothfield, N.F. (1980): Systemic lupus erythematosus in the younger patient: survival studies. *J. Rheumatol.* **7**, 515–522.

Abud-Mendoza, C., Sturbaum, A.K., Vazquez-Compean, R. & Gonzalez-Amaro, R. (1993): Methotrexate therapy in childhood systemic lupus erythematosus. *J. Rheumatol.* **20**, 731–733.

Akashi, K., Nagaswa, K., Mayumi, T., Yokota, E., Oochi, N. & Kusaba, T. (1990): Successful treatment of refractory systemic lupus erythematosus with intravenous immunoglobulins. *J. Rheumatol.* **17**, 375–379.

Alexander, E.L., McNicholl, J., Watson, R.M., Bias, W., Reichlin, M. & Provost, T.T. (1989): The immunogenetic relationship between anti-Ro(SS-A)/La(SS-B) antibody positive Sjogren's/lupus erythematosus overlap syndrome and the neonatal lupus syndrome. *J. Invest. Dermatol.* **93**, 751–756.

Arisaka, O., Obinata, K., Sasaki, H., Arisaka, M. & Kaneko, K. (1984): Chorea as an initial manifestation of systemic lupus erythematosus. A case report of a 10-year-old girl. *Clin. Pediatr. Phila.* **23**, 298–300.

Austin, H.A., Klippel, J.H., Balow, J.E., le-Riche, N.G., Steinberg, A.D., Plotz, P.H. & Decker, J.L. (1986): Therapy of lupus nephritis. Controlled trial of prednisone and cytotoxic drugs. *N. Engl. J. Med.* **314**, 614–619.

Barron, K.S., Person, D.A., Brewer-E.J., J., Beale, M.G. & Robson, A.M. (1982): Pulse methylprednisolone therapy in diffuse proliferative lupus nephritis. *J. Pediatr.* **101**, 137–141.

Beernink, D.H. & Miller, J.J. (1973): Anticonvulsant-induced antinuclear antibodies and lupus-like disease in children. *J. Pediatr.* **82,** 113–117.

Berkman, S.A., Lee, M.L. & Gale, R.P. (1988): Clinical uses of intravenous immunoglobulins. *Semin. Hematol.* **25,** 140–158.

Bruyn, G.W. & Padberg, G. (1984): Chorea and systemic lupus erythematosus. A critical review. *Eur. Neurol.* **23,** 435–448.

Bulkley, B.H. & Roberts, W.C. (1975): The heart in systemic lupus erythematosus and the changes induced in it by corticosteroid therapy. A study of 36 necropsy patients. *Am. J. Med.* **58,** 243–264.

Burgio, G.R. & Martini, A. (1990): Immunological features of diffuse connective tissue diseases. *Eur. J. Pediatr.* **149,** 224–231.

Cassidy, J.T. & Petty, R.E. (2001): *Textbook of pediatric rheumatology* (4th edn.). Philadelphia: W.B. Saunders Co.

Cassidy, J.T., Sullivan, D.B., Petty, R.E. & Ragsdale, C. (1977): Lupus nephritis and encephalopathy. Prognosis in 58 children. *Arthritis Rheum.* **20,** 315–322.

Cathcart, E.S., Idelson, B.A., Scheinberg, M.A. & Couser, W.G. (1976): Beneficial effects of methylprednisolone 'pulse' therapy in diffuse proliferative lupus nephritis. *Lancet* **1,** 163–166.

Celermajer, D.S., Thorner, P.S., Baumal, R. & Arbus, G.S. (1984): Sex differences in childhood lupus nephritis. *Am. J. Dis. Child* **138,** 586–588.

Cerveri, I., Bruschi, C., Ravelli, A., Zoia, M.C., Fanfulla, F., Zonta, L., Pellegrini, G. & Martini, A. (1992): Pulmonary function in childhood connective tissue diseases. *Eur. Respir. J.* **5,** 733–738.

Cerveri, I., Fanfulla, F., Ravelli, A., Zoia, M.C., Ramenghi, B., Spagnolatti, L., Villa, I. & Martini, A. (1996): Pulmonary function in children with systemic lupus erythematosus. *Thorax* **51,** 424–428.

Cheigh, J.S., Kim, H., Stenzel, K.H., Tapia, L., Sullivan, J.F., Stubenbord, W., Riggio, R.R. & Rubin, A.L. (1990): Systemic lupus erythematosus in patients with end-stage renal disease: long-term follow-up on the prognosis of patients and the evolution of lupus activity. *Am. J. Kidney Dis.* **16,** 189–195.

de-Jongste, J.C., Neijens, H.J., Duiverman, E.J., Bogaard, J.M. & Kerrebijn, K.F. (1986): Respiratory tract disease in systemic lupus erythematosus. *Arch. Dis. Child* **61,** 478–483.

Delgado, E.A., Malleson, P.N., Pirie, G.E. & Petty, R.E. (1990): The pulmonary manifestations of childhood-onset systemic lupus erythematosus. *Semin. Arthritis Rheum.* **19,** 285–293.

DelGiudice, G.C., Scher, C.A., Athreya, B.H. & Diamond, G.R. (1986): Pseudotumor cerebri and childhood systemic lupus erythematosus. *J. Rheumatol.* **13,** 748–752.

Dietze, H.J. & Voegele, G.E. (1966): Neuropsychiatric manifestations associated with systemic lupus erythematosus in children. Review of the literature and report of a case. *Psychiatr. Q.* **40,** 59–70.

Donadio-JV, J., Holley, K.E., Ferguson, R.H. & Ilstrup, D.M. (1978): Treatment of diffuse proliferative lupus nephritis with prednisone and combined prednisone and cyclophosphamide. *N. Engl. J. Med.* **299,** 1151–1155.

Donadio-JV, J., Holley, K.E. & Ilstrup, D.M. (1982): Cytotoxic drug treatment of lupus nephritis. *Am. J. Kidney Dis.* **2,** 178–181.

Eberhard, A., Shore, A., Silverman, E. & Laxer, R. (1991a): Bowel perforation and interstitial cystitis in childhood systemic lupus erythematosus. *J. Rheumatol.* **18,** 746–747.

Eberhard, B.A., Laxer, R.M., Eddy, A.A. & Silverman, E.D. (1991b): Presence of thyroid abnormalities in children with systemic lupus erythematosus. *J. Pediatr.* **119,** 277–279.

Emery, H. (1986): Clinical aspects of systemic lupus erythematosus in childhood. *Pediatr. Clin. North Am.* **33,** 1177–1190.

Englund, J.A. & Lucas-R.V., J. (1983): Cardiac complications in children with systemic lupus erythematosus. *Pediatrics* **72,** 724–730.

Feutren, G., Querin, S., Noel, L.H., Chatenoud, L., Beaurain, G., Tron, F., Lesavre, P. & Bach, J.F. (1987): Effects of cyclosporine in severe systemic lupus erythematosus. *J. Pediatr.* **111,** 1063–1068.

Foote, R.A., Kimbrough, S.M. & Stevens, J.C. (1982): Lupus myositis. *Muscle Nerve* **5,** 65–68.

Fruman, L.S. (1977): Diabetes mellitus, islet-cell antibodies, and HLA-B8 in a patient with systemic lupus erythematosus. *Am. J. Dis. Child* **131,** 1252–1254.

Galve, E., Candell, R.J., Pigrau, C., Permanyer, M.G., Garcia-Del, C.H. & Soler, S.J. (1988): Prevalence, morphologic types, and evolution of cardiac valvular disease in systemic lupus erythematosus. *N. Engl. J. Med.* **319,** 817–823.

Garin, E.H., Donnelly, W.H., Fennell, R.S. & Richard, G.A. (1976): Nephritis in systemic lupus erythematosus in children. *J. Pediatr.* **89,** 366–371.

Gillespie, J.P., Lindsley, C.B., Linshaw, M.A. & Richardson, W.P. (1981): Childhood systemic lupus erythematosus with negative antinuclear antibody test. *J. Pediatr.* **98,** 578–581.

Glidden, R.S., Mantzouranis, E.C. & Borel, Y. (1983): Systemic lupus erythematosus in childhood: clinical manifestations and improved survival in fifty-five patients. *Clin. Immunol. Immunopathol.* **29,** 196–210.

Golbus, J. & McCune, W.J. (1994): Lupus nephritis. Classification, prognosis, immunopathogenesis, and treatment. *Rheum. Dis. Clin. North Am.* **20,** 213–242.

Hagge, W.W., Burke, E.C. & Stickler, G.B. (1967): Treatment of systemic lupus erythematosus complicated by nephritis in children. *Pediatrics* **40,** 822–827.

Hardy, J.D., Solomon, S., Banwell, G.S., Beach, R., Wright, V. & Howard, F.M. (1979): Congenital complete heart block in the newborn associated with maternal systemic lupus erythematosus and other connective tissue disorders. *Arch. Dis. Child* **54,** 7–13.

Hess, E.V. (1982): Drug-related lupus. *Arthritis Rheum.* **25,** 857

Hochberg, M.C. (1985): The incidence of systemic lupus erythematosus in Baltimore, Maryland, 1970–1977. *Arthritis Rheum.* **28,** 80–86.

Hochberg, M.C., Boyd, R.E., Ahearn, J.M., Arnett, F.C., Bias, W.B., Provost, T.T. & Stevens, M.B. (1985): Systemic lupus erythematosus: a review of clinico-laboratory features and immunogenetic markers in 150 patients with emphasis on demographic subsets. *Medicine Baltimore* **64,** 285–295.

Ishikawa, S., Segar, W.E., Gilbert, E.F., Burkholder, P.M., Levy, J.M. & Viseskul, C. (1978): Myocardial infarct in a child with systemic lupus erythematosus. *Am. J. Dis. Child* **132,** 696–699.

Jacobs, J.C. (1972): Drug-induced lupus. *JAMA* **222,** 1557

Jacobs, J.C. (1977): Treatment of systemic lupus erythematosus in childhood. *Arthritis Rheum.* **20,** 304–307.

Jacobs, J.C. (1992): *Pediatric rheumatology for the practitioner* (2nd edn.). New York: Springer-Verlag.

Jarrett, M.P., Santhanam, S. & Del-Greco, F. (1983): The clinical course of end-stage renal disease in systemic lupus erythematosus. *Arch. Intern. Med.* **143,** 1353–1356.

Johannessen, A., Gutteberg, T. & Husby, G. (1982): Plasma exchange in the treatment of severe, childhood onset systemic lupus erythematosus. *Acta Paediatr. Scand.* **71,** 347–350.

Kaufman, D.B., Laxer, R.M., Silverman, E.D. & Stein, L. (1986): Systemic lupus erythematosus in childhood and adolescence – the problem, epidemiology, incidence, susceptibility, genetics, and prognosis. *Curr. Probl. Pediatr.* **16,** 545–625.

Kimberly, R.P., Lockshin, M.D., Sherman, R.L., McDougal, J.S., Inman, R.D. & Christian, C.L. (1981): High-dose intravenous methylprednisolone pulse therapy in systemic lupus erythematosus. *Am. J. Med.* **70,** 817–824.

King, K.K., Kornreich, H.K., Bernstein, B.H., Singsen, B.H. & Hanson, V. (1977): The clinical spectrum of systemic lupus erythematosus in childhood. *Arthritis Rheum.* **20,** 287–294.

Kornreich, H.K. & Hanson, V. (1974): The rheumatic diseases of childhood. *Curr. Probl. Pediatr.* **4,** 3–40.

Laaksonen, A.L., Koskiahde, V. & Juva, K. (1974): Dosage of antimalarial drugs for children with juvenile rheumatoid arthritis and systemic lupus erythematosus. A clinical study with determination of serum concentrations of chloroquine and hydroxychloroquine. *Scand. J. Rheumatol.* **3,** 103–108.

Lacks, S. & White, P. (1990): Morbidity associated with childhood systemic lupus erythematosus. *J. Rheumatol.* **17,** 941–945.

Lehman, T.J., Hanson, V., Singsen, B.H., Kornreich, H.K., Bernstein, B. & King, K. (1980): The role of antibodies directed against double-stranded DNA in the manifestations of systemic lupus erythematosus in childhood. *J. Pediatr.* **96,** 657–661.

Lehman, T.J., McCurdy, D.K., Bernstein, B.H., King, K.K. & Hanson, V. (1989): Systemic lupus erythematosus in the first decade of life. *Pediatrics* **83,** 235–239.

Lewis, E.J., Hunsicker, L.G., Lan, S.P., Rohde, R.D. & Lachin, J.M. (1992): A controlled trial of plasmapheresis therapy in severe lupus nephritis. The Lupus Nephritis Collaborative Study Group. *N. Engl. J. Med.* **326,** 1373–1379.

Lippman, S.M., Arnett, F.C., Conley, C.L., Ness, P.M., Meyers, D.A. & Bias, W.B. (1982): Genetic factors predisposing to autoimmune diseases. Autoimmune hemolytic anemia, chronic thrombocytopenic purpura, and systemic lupus erythematosus. *Am. J. Med.* **73,** 827–840.

Magil, A.B., Ballon, H.S. & Rae, A. (1982): Focal proliferative lupus nephritis. A clinicopathologic study using the W.H.O. classification. *Am. J. Med.* **72,** 620–630.

Malleson, P., Petty, R.E., Nadel, H. & Dimmick, J.E. (1988): Functional asplenia in childhood onset systemic lupus erythematosus. *J. Rheumatol.* **15,** 1648–1652.

Martini, A., Lorini, R., Zanaboni, D., Ravelli, A. & Burgio, R.G. (1989): Frequency of autoantibodies in normal children. *Am. J. Dis. Child* **143,** 493–496.

Martini, A., Notarangelo, L.D., Barberis, L. & Plebani, A. (1983): Pancreatitis in systemic lupus erythematosus. *Arthritis Rheum.* **26,** 1173–1173.

Martini, A., Ravelli, A., Viola, S. & Burgio, R.G. (1987): Systemic lupus erythematosus with Jaccoud's arthropathy mimicking juvenile rheumatoid arthritis. *Arthritis Rheum.* **30,** 1062–1064.

McCurdy, D.K., Lehman, T.J., Bernstein, B., Hanson, V., King, K.K., Nadorra, R. & Landing, B.H. (1992): Lupus nephritis: prognostic factors in children. *Pediatrics* **89,** 240–246.

Meislin, A.G. & Rothfield, N. (1968): Systemic lupus erythematosus in childhood. Analysis of 42 cases, with comparative data on 200 adult cases followed concurrently. *Pediatrics* **42,** 37–49.

Miller, J.J. (1977): Drug-induced lupus-like syndromes in children. *Arthritis Rheum.* **20,** 308–311.

Miller, R.W., Salcedo, J.R., Fink, R.J., Murphy, T.M. & Magilavy, D.B. (1986): Pulmonary hemorrhage in pediatric patients with systemic lupus erythematosus. *J. Pediatr.* **108,** 576–579.

Mintz, G., Niz, J., Gutierrez, G., Garcia, A.A. & Karchmer, S. (1986): Prospective study of pregnancy in systemic lupus erythematosus. Results of a multidisciplinary approach. *J. Rheumatol.* **13,** 732–739.

Nadorra, R.L., Nakazato, Y. & Landing, B.H. (1987): Pathologic features of gastrointestinal tract lesions in childhood-onset systemic lupus erythematosus: study of 26 patients, with review of the literature. *Pediatr. Pathol.* **7,** 245–259.

Norris, D.G., Colon, A.R. & Stickler, G.B. (1977): Systemic lupus erythematosus in children: the complex problems of diagnosis and treatment encountered in 101 such patients at the Mayo Clinic. *Clin. Pediatr. Phila.* **16,** 774–778.

Passas, C.M., Wong, R.L., Peterson, M., Testa, M.A. & Rothfield, N.F. (1985): A comparison of the specificity of the 1971 and 1982 American Rheumatism Association criteria for the classification of systemic lupus erythematosus. *Arthritis Rheum.* **28,** 620–623.

Pepys, M.B., Lanham, J.G. & De-Beer, F.C. (1982): C-reactive protein in SLE. *Clin. Rheum. Dis.* **8,** 91–103.

Petri, M., Watson, R. & Hochberg, M.C. (1989): Anti-Ro antibodies and neonatal lupus. *Rheum. Dis. Clin. North Am.* **15,** 335–360.

Petty, R.E., Cassidy, J.T. & Sullivan, D.B. (1977): Serologic studies in juvenile rheumatoid arthritis: a review. *Arthritis Rheum.* **20,** 260–267.

Ravelli, A., Ballardini, G., Viola, S., Villa, I., Ruperto, N. & Martini, A. (1998): Methotrexate therapy in refractory pediatric onset systemic lupus erythematosus. *J. Rheumatol.* **25**, 572–575.

Reilly, P.A., Evison, G., McHugh, N.J. & Maddison, P.J. (1990): Arthropathy of hands and feet in systemic lupus erythematosus. *J. Rheumatol.* **17**, 777–784.

Reynolds, J.C., Inman, R.D., Kimberly, R.P., Chuong, J.H., Kovacs, J.E. & Walsh, M.B. (1982): Acute pancreatitis in systemic lupus erythematosus: report of twenty cases and a review of the literature. *Medicine Baltimore.* **61**, 25–32.

Rothfield, N.F. (1977): Systemic lupus erythematosus. Laboratory studies. *Arthritis Rheum.* **20**, 299–303.

Rush, P.J., Baumal, R., Shore, A., Balfe, J.W. & Schreiber, M. (1986): Correlation of renal histology with outcome in children with lupus nephritis. *Kidney Int.* **29**, 1066–1071.

Schaller, J. (1982): Lupus in childhood. *Clin. Rheum. Dis.* **8**, 219–228.

Scott, J.S., Maddison, P.J., Taylor, P.V., Esscher, E., Scott, O. & Skinner, R.P. (1983): Connective-tissue disease, antibodies to ribonucleoprotein, and congenital heart block. *N. Engl. J. Med.* **309**, 209–212.

Siegel, M. & Lee, S.L. (1973): The epidemiology of systemic lupus erythematosus. *Semin. Arthritis Rheum.* **3**, 1–54.

Silber, T.J., Chatoor, I. & White, P.H. (1984): Psychiatric manifestation of systemic lupus erythematosus in children and adolescents. A review. *Clin. Pediatr. Phila.* **23**, 331–335.

Singsen, B.H., Bernstein, B.H., King, K.K. & Hanson, V. (1976): Systemic lupus erythematosus in childhood: correlations between changes in disease activity and serum complement levels. *J. Pediatr.* **89**, 358–369.

Smith, F.E., Sweet, D.E., Brunner, C.M. & Davis, J.S. (1976): Avascular necrosis in SLE. An apparent predilection for young patients. *Ann. Rheum. Dis.* **35**, 227–232.

Spiera, H. & Rothenberg, R.R. (1983): Myocardial infarction in four young patients with SLE. *J. Rheumatol.* **10**, 464–466.

Steinberg, A.D. and Decker, J.L. (1974): A double-blind controlled trial comparing cyclophosphamide, azathioprine & placebo in the treatment of lupus glomerulonephritis. *Arthritis Rheum.* **17**, 923–937.

Steinberg, A.D. and Steinberg, S.C. (1991): Long-term preservation of renal function in patients with lupus nephritis receiving treatment that includes cyclophosphamide versus those treated with prednisone only. *Arthritis Rheum.* **34**, 945–950.

Tan, E.M., Cohen, A.S., Fries, J.F., Masi, A.T., McShane, D.J., Rothfield, N.F., Schaller, J.G., Talal, N. & Winchester, R.J. (1982): The 1982 revised criteria for the classification of systemic lupus erythematosus. *Arthritis Rheum.* **25**, 1271–1277.

Urman, J.D. & Rothfield, N.F. (1977): Corticosteroid treatment in systemic lupus erythematosus. Survival studies. *JAMA* **238**, 2272–2276.

Wallace, D.J. & Hahn, B.H. (1993): *Dubois' lupus erythematosus* (4th edn.). Philadelphia: Lea & Febiger.

Walravens, P.A. & Chase, H.P. (1976): The prognosis of childhood systemic lupus erythematosus. *Am. J. Dis. Child* **130**, 929–933.

Watson, R.M., Lane, A.T., Barnett, N.K., Bias, W.B., Arnett, F.C. & Provost, T.T. (1984): Neonatal lupus erythematosus. A clinical, serological, and immunogenetic study with review of the literature. *Medicine (Baltimore)* **63**, 362–378.

Wedgwood, R.J. (1977): Prognostic factors in childhood systemic lupus erythematosus. *Arthritis Rheum.* **20**, 295–298.

Wei, N., Klippel, J.H., Huston, D.P., Hall, R.P., Lawley, T.J., Balow, J.E., Steinberg, A.D. & Decker, J.L. (1983): Randomised trial of plasma exchange in mild systemic lupus erythematosus. *Lancet* **1**, 17–22.

Wertheimer, D. & Barland, P. (1976): Clinical significance of immune deposits in the skin in SLE. *Arthritis Rheum.* **19**, 1249–1255.

Yancey, C.L., Doughty, R.A. & Athreya, B.H. (1981): Central nervous system involvement in childhood systemic lupus erythematosus. *Arthritis Rheum.* **24**, 1389–1395.

Chapter 12

Neurological involvement in systemic lupus erythematosus

Andrea Salmaggi, Elena Lamperti, Silvana Zeni* and Flavio Fantini*

Department of Neurology II, Istituto Nazionale Neurologico 'C. Besta', via Celoria 11, 20133 Milan, Italy;
*Department of Rheumatology, University of Milan, Italy

Summary

The clinical presentations of neurological involvement during systemic lupus erythematosus (SLE) are multifaceted, ranging from severe, potentially life-threatening events like major stroke, to subtle neuropsychological disturbances which can go undetected during routine neurological examination.

A good knowledge of the neurologic spectrum in SLE is mandatory in order to reach appropriate diagnosis and provide treatment of these complications.

This chapter will briefly review the available literature evidence concerning prognostic impact of early or late neurologic involvement, main differential diagnoses, and optimal treatment. Pathogenetic mechanisms of neurological involvement will only be briefly outlined, as well as anatomopathological evidences.

Special emphasis will be given to the clinical problem of difficulties in differential diagnosis between disease flare-up and complications of immunosuppressive therapy, since this possibility is becoming increasingly frequent due to the prolonged survival of patients with serious SLE chronically treated with immunosuppressive drugs. A case report will illustrate these difficulties as they present in clinical practice.

Introduction

Neurological involvement in systemic lupus erythematosus (SLE) is a long-known sign of disease activity; despite its multiple well-recognized clinical manifestations, its contribution to a diagnosis of SLE is still limited to occurrence of two main features, i.e. seizures and/or 'psychosis'. These two features are included in the revised American College of Rheumatology (ACR) criteria for SLE diagnosis (Tan et al., 1982).

However, many more manifestations are listed in the reviews about the prevalence of neurological symptoms/signs in SLE; among these, a large study (Kovacs et al., 1993) has reported a 5 per cent prevalence for stroke, a 39 per cent prevalence for headache, a 20 per cent prevalence for neuropathies (either cranial of peripheral), a 7 per cent prevalence for myopathies and a less than 1 per cent prevalence for 'movement disorders' (including chorea, ballismus, athetosis and cerebellar ataxia), aseptic meningitis and transverse myelitis.

Concerning the broad spectrum of clinical manifestations included under the denominations of psychosis, organic brain syndrome (OBS) and cognitive dysfunction, the prevalence of psychosis is reported at 5 per cent, whereas the combined prevalence of OBS and cognitive dysfunction may reach 17 per cent of the SLE population.

These figures must be regarded critically, since they are heavily influenced by potential biases: such confounding factors include, for instance, the definition of 'normal' performance levels for cognitive functions, or the exclusion of non-SLE-related, drug-induced, complication- induced manifestations; last, but not least, a mere concomitance of manifestations has to be excluded (especially with frequent symptoms such as headache).

Rheumatologists, therefore, seem to accept only seizures or psychosis as nervous system-related diagnostic elements in SLE; however, a recent survey (Tincani *et al.*, 1996) performed with the cooperation of 59 centres active in diagnosis and management of SLE, has yielded the following results in terms of the first ten more important signs/symptoms of neurological involvement in SLE: (1) generalized seizures; (2) transverse myelitis; (3) status epilepticus; (4) psychosis; (5) focal seizures; (6) complex partial seizures; (7) stroke; (8) TIA; (9) aseptic meningitis; (10) delusion.

The relevance of transverse myelitis has been further supported by the results of a workshop aiming to delineate a consensus on diagnostic criteria for neuropsychiatric SLE (Singer *et al.*, 1990), which showed the 'top 5' criteria potentially useful for this diagnosis to be:

(1) seizures, primary generalized

(2) psychosis (brief reactive or atypical)

(3) transverse myelitis

(4) global cognitive dysfunction (dementia)

(5) seizures, focal (motor or sensory)

as reported by scientists representing 22 centres active in SLE in North America, Great Britain and Ireland.

However, despite increased awareness of the relevance of other criteria of neurological involvement in the diagnosis of SLE, no changes have been so far made to the 1982 Criteria, except for immunological parameters (Hochberg *et al.*, 1997).

The involvement of the central nervous system at the onset of SLE is not necessarily related to a worse long-term outcome of the disease, as has been proved for kidney involvement; actually, only three of the six studies so far performed have shown such a negative prognostic value, whereas the remaining three have not.

About 20 per cent of patients show an involvement of the CNS at disease onset (Jacobs, 1963; Meislin & Rothfield, 1968; King *et al.*, 1977; Platt *et al.*, 1982; Glidden *et al.*, 1983).

In a recent study (Steinlein *et al.*, 1995), 40 out of 91 patients of paediatric age with SLE were found to display neurological involvement; of these, 19 had shown neurological signs and symptoms at the onset of the disease, but this did not adversely affect short-term outcome, with a 90 per cent rate of 'excellent' recovery from neurological manifestations.

Pathogenetic mechanisms of neurological dysfunction/damage in SLE are still debated: despite SLE being the paradigm for 'autoantibody' disease, the available evidence suggests:

– Antibodies to neuronal proteins (located or not in synaptic endings) are more frequently present in the CSF in SLE patients with psychosis (Bonfa *et al.*, 1987; Schneebaum *et al.*, 1991);

– Immune-complex vasculitis seems to be very rare, with scant evidence for choroid plexus involvement, which moreover seems to be present regardless of evident prior neuropsychiatric involvement (Boyer *et al.*, 1980);

– Antiphospholipid-associated vasculopathy is not a rare event;

– Possibly embolic small vessel brain vasculopathy may be related to Libman-Sacks endocarditis (Devinsky *et al.*, 1988);

– Cytokines released within the CNS during disease activity may induce alterations in neuropsychiatric functioning (Shiozawa *et al.*, 1992).

The relationships between antiphospholipid (aPL) antibodies and neurological manifestations have been the object of extensive investigation (Brey and Escalante, 1998): the neurological manifestations include stroke, TIA, cerebral venous sinus thrombosis, seizures, chorea, transverse myelopathy, 'atypical migrainous-like events', sensorineural hearing loss, transient global amnesia, psychiatric disorders, Guillain-Barré syndrome and orthostatic hypotension.

Antiphospholipid antibodies may actually interfere with the degradation of factor Va by activated protein C, and/or induce expression of adhesion molecules on the surface of endothelial cells (McNeil *et al.*, 1991; Del Papa *et al.*, 1997).

Experimental data (Kent *et al.*, 1997) showing that aPL bind to cat brain may be assumed as indirect evidence for the role aPL play in seizures as well as in acute psychotic manifestations (Schwartz *et al.*, 1998), in which a transient alteration of normal brain functioning is supposed to take place in the absence of vascular involvement; however, interpretations are made difficult by the loose associations detected between aPL and these clinical aspects (Brey *et al.*, 1990).

This holds true also for migraine, except perhaps for the uncommon complication of migrainous infarction (Silvestrini *et al.*, 1994). The association with aPL antibodies is probably stronger in the case of transverse 'myelitis' and chorea, even if also in these it is far from absolute.

Few neuropathological studies have been published in the last years dealing with neurological involvement in SLE. In the investigation by Hanly and colleagues (Hanly *et al.*, 1992), frequent cerebral micro-infarcts were detected in 10 patients with SLE (seven of whom had shown neuropsychiatric manifestations during life, with an interval of the last clinical neuropsychiatric event to death ranging from 3 to 730 days), in association with either fibrinoid sclerosis of the vessel wall or lupus endocarditis or endovascular thrombi. On the other hand, evidence for presence of immune complexes was extremely rare. The authors stated 'no source of emboli is identified in our cases ... we favour a primary small vessel vasculopathy as the precipitating event'.

In the study by Devinsky and colleagues (Devinsky *et al.*, 1988) 37 out of 50 patients studied neuropathologically at necropsy had displayed neurological and/or psychiatric involvement: of these, 13 had a normal neuropathological brain examination; in the remaining patients, the most common neuropathological abnormalities included (presumably) embolic infarctions, evidence of infection and/or microglial nodules, fibrin-platelet thrombi. At variance with the data later reported by Hanly, in this study cerebral small-sized infarctions were often concomitant with

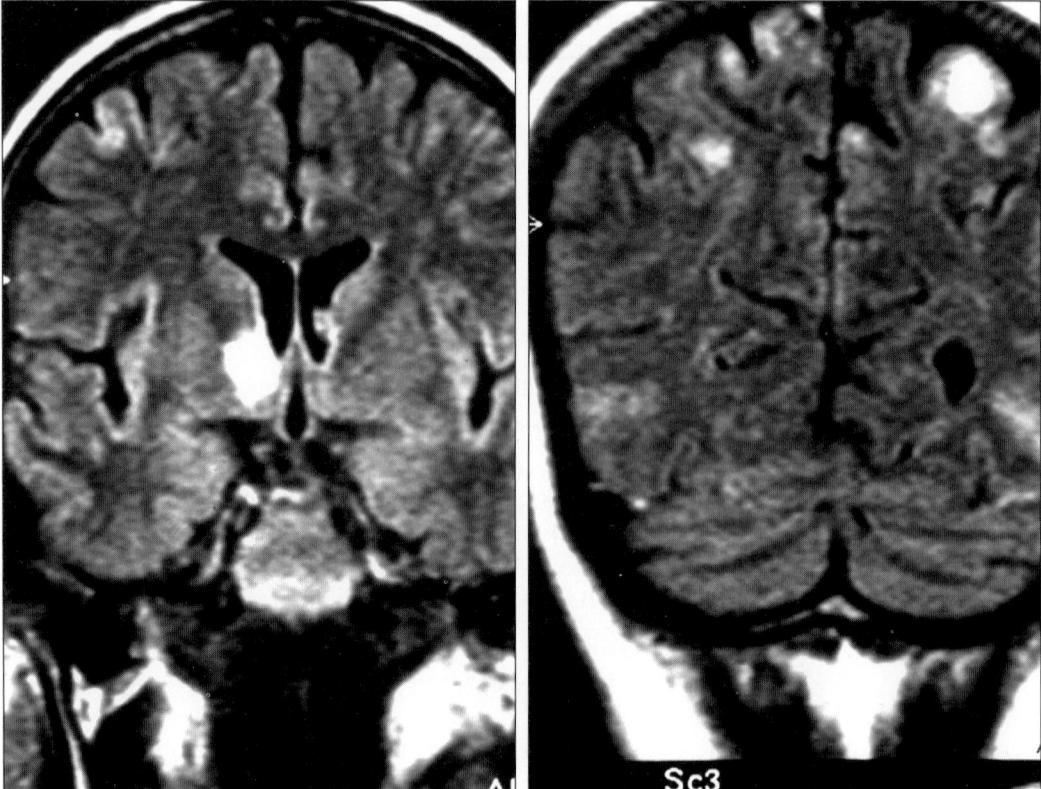

Fig.1. Coronal FLAIR sequences at the temporal (A) and parietal (B) levels.
A (left): Hyperintensity in the lower portion of right internal capsule and pallidum;
B (right): Multiple hyperintensities in the cortical-subcortical left parietal, right interhaemispheric and left occipitoparietal regions.
The location and features of MRI alterations are strongly suggestive of multiple ischaemic lesions.

endocarditis (mitral 'valvulitis' was detected in 23 patients, but those with endoluminal vegetations and/or endoluminal thrombus had a higher frequency of brain infarction).

Neuropathological alterations consistent with thrombotic thrombocytopenic purpura were detected in seven patients.

Imaging of central nervous system SLE

The presently available neuroradiological tools to assess neurological involvement in SLE include computed tomography (CT), magnetic resonance imaging (MRI), single photon emission computed tomography (SPECT), spectro-MRI. Practically all hospitals have CT facilities; many have MRI. Only a few research centres use SPECT and spectro-MRI.

The usefulness of CT in SLE-related CNS involvement – as in other clinical situations – is mostly related to its speed of execution (which makes it a suitable test in agitated, confused patients, as well as in claustrophobic individuals), and to its ability to exclude or confirm haemorrhage (either intracerebral or subarachnoid) or lesions with a mass effect.

CT may yield negative results in the very early phases of stroke and is usually scarcely informative in CNS infections (although contrast enhancement may be detected at the meningeal level in meningitis).

In SLE, CT studies have shown as most frequent abnormality a picture of cerebral atrophy, associated or not with ventricular enlargement; this finding may be detected in up to 50 per cent of the patients (Miguel et al., 1994); opinions diverge as to whether this atrophy is related to concomitant steroid therapy and/or disease duration and/or previous or present clinical/subclinical CNS SLE-related disease activity (Miguel et al., 1994; Carette et al., 1982; Ostrov et al., 1982).

Brain CT is also the technique of choice to show cerebral calcifications, which may go undetected by MRI; however, cerebral calcifications are also an unspecific feature. Brain MRI has a much more powerful resolution as compared with CT; it also better visualizes structures in the posterior fossa; but it is more time-consuming.

Both diffuse and focal alterations have been described by MRI in SLE brains; in the paper by Bell (Bell et al., 1991), the authors have proposed a distinction between two main types of CNS involvement in SLE based upon neuroradiological (MRI), immunological (anti-neurofilament and anti-cardiolipin antibodies) and clinical (i.e. response to steroid treatment) criteria: patients with diffuse clinical and neuroradiological alterations usually had elevated anti-neurofilament antibodies and were good responders to steroids, whereas patients with focal clinicoradiological disease had elevated anticardiolipin antibodies and were poor responders to steroids. On the other hand, no differences were reported by a group (Gonzalez-Crespo et al., 1995), which detected similar frequency and type of MRI alterations (i.e. multiple small punctate areas of increased signal at periventricular or subcortical white matter of both cerebral hemispheres) in SLE patients with past or active CNS involvement or no such involvement; the lesions were associated with age and disease duration.

Refinements of conventional MRI include the use of diffusion-perfusion imaging; as a matter of fact, hypoperfusion can be evaluated in microcirculation by perfusion imaging, while diffusion imaging can detect early ischaemia and infarction with higher sensitivity as compared with conventional MRI; the use of such techniques needs expertise and is best performed in research centres (Yuh et al., 1998).

Also MRI-spectroscopy is informative as far as chemical composition of the tissues is concerned; loss of axons and/or neurons leads to a decreased N-acetyl-aspartate peak, and lactate as well as phosphocreatine may also be measured by this technique.

SPECT gives information on the cerebral blood flow and may therefore be altered in cases with normal MRI. Of interest, abnormalities in blood flow can be detected by SPECT in SLE patients with minor clinical features, such as headache, anxiety and slight cognitive disturbances (Rubbert et al., 1993)

Finally, PET with the use of F-18-fluoro-2-deoxy-D-glucose has been reported to provide a sensitive tool in CNS involvement in SLE also in cases with normal MRI, by showing significant hypometabolism in regions of the brain producing clinical symptomatology, and by showing regression of this hypometabolism after therapy (Otte et al., 1998)

Differential diagnosis

The differential diagnosis of SLE-related CNS involvement encompasses a great part of clinical neurology. The most frequent issues to deal with in order to rule out 'secondary' CNS disease are metabolic alterations (due to organ failure and/or to therapy), direct therapy-related complications (for instance, mood alterations related to steroid treatment), and infections (both in untreated and more commonly in heavily immunosuppressed patients).

Accuracy of differential diagnosis and effective treatment of complications are therefore connected with clinical expertise and depend on extensive search for possible infectious agents in doubtful cases (see case report).

Bacterial infections are not the most common complications in the setting of long-standing immunosuppression, being outweighed by viral, fungine, and parasitic infections. Protozoal infections may also take place.

Differential diagnosis between multiple sclerosis (MS) and neurological involvement in SLE may sometimes be difficult, in that at MRI multiple areas of increased signal in T2-weighted images of brain white matter may be detected in both diseases; however, lesions involving the corpus callosum are highly specific for MS (Miller et al., 1987). On the other hand, no such specificity can be expected from other tests, such as oligoclonal bands in the CSF (which can be found in both MS and SLE).

Lupus 'cerebritis' may mimic the neuroradiological aspects of progressive multifocal leukoencephalopathy (PML), a rare viral disease of the white matter caused by the JC virus in immunocompromised hosts (Kaye et al., 1992). In PML, widespread signal increase in T2-weighted images at MRI are detected in the white matter of the cerebral hemispheres; intranuclear viral inclusions are seen in oligodendrocytes in electron microscopy, even if recent studies suggest that detection of genomic sequences of JC virus in the CSF may be sufficient for *in vivo* diagnosis (Cinque et al., 1996).

Cytomegalovirus infection of the brain and toxoplasmosis usually have distinct features which allow differentiation from lupus cerebritis.

Chorea and tranverse myelitis may be the first signs/symptoms of SLE (Kuroe et al., 1994; Salmaggi et al., 1994); the detection of antiphospholipid antibodies is frequent in SLE-associated chorea, but much less so in myelitis. Therefore, clinical differential diagnosis (for chorea involving mostly Sydenham's chorea and less likely Huntington's disease) depends on the degree of awareness of this possibility.

In myelitis, the most likely alternative diagnosis is of infectious myelitis (often due to *Herpes zoster* virus).

Psychosis in the course of SLE may be due to disease activity in the brain or leading to organ failure, or to the effects of treatment (steroids) or else to complications (CNS infections).

Ancillary tests (MRI, CSF) may provide answers to these questions; if steroid-induced psychosis is the differential diagnosis of highest likelihood, then a tapering of the dosage is required, with concomitant close monitoring for detection of SLE reactivation.

Seizures in the course of SLE should be carefully observed; in many cases, brain imaging and CSF analysis have to be performed for appropriate diagnosis and treatment.

Therapy

No large properly conducted trials have so far been published on the optimal therapy for SLE-related CNS involvement; it is interesting to consider the responses to the questionnaire by Tincani (Tincani et al., 1996); steroids and cyclophosphamide were used in 54 per cent and

13 per cent, respectively, of SLE patients with generalized seizures, and in 41.5 per cent and 25 per cent of patients with status epilepticus.

In the management of stroke, 49 per cent of patients were treated with anticoagulants, 22 per cent with anti-platelet agents, 42 per cent with steroids, 6.5 per cent with cyclophosphamide. Psychosis was managed by steroids in 60 per cent of cases, with symptomatic therapy in 62.5 per cent.

Concerning the selected modality of steroid delivery, low-dose steroids seem to be the least popular, whereas bolus or high-dose daily therapy were equally chosen by the responding centres.

A reasonable approach could be the one suggested by Ramos (Ramos *et al.*, 1996): in their study, it was reported by a retrospective analysis that 24 out of 25 SLE patients with CNS involvement, nonresponders to methylprednisolone boli and without APA or LA, were effectively treated by cyclophosphamide 500 mg/week i.v., for at least three times, reaching the clinical effect after a mean delay of 11 days.

In addition to immunosuppressive therapy and to anticoagulant or anti-platelet therapy when indicated, there have been reports of effectiveness of plasma exchange and/or immunoglobulin; even if based on case reports, these may represent a worthwhile option, for instance, in chorea (Nectoux *et al.*, 1992), or else in cases failing to positively respond to immunosuppression.

Case report

A left-handed 27-year-old female, with familiarity for autoimmune disease (father with rheumatoid arthritis, mother with psoriatic arthritis, an uncle with seronegative spondyloarthritis) but no family neuropsychiatric disease, had been suffering from SLE since the age of 10.

Initial disease symptomatology had included fever, joint and skin involvement; laboratory examinations had disclosed antinuclear antibodies and positive LE-cells. The patient was treated for various years with prednisone (10–25 mg every other day), non-steroidal anti-inflammatory drugs, and hydroxychloroquine. At the age of 16, haemolytic anaemia with positive Coombs' test responded to an increase in steroid therapy.

At the age of 17, peritoneal serositis was diagnosed by echography. At the age of 18, the patient showed proteinuria (1 g/24 h); no kidney biopsy was performed; treatment was with three methylprednisolone pulses of 750 mg each and increase in prednisone dosage from 10 mg to 25 mg every other day.

At the age of 19, the patient displayed fever, arthromyalgias, and appearance of hypostenia and hypoaesthesia in lower limbs, sensory loss at mid-thoracic level, difficulties in emptying the bladder, diplopia and signs of left hemispheric cerebellar dysfunction.

Laboratory evaluation at this time showed low C3 and C4 levels, normochromic anaemia, leukopenia, increased ESR (58), increased creatinine (1.76, normal values 0.8–1.2), weak positivity of anti-DNA antibodies, presence of ANA and anticytoplasmic antibodies; Coombs' test was negative, LA, VDRL and ACA were negative.

Brain MRI showed slightly enlarged sulci and lateral ventricles, an alteration in peri-acqueductal signal and small alterations in signal in the white matter of the cerebral hemispheres. Dorsal MRI was normal.

The patient was treated with i.v. methylprednisolone (1000 mg/day for 3 days, 500 mg/day for 3 days, 250 mg/day for 3 days and 125 mg/day for 3 days) with slow recovery.

Since the relapse at age 19, the patient received treatment with cyclophosphamide (overall, one bolus every 3 months for 3 years, followed by two boli at a distance of 6 months) together with prednisone 25 mg every other day, with satisfactory clinical control of disease activity (fluctuating rash and arthralgias).

At the age of 23, the patient suffered from fever, sudden sharp left supraorbital pain, diplopia, dysphagia, paraesthesias on the right side of the face and of the right upper limb; neurological examination disclosed a deficit of the right 6th and 7th cranial nerves, a reduction in left-sided conjugate gaze, superficial hypoaesthesia in the right hemisoma, hypomobility of the soft palate on the left side and internuclear ophtalmoplegia on right-sided gaze.

Brain MRI showed an alteration of signal of probable ischaemic origin in the left paramedian medulla, extending cranially up to the bulbo-pontine junction near the floor of the 4th ventricle.

Treatment with i.v. methylprednisolone, cyclophosphamide and plasmapheresis was started, with incomplete clinical recovery; residua included right hemisoma superficial sensory loss and nystagmus on both horizontal gaze directions.

The patient has since been treated with steroids (prednisone 25 mg every other day) and anti-platelet therapy. At age 24, hyperpirexia developed; haemoculture was positive for *Salmonella*; amoxicyllin treatment for 10 days treated the infection.

At the age of 25, the patient was again hospitalized for relapse with rash, diffuse arthralgias, anaemia with negative Coombs, and treated with methylprednisolone and cyclophosphamide boli. At the age of 26, the patient was on treatment with cyclophosphamide 500 mg every 15 days for 6 months. At the age of 27, the patients had dorsolumbar pain, followed by paraesthesia-hypoaesthesia in the sacral region; methylprednisolone did not give clinical benefit.

In the following weeks, retrosternal pain appeared, which was worsened by respiratory efforts, but without evidence of pleurisy or pericarditis from echocardiography; moreover, a right iridocyclitis appeared, followed 10 days later by lower limb hypostenia and reduced sensitivity to stool transit.

A first dorsolumbar MRI was normal. Seven days later, neurological examination showed paraparetic gait, brisk tendon reflexes except for a weak right tricipital reflex in the lower limbs, bilateral Babinski sign, hypoaesthesia for touch and pain at the posterior face of thigh and leg bilaterally and in the sellar region.

Dorsolumbar MRI with gadolinium was repeated, showing a slight enhancement of a descending root on the right side in the cauda equina and a small signal hyperintensity in T2-weighted images at the D7 level on the left dorsolateral part of the cord.

Concomitantly, a slight bilateral pleural effusion was reported. Laboratory examinations showed leukopenia (WBC 2.200), low levels of C3, ESR 45; ACA and antinuclear antibodies were not detected.

Cerebrospinal fluid examination showed slight lymphocytic pleocytosis (19 cells/mm^3), increase in IgG-index (0.96); oligoclonal bands were present at isoelectric focusing. Cultures for bacteria were negative; the search of Mycobacterium Tuberculosis genome by PCR was negative. Cryptococcal antigen was absent.

Antibodies anti-Cytomegalovirus, -Toxoplasma, -HSV, -HIV, anti-Echo- and Coxsackie-virus were absent, while a slight positivity was found for anti-EBV antibodies. Antibodies to varicella-Zoster virus (VZV) were detected both in serum and in CSF, with negative C-reactive protein. Cryoglobulins were absent. Antinuclear antibodies were repeated and found slightly positive.

After 5 days, the patient suffered from a partial motor epileptic seizure, involving the right upper limb, followed by generalization with loss of consciousness and post-critic confusion.

EEG showed right temporo-parieto-occipital epileptiform discharges (sharp waves) during hyperapnea.

Brain MRI showed the presence of many areas of increased signal in T2-weighted images with cortico-subcortical involvement, in agreement with multiple ischaemic lesions. The lesions were present in both frontal and parietal regions, in the left temporal lobe, in the left thalamus, in the right internal capsule, in pons and in midbrain.

The patient started treatment with phenobarbital, 100 mg/day, and antiplatelet treatment; 4 days later, the patient displayed three episodes of a few hours characterized by sudden onset of aphasia and paresis of right lower limb.

At CT, no signs of haemorrhages and no new ischaemic lesions were visible. Shortly thereafter, the patient had a sudden onset of right brachiocrural paresis. Anti-coagulant therapy was then started.

Together with anticoagulant therapy, we started treatment with anti-viral agents, in view of the results of CSF and serum anti-VZV antibodies quantitation.

The patient has since been slowly recovering, but after 18 months, still needs the help of a cane to walk.

This case represents the difficulties in the practical management of neurological involvement in SLE, particularly in the differential diagnosis between disease flare-ups and – on the contrary – complications (most notably infectious) related to long-standing immunosuppression.

In our case, the suspicion of *Herpes zoster* myelitis, heralded possibly by iridocyclitis, and followed by granulomatous angiitis of the brain vessels leading to multiple areas of cerebral infarction, is supported by the marked immunosuppression present in our patient; a definite confirmation of the diagnosis could have been attained only by brain biopsy, but this procedure was considered too risky in the context of a patient embarked on long-term anticoagulant therapy. Therefore, the diagnosis remains presumptive; however, *Herpes zoster* myelitis during treatment for SLE has already been described in the literature (Ebo *et al.*, 1996); moreover, the presence of a typical zoster rash is not always seen (Puchhammer-Stockl *et al.*, 1991).

As far as CNS vessel involvement is concerned, the association of *Herpes zoster* infection with vasculitis of the CNS has been reported since a long time (Younger *et al.*, 1988).

The issue of the difficulties in this differential diagnosis has strong implications on the correct choice of treatment; as a matter of fact, in our case, increased ESR, low C3 levels and the detection of pleural effusion could suggest a flare-up of SLE; the low level of WBC (with an even lower level of lymphocytes, 15 per cent of the total) could have been ascribed both to prolonged immunosuppression and to disease activity; iridocyclitis is not a clinical manifestation of SLE.

Concerning the neurological manifestations, SLE-related myelitis only rarely implies involvement of spinal roots; multiple brain ischaemic lesions may indeed be present in SLE, but are often associated either with antiphospholipid antibodies or with Libman-Sacks endocarditis.

Herpes zoster-related neurological involvement should always be suspected in cases of CNS disorders in the context of SLE, especially in long-standing immunosuppression.

References

Bell, C.L., Partington, C., Robbins, M., Graziano, F., Turski, P. & Kornguth, S. (1991): Magnetic resonance imaging of central nervous system lesions in patients with lupus erythematosus. Correlation with clinical remission and antineurofilament and anticardiolipin antibody titers. *Arhtritis Rheum.* **34**, 432–441.

Bonfa, E., Golombek, S.J., Kaufman, L.D., Skelly, S., Weissbach, H., Brot, N. & Elkon, K.B. (1987): Association between lupus psychosis and anti-ribosomal P protein antibodies. *N. Engl. J. Med.* **317**, 265–271.

Boyer, R.S., Sun, N.C.J., Verity, A., Nies, K.M., Louie, J.S. (1980): Immunoperoxidase staining of the choroid plexus in systemic lupus erythematosus. *J. Rheumatol.* **7**, 645–650.

Brey, R.L. & Escalante, A. (1998): Neurological manifestations of antiphospholipid antibody syndrome. *Lupus* **7** (Suppl.2), S67–S74.

Brey, R.L., Hart, R.G., Sherman, D.G. & Tegeler, C.T. (1990): Antiphospholipid antibodies and cerebral ischemia in young people. *Neurology* **40**, 1190–1196.

Carette, S., Urowitz, M.B., Grosman, H. & St.Louis, E.L. (1982): Cranial computerized tomography in systemic lupus erythematosus. *J. Rheumatol.* **9**, 855–859.

Cinque, P., Vago, L., Dahl, H., Brytting, M., Terreni, M.R., Fornara, C., Racca, S., Castagna, A., D'Arminio Monforte, A., Wahren, B., Lazzarin, A. & Linde, A. (1996): Polymerase chain reaction on cerebrospinal fluid for diagnosis of virus-associated opportunistic diseases of the central enrvous system in HIV-infected patients. *AIDS* **10**, 951–958.

Del Papa, N. , Guidali, L., Sala, A., Buccellati, C., Khamashta, M.A., Ichikawa, K., Koike, T., Balestrieri, G., Tincani, A., Hughes, G.R. & Meroni, P.L. (1997): Endothelial cells as target for antiphospholipid antibodies. Human polyclonal and monoclonal anti-beta-2-glycoprotein I antibodies react *in vitro* with endothelial cells through adherent beta-2-glycoprotein I and induce endothelial activation. *Arthritis Rheum.* **40**, 551–561.

Devinsky, O., Petito, C.K. & Alonso, D.R. (1988): Clinical and neuropathological findings in systemic lupus erythematosus: the role of vasculitis, heart emboli, and thrombotic thrombocytopenic purpura. *Ann. Neurol.* **23**, 380–384.

Ebo, D.G. , DeClerck, L.S., Stevens, W.J., Ieven, M., Ursi, D., Van Goethem, J.W. & Couttenye, M.M. (1996): Herpes zoster myelitis occurring during treatment for systemic lupus erythematosus. *J. Rheumatol.* **23**, 548–550.

Glidden, R.S., Mantzouranis, E.C. & Borel, Y. (1983): SLE in childhood: clinical manifestations and improved survival in 55 patients. *Clin. Immunol. Immunopathol.* **29**, 196–210.

Gonzalez-Crespo, M.R., Blanco, F.J., Ramos, A., Ciruelo, E., Mateo, I., Lopez-Pino, M.A. & Gomez-Reino, J.J. (1995): Magnetic resonance imaging of the brain in systemic lupus erythematosus. *Br. J. Rheumatol.* **34**, 1055–1060.

Hanly, J.G., Walsh, N.M.G. & Sangalang, V. (1992): Brain pathology in systemic lupus erythematosus. *J. Rheumatol.* **19**, 732–741.

Hochberg M.C. (1997): Updating the American College of Rheumatology revised criteria for the classification of SLE. *Arthr. Rheum.* **40**(9), 1725.

Jacobs, J.C. (1963): Systemic lupus erythematosus in childhood. *Pediatrics* **32**, 257–259.

Kaye, B.R., Neuwelt, C.M., London, S.S. & De Armond, S.J. (1992): Central nervous system systemic lupus erythematosus mimicking progressive multifocal leukoencephalopathy. *Ann. Rheum.* **51**, 1152–1156.

Kent, M., Vogt, E. & Rote, N.S. (1997): Monoclonal antiphosphatidylserine antibodies react directly with feline and murine central nervous system. *J. Rheumatol.* **24**, 1725–1733.

King, K.K., Kornreich, H.K., Bernstein, B.H., Singsen, B.H. & Hanson, V. (1977): The clinical spectrum of SLE in childhood. *Arthr. Rheum.* **20**, 287–294.

Kovacs, J.A.J., Urowitz, M.B. & Gladman, D.D. (1993): Dilemmas in neuropsychiatric lupus. In: Neurologic aspects of rheumatic diseases. *Rheumatic Disease Clinics of North America* **19** (4), 795–814.

Kuroe, K., Kurahashi, K., Nakano, I., Morimatsu, Y. & Takemori, H. (1994): A neuropathological study of a case of lupus erythematosus with chorea. *J. Neurol. Sci.* **123**, 59–62.

McNeil, H.P., Chesterman, C.N. & Krilis, S.A. (1991): Immunology and clinical importance of antiphospholipid antibodies. *Adv. Immunol.* **49**, 193–280.

Meislin, A.G. & Rothfeld, N (1968): Systemic lupus in childhood. *Pediatrics* **42**, 37–49.

Miguel, E.C., Pereira, R.M., Pereira, CA., Baer, L., Gomes, R.E., de Sa, L.C., Hirsch, R., de Barros, N.G., de Navarro, J.M. & Gentil, V. (1994): Psychiatric manifestations of systemic lupus erythematosus: clinical features, symptoms and signs of central nervous system activity in 43 patients. *Medicine* **73**, 224–232.

Miller, D.H., Ormerod, J.E., Gibson, A., du Boulay, E.P.G.H., Rudge, P. & McDonald, W.I. (1987): MRI brain scanning in patients with vasculitis: differentiation from multiple sclerosis. *Neuroradiology* **29**, 226–231.

Nectoux, F., Euller-Ziegler, L., Grisot, C., Quaranta, J.F. & Duplay, H. (1992): Lupus chorea revealing. Study in magnetic resonance imaging. Success of plasma exchange after resistence to pulsed cortisone. *Rev. Rhum. Malad. Ostéo-Articulaires* **59**, 436.

Ostrov, S.G., Quencer, R.M., Gaylis, M.B. & Altman, R.D. (1982): Cerebral atrophy in systemic lupus erythematosus: corticosteroid or disease-induced phenomenon? *AJNR* **3**, 21–23.

Otte, A., Weiner, S.M., Hoegerle, S., Wolf, R., Jungling, F.D., Peter, H.H. & Nitzsche, E.U. (1998): Neuropsychiatric systemic lupus erythematosus before and after immunosuppressive treatment: a FDG PET study. *Lupus* **7**, 57–59.

Platt, J.L., Burke, B.A., Fish, A.J., Kim, Y. & Michael, A.F. (1982): SLE in the first two decades of life. *Am. J. Kidney Dis.* **2** (Suppl. 1), 212–222.

Puchhammer-Stockl, E., Popow-Kraupp, T., Heinz, F.X., Mandl, C.W. & Kunz, C (1991): Detection of varicella-zoster virus DNA by polymerase chain reaction in the cerebrospinal fluid of patients suffering from neurological complications associated with chicken pox or herpes zoster. *J. Clin. Microbiol.* **29**, 1513–1516.

Ramos, P.C., Mendez, M.J., Amer, P.R.J., Khamashta, M.A & Hughes, G.R.V. (1996): Pulse cyclophosphamide in the treatment of neuropsychiatric SLE. *Clin. Exp. Rheumatol.* **14**, 295–299.

Rubbert, A., Marienhagen, J., Pirner, K., Manger, B., Grebmeier, J., Engelhardt, A., Wolf, F. & Kalden, J.R. (1993): Single photon emission computed tomography analysis of cerebral blood flow in the evaluation of central nervous system involvement in patients with systemic lupus erythematosus. *Rheum.* **36**, 1253–1262.

Salmaggi, A., Lamperti, E., Eoli, M., Venegoni, E., Bruzzone, M.G., Riccio, G. & La Mantia, L. (1994): Spinal cord involvement and systemic lupus erythematosus: clinical and magnetic resonance findings in 5 patients. *Clin. Exp. Rheumatol.* **12**, 389–394.

Schneebaum, A.B., Singleton, J.D., West, S.G., Blodgett, J.K., Allen, L.G., Cheronis, J.C. & Kotzin, B.L. (1991): Association of psychiatric manifestations with antibodies to ribosomal P proteins in systemic lupus erythematosus. *Am. J. Med.* **90**, 54–62.

Schwartz, M., Rochas, M., Weller, B., Sheinkman, A., Tal, I., Golan, D., Toubi, N., Eldar, I., Sharf, B. & Attias, D. (1998): High association of anticardiolipin antibodies with psychosis. *J. Clin. Psychiatry* **59**, 20–23.

Shiozawa, S., Kuroki, Y., Kim, M., Hirohata, S. & Ogino, T. (1992): Interferon-alpha in lupus psychosis. *Arthr. Rheum.* **35**, 417–422.

Silvestrini, M., Matteis, M., Troisi, E., Cupini, L.M., Zaccari, G. & Bernardi, G. (1994): Migrainous stroke and the antiphospholipid antibodies. *Eur. Neurol.* **34**, 316–319.

Singer, J., Denburg, J.A. & The Ad Hoc Neuropsychiatric Lupus workshop Group (1990): Diagnostic criteria for neuropsychiatric systemic lupus erythematosus: the results of a consensus meeting. *J. Rheumatol.* **17**, 1397–1402.

Steinlein, M.I., Blaser, S.I., Gilday, D.L., Eddy, A.A., Logan, W.J., Laxer, R.M. & Silverman, E.D. (1995): Neurologic manifestations of pediatric systemic lupus erythematosus. *Pediatr. Neurol.* **13,** 191–197.

Tan, E.M., Cohen, A.S., Fries, J.F., Masi, A.T., McShane, D.J., Rothfield, N.F., Schaller, J.G., Talal, N. & Winchester, R.J. (1982): The 1982 revised criteria for the classification of SLE. *Arthr. Rheum.* **25,** 1271–1277.

Tincani, A., Brey, R., Balestrieri, G., Vitali, C., Doria, A., Galeazzi, M., Meroni, P.L., Migliorini, P., Neri, R., Tavoni, A. & Bombardieri, S. (1996): International survey on the management of patients with SLE. II. The results of a questionnaire regarding neuropsychiatric manifestations. *Clin. Exp. Rheumatol.* **14** (Suppl. 16), S23–S29.

Younger, D.S., Hays, A.P., Brust, J.C.M. & Rowland, L.P. (1988): Granulomatous angiitis of the brain. An inflammatory reaction of diverse etiology. *Arch. Neurol.* **45,** 514–518.

Yuh, W.T.C., Ueda, T. & Maley, J.E. (1998): Perfusion and diffusion imaging: a potential tool for improved diagnosis of CNS vasculitis. *AJNR* January 1998, 87–89.

Note: In 1999, the American College of Rheumatology (ACR) Ad Hoc Committee on neuropsychiatric lupus nomenclature has produced a document which takes into account several manifestations (in all, 19) in the diagnosis of neuropsychiatric SLE (*Arthr. Rheum.* 1999, **42**, 599–608).

Chapter 13

Pathogenetic mechanisms of the antiphospholipid syndrome

Marco Taglietti, Chiara Biasini, Micol Frassi, Massimo Cinquini,
Genesio Balestrieri and Angela Tincani

Clinical Immunology Service, Spedali Civili di Brescia, P.le Spedali Civili 1, 25125 Brescia, Italy

Summary

In 1983, the combination of stroke and miscarriages in presence of LAC (Lupus anticoagulant) was described as a clinical syndrome by Graham Hughes and a radioimmunoassay for the detection of anticardiolipin antibodies (aCL) was developed by Harris *et al.* (1983) in the same group. Converted to an enzyme-linked immunosorbent assay (ELISA), the aCL assay became a new tool for the study of the antiphospholipid antibodies.

Nevertheless, conclusive proofs that the clinical features of the antiphospholipid syndrome (APS) were mediated by antiphospholipid antibodies were not obtained until animal models for the syndrome itself became available. As in humans, APS occurs also in lupus-prone mice and can be induced in normal mice. Following reports of APS in patients with SLE, studies were conducted in various strains of lupus-prone mice in order to look for antiphospholipid antibodies and for manifestations consistent with APS. Animal models supported the close relationship existing between antiphospholipid antibodies and clinical features of the syndrome itself.

In vitro experiments show that autoantibodies to phospholipid-binding plasma proteins play a significant role in the pathogenetic mechanisms of thrombosis and foetal loss, also by impairing the thrombo-modulatory function of annexin-V.

Introduction: a brief history

The antiphospholipid antibodies syndrome was born as a clinical entity, characterized by arterial and/or venous thrombosis, recurrent foetal losses and autoimmune thrombocytopenia associated with high levels of antiphospholipid antibodies at the dawn of the 1980s (Hughes, 1983), even if antiphospholipid antibodies (aPL) were first observed in nontreponemal serological tests for syphilis (STS), in the early part of last century.

In 1942, Mary Pangborn identified the critical antigen in these reactions as a novel anionic phospholipid, named *cardiolipin* (Pangborn, 1942). During the 1950s, a number of patients with chronically false positive STS who subsequently developed systemic lupus erythematosus

(SLE) was described (Moore & Lutz, 1955). During the same period, several case-reports underlined the association of chronic false positive STS and an *in vitro* coagulation defect, characterized by the prolongation of phospholipid-dependent coagulation reactions (Laurell & Nilsson, 1957). This defect, called '*lupus anticoagulant*' (LA), appeared to be due to phospholipid-binding antibodies (Lee & Sanders, 1955; Laurell & Nilsson, 1957). Interestingly, despite its *in vitro* anticoagulant activity, LA was described in women with unexplained foetal losses (Laurell & Nilsson, 1957; Nilsson *et al.*, 1975), in patients with SLE suffering from repeated thrombotic episodes (Bowie *et al.*, 1963; Alarçon-Segovia & Osmundson, 1965) and in patients with both features, i.e. repeated miscarriages and thrombosis (Alagille *et al.*, 1956; Soulier and Boffa, 1980).

In 1983, the combination of stroke and miscarriages in presence of LA, was described as a clinical syndrome by Graham Hughes and a radioimmunoassay for the detection of anticardiolipin antibodies (aCL) was developed by Harris *et al.* (1983) in the same group. Converted to an enzyme-linked immunosorbent assay (ELISA) (Loizou *et al.*, 1985), the aCL assay became a new tool for the study of the antiphospholipid antibodies and clinical manifestation associated with them.

Widespread use of the aCL ELISA in large series of patients, together with clinical observation, led to the generally accepted definition of the antiphospholipid syndrome (APS) (Asherson *et al.*, 1989; Alarçon-Segovia & Sanchez-Guerrero, 1989; Roubey, 1997). aCL were considered as the major serological marker of APS (Hughes, 1985), although the broad cross-reactivity of these antibodies with most anionic phospholipid soon became evident (Harris *et al.*, 1985). Although aCL and LA appeared to have similar specificities (Thiagarjan *et al.*, 1980), the relationship between the two assays was not straightforward. The majority of patients with APS were both LA and aCL positive; however, some were found positive in just one of these tests (McNeil *et al.*, 1991). Furthermore, aPL associated with APS seemed to differ from those associated with syphilis. Antibodies from syphilis patients are frequently found to react with cardiolipin, even if they do not cross-react with other anionic phospholipids (Harris *et al.*, 1988). LA assays are usually, although not always, negative in patients with syphilis (Johansson and Lassus, 1974).

In 1990, three groups discovered independently that the binding of highly purified aCL to cardiolipin required the presence of serum or plasma (Galli *et al.*, 1990; McNeil *et al.*, 1990; Matsuura *et al.*, 1990). The relevant serum component, named aCL 'cofactor', was identified in the β2-glycoprotein I (β2GPI), a 50 kD glycoprotein present in normal human plasma and serum at a concentration of ~ 200 μg/ml (Schultze *et al.*, 1961). *In vitro*, β2GPI binds to negatively charged phospholipids (Wurm, 1984) and other anionic molecules, such as DNA and heparin and displays a number of anticoagulant properties (Nimpf *et al.*, 1986; Schousboe, 1985; Nimpf *et al.*, 1987).

The aCL in patients with APS binds to a complex of β2GPI and negatively charged phospholipids, in contrast to the aCL present in patients with infectious diseases, which recognizes cardiolipin, independent of β2GPI. It is now considered that the major antigenic target for 'pathogenic' aCL resides on β2GPI itself.

Studies have shown that measurement of anti-β2GPI may be of value in determining the risk of thrombotic episodes in patients with autoimmune diseases, and that the anti-β2GPI assays may have better specificities than do the aCL assays (Tincani *et al.*, 1998a).

Experimental models

Conclusive proof that the clinical features of the antiphospholipid syndrome were mediated by antiphospholipid antibodies was not obtained until animal models for the syndrome itself became available. APS can occur as a primary disorder in otherwise healthy subjects, or as a secondary disorder in patients with systemic autoimmune disease, mainly SLE.

Similarly, APS occurs in lupus-prone mice and can be induced in normal mice.

Following reports of APS in patients with SLE, studies were conducted in various strains of lupus-prone mice in order to look for antiphospholipid antibodies and for manifestations consistent with antiphospholipid syndrome.

In 1989, Gharavi et al. (1989) were the first to report anticardiolipin antibodies in MLR/lpr mice. NZBxWF1 mice that had a similar lupus-like disease associated with high titres of anti-double-stranded DNA antibodies, were negative for anticardiolipin antibodies. Interestingly, clinical evidence of APS such as decreased platelet count and a decreased litter size were also observed in MLR/lpr mice, suggesting a possible pathogenic role of aPL.

Other studies focused on the central nervous system disease of MLR/lpr mice, occurring in association with aCL antibodies; they described histological evidence of cerebral thrombosis as well as cognitive and motor abnormalities and came to the conclusion that MLR/lpr can be taken as a good model of the different aspects of secondary APS described in humans (Hess et al., 1993; Brey & Teale, 1992). The finding of an altered prostacyclin-thromboxane ratio gives a brilliant biological support to the thrombogenic tendency of this strain of mice (Schorer, 1997).

Myocardial infarction, thrombocytopenia and aCL antibodies have been recorded in NZB x BXSB F1 mice suffering from immune-complex lupus nephritis (Hashimoto et al., 1992). These antibodies, whose titres increase with the age of the mice, were found to have the same reactivity pattern of those seen in humans, including the so-called $\beta 2$-glycoprotein I dependency. Recently, a Japanese group described in these mice fundus lesions including choricapillaris thrombosis, possibly contributing to the elucidation of another aspect of APS (Nakamura et al., 1998).

A peculiar kind of aPL antibodies directed to zwitterionic phospholipid such as phosphatidylcoline (PC) were recorded in patients with autoimmune haemolytic anaemia (both idiopathic and within SLE) that therefore was regarded as a peculiar aspect of APS (Cabral et al., 1990). It is of extreme interest that NZB mice, known to develop during their life an autoimmune haemolytic anaemia, were found to have high titre of IgM antiphosphatidylcholine antibodies, therefore representing the exact equivalent of the human disease (Cabiedes et al., 1994).

All the above quoted models supported the close relationship existing between systemic autoimmunity and APS within a defined genetic background; however on this basis a direct responsibility of antibodies in causing foetal loss or thrombosis cannot be established because, at least theoretically, other pathogenic mechanisms could be responsible for these events in the context of systemic lupus.

The difficulty to understand whether aPL could be considered the cause or the epiphenomenon of the disease was almost completely overcome by the study of healthy mice in which antibodies were artificially induced thus allowing a recording of the direct effect of their presence. This result can be achieved by two different procedures: the infusion of human or murine aPL antibodies in mice (*passive immunization*) or the stimulation of animals to produce their own antibodies (*active immunization*).

Passive immunization

Different strains of normal mice (BALB/c, ICR, CD1) were used to verify the effect of the infusion of purified immunoglobulin fractions from patients with APS (Branch *et al.*, 1990; Blank *et al.*, 1991, 1994a; Piona *et al.*, 1995). When the infusion was performed in pregnant mice it caused foetal resorptions (equivalent to the abortion in humans), decrease in placental weights and placental thromboses. In addition the mice were shown to have a low platelet count and a prolonged PTT, an indication for the induction of lupus anticoagulant activity. CD1 mice were used for the study of thrombosis model (Pierangeli & Harris, 1994). For this purpose the femoral vein was exposed and a mechanical standardized thrombogenic stimulus was applied. When mice were infused with immunoglobulins from APS patients, increased thrombus size and slower dissolution time were recorded (Pierangeli *et al.*, 1995).

Taken together, these groups of experiments, although suggesting a linkage between aPL and some pathological events observed in human disease, are not completely satisfactory, because they were performed by infusing the animals with whole immunoglobulin fractions potentially containing different autoantibody populations often described as associated to aPL. Moreover even in the same patient the so called aPL antibodies can include autoantibodies with different reactivity such as the β2GPI-dependent and the β2GPI-independent aCL antibodies.

In this respect the studies designed employing monoclonal antibodies with well-defined specificity or autoantigen-affinity purified antibody populations were more useful.

Interestingly, the impairment of normal pregnancy outcome has been obtained infusing antibodies with a different specificity. In fact in 1991, Blank *et al.* (1991) infusing a β2GPI independent anticardiolipin murine monoclonal antibody were able to show increased number of foetal resorptions together with decreased placental and embryo weights. In 1998, Ikematsu *et al.* (1998), using two β2GPI-independent human monoclonal aCL confirmed the previous results and, in addition, showed the antibody deposition in the placenta with the occurrence of a significant number of placental thromboses. However the same effect was also obtained by infusion of a murine monoclonal antiphosphatidylserine antibody, not reacting with cardiolipin, but able to bind the trophoblastic cells (Vogt *et al.*, 1996). In addition, IgM anti β2GPI human monoclonal antibodies (George *et al.*, 1998a) as well as polyclonal affinity purified anti β2GPI IgG (observations from our group), when infused in normal pregnant mice, were able to impair the normal pregnancy outcome. Finally, in an elegant model of molecular biology, Radic *et al.* (1995) showed that the induction in transgenic mice of antibody directed to DNA/CL, was able to reduce the number of pups significantly and to prolong clotting time.

In conclusion, a large number of the so called aPL antibodies with sometimes well-defined different specificity, when passively infused, were pathogenetic in the pregnancy model, suggesting that the same effect could be produced by different mechanisms mediated by autoantibodies directed to different autoantigens.

Murine monoclonal antibodies directed to CL, or alternatively to β2GPI were also studied in the thrombosis formation model. The thrombus formation in the mice femoral vein was not affected by infusion of monoclonal anti-β2GPI while monoclonals directed to cardiolipin itself or to the complex CL-β2GPI were capable of modifying it (Olee *et al.*, 1996).

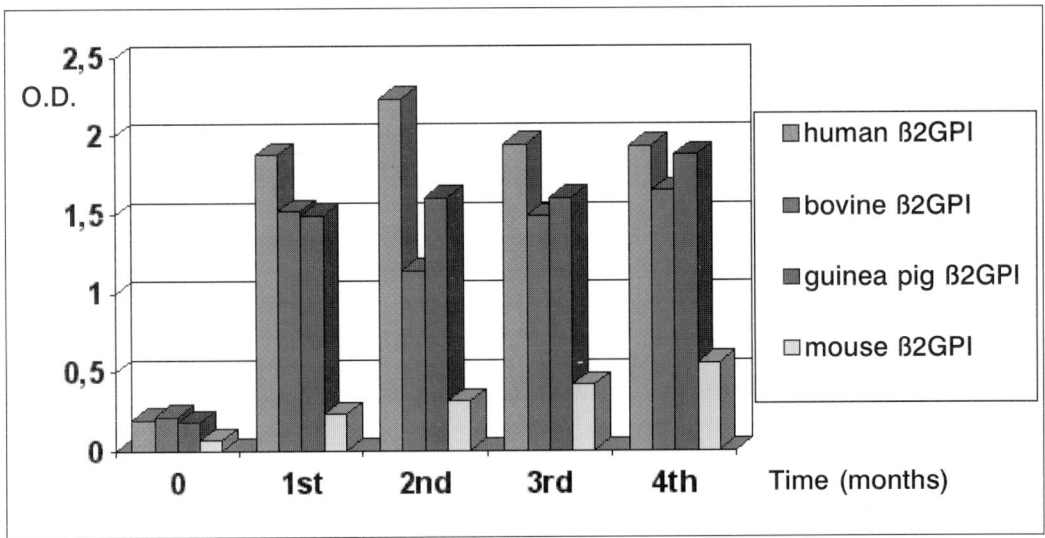

Fig. 1. Reactivity to human, bovine, guinea pig and murine β2GPI of BALB/c mice immunized with human β2GPI.

Active immunization

Antigen stimulation can be used to induce antibody production in normal animals. However since PL are rather difficult antigens, most of the active immunization experiments were performed by stimulating animals either with aPL antibodies or with β2GPI.

In the first case the procedure was based on the idiotype/anti-idiotype network theory and it was already used to induce anti-DNA antibodies as well as features of systemic lupus in normal mice (Mendlovic et al., 1988). The injection of monoclonal and polyclonal aCL antibodies in complete Freund's adjuvant into the foot-pads of normal mice, resulted in the production of autologous aCL antibodies associated with a prolonged PTT (Bakimer et al., 1992). When observed long enough, these animals were shown to have the full-blown picture of APS with decreased fecundity, high rate of resorption index of the foetuses and low weights of embryos and placentas. Recently, neurological and behavioural defects were shown in BALB/c mice immunized with a human aCL monoclonal (H3), who developed APS, with aCL, anti-β2GPI and also anti-endothelial cell antibodies (Ziporen et al., 1997).

Interestingly, active immunization with aPL antibodies induces different pathological pictures according to the different stimulating antibodies used: in fact lupus features (anti-DNA antibodies, proteinuria etc.) associated with APS were seen in the mice when they were immunized with an anti-DNA/CL antibody carrying the 16/6 idiotype (Blank et al., 1992), while the primary syndrome is produced by immunization with monoclonal antibodies specific for CL (Cohen et al., 1994).

The discovery in 1990 that β2GPI, the so called 'cofactor', was a very important part of the antigenic complex recognized by antibodies in aCL ELISA, allowed a new way of active immunization induction model. β2GPI was in fact used as an immunizing antigen for mice and rabbits in a number of different studies, starting from the first performed by Gharavi et al. (1992). A common finding of the different papers reporting these experiments was the detection, in the immunized animals, of antibodies reactive in both anti-β2GPI and aCL ELISA

(Gharavi et al., 1992; Pierangeli & Harris, 1993; Blank et al., 1994b). However, all these data do not clarify the real relationship existing between the antibodies detected in the two assays and do not elucidate whether immunized mice may lose tolerance starting to react with their own β2GPI.

Some findings from our group have shown that BALB/c mice immunized with human β2GPI first produce antibodies to *human* β2GPI, followed later by antibodies directed to β2GPI from different sources, including *murine* (Tincani et al., 1998b) (see Fig. 1). These antibodies directed to epitopes preserved in the species' evolution appear identical to those seen in the spontaneous human disease (Tincani *et al.*, 1996).

Animals immunized with β2GPI also develop pathological manifestations within the APS spectrum. In MLR/++ mice immunized with human β2GPI, an accelerated autoimmune disease was observed prior to 18 months of age, when it usually occurs.

The disease is characterized by neurological and renal dysfunction, increased foetal resorptions and thrombocytopenia (Aron *et al.*, 1995). APS manifestations were also described in BALB/c and PL/J mice immunized with β2GPI (Blank *et al.*, 1992; Garcia *et al.*, 1997). Interestingly, this disease was observed 3 or 4 months after immunization, when also anti-murine β2GPI are detected in the serum of the mice (Tincani *et al.*, 1998b).

Recently a different animal model was described suggesting a possible role of anti-β2GPI antibodies in atherosclerosis (George *et al.*, 1998b). Immunization of low-density lipoprotein (LDL) receptor-deficient mice with β2GPI resulted in an enhanced atherosclerosis occurrence. Oxidized LDL were shown to be involved in the development and progression of atherosclerosis and aCL were recently reported to cross-react with anti-oxidized LDL. Autoantibodies to β2GPI may be responsible of this cross-reactivity, since β2GPI binds both CL and oxidized LDL. If this is true, anti-β2GPI antibodies may be involved in the development of premature atherosclerosis of SLE patients.

Furthermore, the atherosclerotic lesion of spiral artery, that is considered the patognomonic lesion of preeclampsia/eclampsia, might be mediated by the presence of aPL or more specifically anti-β2GPI antibodies.

The pathogenesis of thrombosis

A growing body of circumstantial and direct evidence suggests that autoantibodies are not only serological markers of APS, but directly contribute to the development of thrombosis and other clinical manifestations.

Thrombosis in APS appears to be a 'two-hit' phenomenon. Autoantibodies (the first 'hit') are continually present in the circulation, yet a local trigger (the second 'hit') is required in order to induce thrombus formation at a particular site in the vasculature at a particular time. It is hypothesized therefore that autoantibodies cause a prothrombotic state in which thrombosis is triggered by local stimuli that would not normally be sufficient to do so.

There are a limited number of general mechanisms by which autoantibodies to phospholipid-binding plasma proteins, such as β2GPI or prothrombin, could act.

Four such possibilities are:

(1) High affinity neutralizing autoantibodies may directly inhibit an antigen's function and/or decrease plasma antigen levels via clearance of antigen-antibody complexes. Examples of

this type of autoantibody are acquired inhibiting factors. With the exception of the small subset of patients with *lupus anticoagulant* and hypoprothrombinaemia, antibodies associated with APS tend to be of relatively low affinity and do not decrease plasma antigen levels.

(2) Autoantibodies may form immune complexes that are deposited in vessel walls leading to inflammation and tissue injury. This mechanism occurs in serum sickness and many vasculitides, but does not appear to occur with either acquired factor inhibitors or APS autoantibodies.

(3) Autoantibodies may cross-link membrane-bound antigens, causing dysregulation of phospholipid-dependent reactions.

(4) Antibody cross-linking or antigens bound to cell surfaces or cell surface receptors may trigger signal transduction and cellular activation.

Because the latter two mechanisms involve antibody binding to membrane-bound antigens, they may be particularly relevant for low affinity antibodies and antibodies that are specific for epitopes on membrane-bound antigens.

A major paradox involving antiphospholipid antibodies is the fact that these antibodies act as anticoagulant *in vitro*, whereas they are procoagulant *in vivo*. The mechanisms of *lupus anticoagulant* activity, although not of direct pathophysiological relevance, may serve as examples of the sort of antibody-antigen interaction that may occur *in vivo*. For example, high concentration of β2GPI inhibits prothrombinase activity *in vitro*, by binding to anionic phospholipids, thereby decreasing the availability of the phospholipid surface upon which the prothrombinase complex may assemble (Roubey *et al.*, 1992). At physiological concentration of β2GPI, this inhibitory activity is weak. Anti-β2GPI antibodies potentiate β2GPI's inhibitory activity by crosslinking membrane-bound β2GPI thereby markedly enhancing the avidity of the β2GPI-phospholipid interaction (Willems *et al.*, 1996; Arnout *et al.*, 1998). *In vivo*, β2GPI/anti-β2GPI antibodies could similarly inhibit any phospholipid-dependent reactions, including those of the anticoagulant protein C pathway. The *lupus anticoagulant* activity of non-neutralizing autoantibodies to prothrombin may be due to several mechanisms. These autoantibodies may inhibit prothrombinase activity by slowing the dissociation of the prothrombinase complex and the release of thrombin from the membrane surface. Cross-linking of membrane-bound prothrombin could also inhibit assembly of the prothrombinase complex.

Based on the discussion above, mechanisms of thrombosis in APS may be broadly grouped as those involving antibody interference with haemostatic reactions (physiological anticoagulant reactions, fibrinolysis) and those involving cell-mediated events (endothelial cells, monocytes, platelets).

Among the many thrombogenic mechanisms associated with APS, some of the most consistent and reproducible data involve the inhibition of protein C pathway.

Protein C is a vitamin K-dependent plasma glycoprotein that circulates as a precursor to a serine protease. Activation of protein C occurs when thrombin binds to thrombomodulin, a constitutively expressed protein on the surface of vascular endothelial cells. On binding to thrombomodulin, thrombin's procoagulant activities (for example, cleavage of fibrinogen, activation of platelets) are inhibited, while its ability to activate protein C is markedly enhanced. When activated, protein C acts as an anticoagulant by proteolytically inactivating factors Va and VIIa, thereby limiting the rate of thrombin generation. The most efficient inactivation of factors Va and VIIa requires the cofactor activity of protein S, another vitamin K-dependent plasma glycoprotein. Protein S circulates in plasma both as a free protein and in a bi-molecular complex with the complement regulatory protein C4-b binding protein. Only free protein S acts as cofactor activity for activated protein C.

Inhibition of both protein C activation and the function of activated protein C has been observed in association with APS (Comp et al., 1983; Marciniak & Romond, 1989; Malia et al., 1990; Oosting et al., 1993). Marciniak and Romond (1989) reported a decreased rate of factor Va degradation in the plasma of 15 patients with lupus anticoagulant (LA). Malia et al. (1990) found that the IgG fractions from certain patients prevented Va degradation only in the presence of protein S, while others inhibited equally well with and without protein S. Similar results were obtained by Oosting et al. (1993), who further demonstrated that the antibodies responsible for inhibiting Va degradation were directed against phospholipid-bound protein C or protein S. Plasmas and purified IgG fractions from APS patients may reduce the effect of activated protein C in functional assays for activated protein C resistance, mimicking the inherited resistance to activated protein C (Halbmayer et al., 1994).

Data regarding the effect of β2GPI and anti-β2GPI antibodies on the protein C pathway are equivocal. Although β2GPI can inhibit protein C activation by thrombomodulin incorporated in cardiolipin vesicles (Keeling et al., 1991), it has little or no effect on the endothelial cell-mediated activation of protein C in presence or absence of anti-β2GPI autoantibodies (Oosting et al., 1991). Matsuda et al. (1995) reported that polyclonal rabbit anti-human β2GPI inhibited the activation of factor Va by activated protein C. Although autoantibodies to prothrombin per se would probably not affect the protein C pathway, it is likely that a subset of antiprothrombin antibodies also recognizes thrombin. Such antibodies could have various effects, including the inhibition of protein C activation by thrombin.

Antithrombin III (AT III), a serine protease inhibitor, is the major inhibitor of factors IXa, Xa and thrombin. In order to optimally inhibit these factors, AT III must bind to heparin sulphate expressed on vascular endothelium. Autoantibodies to vascular heparin sulphate proteoglycan and/or heparin, could contribute to a thrombotic tendency by blocking the activation of AT III (Shibata et al., 1994). In view of the fact that β2GPI binds to heparin, anti-β2GPI antibodies could have a similar effect.

It is possible that autoantibodies to β2GPI could inhibit a putative anticoagulant function of this protein. Despite some in vitro data suggesting that β2GPI may be a physiological anti- coagulant, clinical data supporting such a function are lacking. Importantly, the interaction of β2GPI with phospholipid membranes under physiological conditions is too weak to be the basis for an anticoagulant function.

Shi et al. (1993) found that β2GPI inhibited the ability of the platelet surface to support factor Xa generation, and that anti-β2GPI antibodies blocked this effect, leading to increased factor Xa generation.

Considering another intriguing theory of the pathogenesis of thrombosis in APS, a disruption of endothelial cell (EC) function is an attractive hypothesis, because this could explain the non-inflammatory vasculopathy present in APS patients. Furthermore, a large body of evidence indicated that aPL antibodies bind to ECs (Del Papa et al., 1995; Cervera et al., 1991). Hence, antibody-EC mediated injury and EC activation has been identified as a significant potential factor that may be involved in the pathogenesis of thrombosis by aPL. The conversion of a normal anti-thrombotic state into a prothrombotic state may be the primary pathophysiological event in acquired hypercoagulable state, including the APS (Reverter *et al.*, 1996; Bachman & Silverstein, 1993). Some of the most provocative data indicate that aPL activate ECs and induce upregulation of EC adhesion molecules (Del Papa *et al.*, 1995, 1997; Simantov *et al.*, 1995). Actually, endothelial adhesion is able *per se* to induce leukocyte activation and it is widely accepted that activated monocytes, for example, are able to display a procoagulant activity (Reverter *et al.*, 1996). Del Papa *et al.* were the first to demonstrate that aPL or anti-β2GPI antibodies upregulate EC adhesion molecules; this effect is directly related to EC binding of the antibodies and IL-1a and induces an increase of interleukin-6, accompanied by production of IL-1b, which in turn affects the adhesion molecule expression (Del Papa *et al.*, 1995, 1997). In addition, the same group showed that anti-β2GPI antibodies also induced a dose-dependent increase in the endothelial production of 6-keto prostaglandin F (Del Papa *et al.*, 1997). The findings of Del Papa *et al.* were confirmed by Simantov *et al.* (1995), who showed upregulation of adhesion molecules (ICAM-1; VCAM-1 and E-selectin) on HUVEC and increased adhesion of monocytes to ECs by aPL antibodies in presence of β2GPI *in vitro* (Simantov *et al.*, 1995). As further support to the hypothesis that aPL antibodies activate ECs, one recent study indicated that the levels of soluble VCAM-1 were significantly increased in the plasma of patients with APS and recurrent thrombosis (Kaplanski *et al.*, 2000). In a recent study, George *et al.* (1998c) showed that the upregulation of ICAM-1, VCAM-1 and e-selectin on HUVEC *in vitro* by some, but not all, murine monoclonal aPL preparation correlated with increased foetal resorptions in mice *in vivo*. In another recent study proposed by Silvia Pierangeli *et al.* (1999), five out of six affinity-purified aPL antibodies from patients with APS upregulated expression of ICAM-1, VCAM-1 and e-selectin *in vitro*, and these effects correlated with enhanced thrombosis and leukocytes adhesion *in vivo*.

Pregnancy losses pathogenesis: the role of annexin-V

Annexin-V is a member of a family of proteins which were recognized in 1990 (Crumpton *et al.*, 1990). Thus far, the genes for several hundred different annexins, including 10 in mammalian cells, have been described (for a brief review see Rand, 1999). The remainder have been described in other organisms including a wide range of plants (Morgan *et al.*, 1997). Their canonical structure is composed of repetitive homologous domains consisting of sequences about 70 aminoacids, with almost all of the annexins having four of these domains. annexin-V had been independently isolated from human placenta (Tait *et al.*, 1988), blood vessels (Reutelingsperger *et al.*, 1988), among other sites. The protein, which was designated annexin-V in 1992 (Creutz, 1992), has potent anticoagulant activity *in vitro*, which is based on its high affinity for anionic phospholipids and its capacity to displace coagulation factors from phospholipid surfaces (Andree *et al.*, 1992). Interestingly, annexin-V clusters on exposed phospholipid and forms two-dimensional crystalline arrays on this surface (Voges *et al.*, 1994; Mosser *et al.*, 1991). Its potent anticoagulant properties are the consequence of this process, which forms a protective shield of annexin-V over the phospholipid surface, blocking it from availability for coagulation reactions.

There are significant data to support a thrombomodulatory function for annexin-V *in vivo*. Annexin-V is highly expressed by placental trophoblasts, in an apparently constitutive manner (Krikun *et al.*, 1994). The protein is abundant on the apical surfaces of microvilli of syncytiotrophoblasts (Krikun *et al.*, 1994). There is strong evidence that the apical membranes of syncytialized trophoblasts expose phosphatidyl-serine, as detected by monoclonal antiphosphatidyl-serine antibodies (Lyden et al., 1992) and by the localization of annexin-V (Krikun et al., 1994; Vogt et al., 1997). Removal of annexin-V from the cell surface by treatment with EGTA exposes the apical membrane to circulating blood and accelerates the coagulation of plasma exposed to the cells (Rand et al., 1997). In a mouse model, annexin-V has been shown to be necessary for maintenance of placental integrity; infusion with anti-annexin-V antibodies resulted in placental infarction and pregnancy wastage (Wang et al., 1999). It was recently reported that annexin-V expression is decreased on trophoblasts of preeclamptic placentas and that the degree of the decrease correlates with elevation of markers for activation of blood coagulation (Wang et al., 1999). Taken together, the available data support the hypothesis that annexin-V has a thrombomodulatory function on the surfaces which line the intervillous space through which the maternal blood circulates. In addition, the expression of annexin-V by endothelial cells indicates that annexin-V may play a similar role at the vascular-blood interface of the systemic circulation.

Since both aPL antibodies and annexin-V have affinity for anionic phospholipids, it has been hypothesized that the aPL antibodies might interfere with the formation of the antithrombotic annexin-V shield over phospholipids on apical cytoplasmic membranes. It has been shown that aPL antibodies reduce the quantity of annexin-V on cultured placental trophoblasts and endothelial cells.

According to this hypothesis, Rand et al. (1997, 1994) have proposed that autoantibodies may inhibit the physiological anticoagulant activity of annexin-V, based on the observation that decreased amounts of annexin-V are present on placental membranes from women with APS. These investigators proposed that annexin-V on placental membranes acts as a natural anticoagulant by blocking the binding of coagulation factors to these membranes. In APS patients, antibodies and/or antibody-antigen complexes competitively inhibit the binding of annexin-V to cell membranes. One problem with this hypothesis is, however, that if antibodies or antibody-antigen complexes bind to membranes with high enough affinity to displace annexin-V, then such antibody complexes would also effectively block the binding of coagulation factor.

On the other hand, in the presence of annexin-V, an aPL-mediated increase of prothrombin binding to trophoblasts as well as an acceleration of the prothrombinase reaction were reported. This finding seems to confirm the above quoted interference of aPL bound to phospholipid or to protein-phospholipid complexes (containing β2GPI, prothrombin or other proteins) with the membrane-bound annexin-V, resulting in an increased availability of phospholipids for coagulation reactions, apparently not impaired by the high-affinity binding of the antibody complexes.

References

Alagille, D., Crosnier, J. & Soulier, J.P. (1956): Anticoagulant circulant à activité antithromboplastique. *Rev. Franç. et Clin. Biol.* **1**, 335–345.

Alarçon-Segovia, D. & Osmundson, P.J. (1965): Peripheral vascular syndromes associated with systemic lupus erythematosus. *Ann. Intern. Med.* **62**, 416–430.

Alarçon-Segovia, D. & Sanchez-Guerrero, J. (1989): Primary antiphospholipid syndrome. *J. Rheumatol.* **16**, 482–484.

Andree, H.A.M. et al. (1992): Displacement of factor Va by Annexin-V. In: *Phospholipid binding and anticoagulant action of Annexin-V*, pp. 73–85. The Netherlands: Universitaire Pers Maastricht.

Arnout, J. et al. (1998): Beta 2-glycoprotein I-dependent lupus anticoagulants form stable bivalent antibody beta 2-glycoprotein I complexes on phospholipid surfaces. *Thromb. Haemost.* **79**, 79–86.

Aron, A.L., Cuellar, R.L., Brey, R.L., Meceown, S., Espinoza, L.R. & Shoenfeld, Y. (1995): Early onset of autoimmunity in MRL/++ mice following immunization with beta 2-glycoprotein I. *Clin. Exp. Immunol.* **101**, 68.

Asherson, R.A., Khamashta, M.A. & Ordi-Ros, J. (1989): The 'primary' antiphospholipid syndrome: major clinical and serological features. *Medicine* **68**, 366–374.

Bachman, R.L. & Silverstein, R.L. (1993): Hypercoagulable states. *Ann. Intern. Med.* **119**, 819–827.

Bakimer, R., Fishman, P., Blank, M., Sredni, B., Djaldetti, M. & Shoenfeld, Y. (1992): Induction of primary antiphospholipid syndrome in mice by immunization with human monoclonal anticardiolipin antibodies (H3). *J. Clin. Invest.* **89**, 1558–1563.

Blank, M., Cohen, J., Toder, V. & Shoenfeld, Y. (1991): Induction of antiphospholipid syndrome in naive mice with mouse lupus monoclonal and human polyclonal anti-cardiolipin antibodies. *Proc. Natl. Acad. Sci. USA* **88**, 3069–3073.

Blank, M., Krause, L., Ben-Bassat, M. & Shoenfeld, Y. (1992): Induction of experimental antiphospholipid syndrome associated with SLE following immunization with human monoclonal pathogenic anti-DNA idiotype. *J. Autoimmun.* **5**, 495–509.

Blank, M., Tincani, A. & Shoenfeld, Y. (1994a): Induction of experimental antiphospholipid syndrome in naive mice with purified IgG antiphosphatidylserine antibodies. *J. Rheumatol.* **21**, 100–104.

Blank, M., Faden, D., Tincani, A., Kopolovic, J., Goldberg, I., Gilburd, B., Allegri, F., Balestrieri, G., Valesini, G. & Shoenfeld, Y. (1994b): Immunization with anticardiolipin cofactor (beta 2-glycoprotein I) induces experimental antiphospholipid syndrome in naive mice. *J. Autoimmun.* **7**, 441–455.

Bowie, E.J., Thompson, J.H. Jr. & Pascuzzi, C.A. Jr. (1963): Thrombosis in systemic lupus erythematosus despite circulating anticoagulants. *J. Lab. Clin. Med.* **62**, 416–430.

Branch, D.W., Dudley, D.J., Mitchell, M.D., Creighton, K.A., Abbot, T.M., Hammond, E.H. & Daynes, R.A. (1990): Immunoglobulin G fraction from patients with antiphospholipid antibodies cause fetal death in BALB/c mice: a model for autoimmune fetal loss. *Am. J. Obstet. Gynecol.* **163**, 210–216.

Brey, R.L. & Teale, J.M. (1992): Nervous system pathology in MRL/lpr and MRL/++ mice. *Clin. Exp. Rheumatol.* **10**, 641.

Cabiedes, J., Cabral, A.R., Alarçon-Riquelme, M. & Alarçon-Segovia, D. (1994): Overt and hidden aCL and antiphosphatidylcholine antibodies in BALB/c and NZB mice. *Lupus* **3** (Suppl. 4), 340.

Cabral, A.R., Cabiedes, J. & Alarçon-Segovia, D. (1990): Haemolytic anemia related to an IgM autoantibody to phosphatidylcholine that binds *in vitro* to stored and bromeline-treated erythrocyte. *J. Autoimmunity* **3**, 773–787.

Cervera, A., Khamashta, M.A., Font, J. *et al.* (1991): Anti-endothelial cell antibodies in patients with the antiphospholipid syndrome. *Autoimmunity* **11**, 1–6.

Cohen, J., Bakimer, R., Blank, M., Valesini, G. & Shoenfeld, Y. (1994): Pathogenic natural anti-cardiolipin antibodies: the experience from monoclonal gammopathy. *Clin. Exp. Immunol.* **97**, 181–186.

Comp, P.C., DeBault, L.E. *et al.* (1983): Human thrombomodulin is inhibited by IgG from two patients with non-specific anticoagulants. *Blood* **62** (Suppl. 1), 299a (Abstract).

Creutz, C.E. (1992): The annexins and exocytosis. *Science* **258**, 924–931.

Crumpton, M.J. *et al.* (1990): Protein terminology tangle. *Nature* **345**, 212.

Del Papa, N. *et al.* (1995): Relationship between antiphospholipid and anti-EC antibodies: β2-glycoprotein I mediates the antibody binding to endothelial membranes and induces the expression of adhesion molecules. *Clin. Exp. Rheumatol.* **13**, 179–185.

Del Papa, N. *et al.* (1997): Endothelial cells as target for antiphospholipid antibodies. Human polyclonal and monoclonal anti-β2 glycoprotein I antibodies react *in vitro* with endothelial cells through adherent β2-glycoprotein I and induce endothelial activation. *Arthritis Rheum.* **40**, 551–561.

Galli, M., Confurius, P., Maassen, C. *et al.* (1990): Anticardiolipin antibodies directed not to cardiolipin but to a plasma protein cofactor. *Lancet* **335**, 1544–1547.

Garcia, C.O., Kanbourshakir, A., Tang, A., Espinoza, L.R. & Gharavi, A.E. (1997): Induction of experimental antiphospholipid syndrome in PL/J mice following immunization with beta 2-glycoprotein I. *Am. J. Reprod. Immunol.* **37**, 118–124.

George, J., Blank, M., Levy, Y., Meroni, P.L., Damianovich, M., Tincani, A. & Shoenfeld, Y. (1998a): Differential effect of anti-ß2-glyocoprotein I antibodies on endothelial cells and on the manifestations of experimental antiphospholipid syndrome. *Circulation* **97**, 900–906.

George, J., Afek, A., Gilburd, B., Blank, M., Aron-Maor, A., Levy, Y., Levkoviz, H., Shaish, A., Goldberg, I., Kopolovic, J., Harats, D. & Shoenfeld, Y. (1998b): Induction of early atherosclerosis in LDL-receptor deficient mice immunized with beta 2-glycoprotein I. *Circulation* **98** 5(11), 1108–1115.

George, J. *et al.* (1998c): Differential effects of anti-β2-glycoprotein I antibodies on endothelial cells and on the manifestations of experimental antiphospholipid syndrome. *Circulation* **97**, 900–906.

Gharavi, A.E., Mellors, R.C. & Elkon, K.B. (1989): IgG anticardiolipin antibodies in murine lupus. *Clin. Exp. Immunol.* **78**, 233–238.

Gharavi, A.E., Sammaritano, L., Wen, J. & Elkon, K.B. (1992): Induction of antiphospholipid autoantibodies by immunization with beta 2-glycoprotein I (apolipoprotein H). *J. Clin. Invest.* **90**, 1105–1109.

Halbmayer, W.-M., Haushofer, A. *et al.* (1994): Influence of lupus anticoagulant on a commercially available kit for APC-resistance. *Thromb. Haemost.* **72**, 645–646.

Harris, E.N., Gharavi, A.E., Boey, M.L. *et al.* (1983): Anticardiolipin antibodies: detection by radioimmunoassay and association with thrombosis in systemic lupus erythematosus. *Lancet* **2**, 1211–1214.

Harris, E.N., Gharavi, A.E., Loizou, S. *et al.* (1985): Cross-reactivity of antiphospholipid antibodies. *J. Clin. Lab. Immunol.* **16**, 1–6.

Harris, E.N., Gharavi, A.E., Wasley, G.D. & Hughes, G.R.V. (1988): Use of enzyme-linked immunosorbent assay and of inhibition studies to distinguish between anticardiolipin antibodies from patients with syphilis or autoimmune disorders. *J. Infect. Dis.* **157**, 23–31.

Hashimoto, Y., Kawamura, M., Ichicawa, K.K., Suzuki, T., Sumida, T., Yoshida, S., Matsuura, E., Ikehara, S. & Koike, T. (1992): Anticardiolipin antibodies in NZW x BXSB F1 mice. *J. Immunol.* **149**, 1063–1068.

Hess, D.C., Taormina, M. & Thompson, J. (1993): Cognitive and neurologic deficit in MRL/lpr mouse: a clinicopathologic study. *J. Rheumatol.* **20**, 610–617.

Hughes, G.R.V. (1983): Thrombosis, abortion, cerebral disease and lupus anticoagulant. *Br. Med. J.* **287**, 1088–1089.

Hughes, G.R.V. (1985): The anticardiolipin syndrome. *Clin. Exp. Rheumatol.* **3**, 285–286.

Ikematsu, W., Luan, F.L., La Rosa, L., Beltrami, B., Nicoletti, F., Buyon, J., Meroni, P.L., Balestrieri, G. & Casali, P. (1998): Human anticardiolipin monoclonal autoantibodies cause placental necrosis and fetal loss in BALB/c mice. *Arthritis Rheum.* **41**, 1026–1039.

Johansson, E.A. & Lassus, A. (1974): The occurence of circulating anticoagulants in patients with syphilitic and biologically false positive antilipoidal antibodies. *Ann. Clin. Res.* **6**, 105–108.

Kaplanski, G. *et al.* (2000): Increased soluble vascular cell adhesion molecule 2 concentrations in patients with primary or systemic lupus erythematosus-related antiphospholipid syndrome: correlation with the severity of thrombosis. *Arthritis Rheum.* **43**, 55–60.

Keeling, D.M. *et al.* (1991): β2-glycoprotein I inhibits the thrombin/thrombomodulin-dependent activation of protein C. *Blood* **78**, 184a (Abstract).

Krikun, J. *et al.* (1994): The expression of the placental anticoagulant protein, annexin-V, by villous trophoblasts: immunolocalization and *in vitro* regulation. *Placenta* **15**, 601–612.

Laurell, A.B. & Nilsson, I.M. (1957): Hypergamma-globulinemia, circulating anticoagulant and biologic false positive Wassermann reaction: a study of 2 cases. *J. Lab. Clin. Med.* **49**, 694–707.

Lee, S.L. & Sanders, M. (1955): A disorder of blood coagulation in systemic lupus erythematosus. *J. Clin. Invest.* **34**, 1814–1822.

Loizou, S., McCrea, J.D., Rudge, A.C., Reynolds, R., Boyle, C.C. & Harris, E.N. (1985): Measurement of anticardiolipin antibodies by an enzyme-linked immunosorbent assay (ELISA): standardization and quantitation of result. *Clin. Exp. Immunol.* **62**, 738–745.

Lyden, T.W. et al. (1992): Monoclonal antiphospholipid antibody reactivity against human placental trophoblast. *J. Reprod. Immunol.* **22**, 1–14.

Malia, R.G. et al. (1990): Inhibition of activated protein C and its cofactor protein S by antiphospholipid antibodies. *Br. J. Haematol.* **79**, 101–107.

Marciniak, E. & Romond, E.H. (1989): Impaired catalytic function of activated protein C: a new *in vitro* manifestation of lupus anticoagulant. *Blood* **74**, 2426–2432.

Matsuda, J. et al. (1995): Inhibitory activity of anti-β2-glycoprotein I antibody on factor Va degradation by activated protein C and its cofactor protein S. *Am. J. Hematol.* **49**, 89–91.

Matsuura, E., Igarashi, Y., Fujimoto, M., Ichikawa, K. & Koike, T. (1990): Anticardiolipin cofactor(s) and differential diagnosis of autoimmune disease. *Lancet* **336**, 177–178.

McNeil, H.P., Simpson, R.J., Chesterman, C.N. & Krilis, S.A. (1990): Antiphospholipid antibodies are directed against a complex antigen that includes a lipid-binding inhibitor of coagulation: β2-glycoprotein I (apolipoprotein H). *Proc. Natl. Acad. Sci. USA* **87**, 4120–4124.

McNeil, H.P., Chesterman, C.N. & Krilis, S.A. (1991): Immunology and clinical importance of antiphospholipid antibodies. *Adv. Immunol.* **49**, 193–280.

Mendlovic, S., Brocke, S., Shoenfeld, Y., Ben-Bassat, M., Meshorer, A., Bakimer, R. & Mozes, E. (1988): Induction of systemic lupus erithematosus-like disease in mice by a common human anti-DNA idiotype. *Proc. Natl. Acad. Sci. USA* **85**, 2260–2264.

Moore, J.E. & Lutz, W.B. (1955): The natural history of systemic lupus erythematosus: an approach to its study through chronic biologic false positive reaction. *J. Chronic. Dis.* **48**, 798.

Morgan, R.O. et al. (1997): Distinct annexin subfamilies in plants and protists diverged prior to animal annexins and from a common ancestor. *J. Mol. Evol.* **44**, 178–188.

Mosser, J. et al. (1991): Sub-domain structure of lipid-bound annexin-V resolved by electron image analysis. *J. Mol. Biol.* **217**, 241–245.

Nakamura, A., Yokoyama, T., Kodera, S., Zhang, D. & Hirose, S. (1998): Ocular fundus lesions in systemic lupus erythematosus model mice. *Nippon Ganka Gakkai Zasshi* **102**, 8–14.

Nilsson, I.M., Astedt, B. & Hedner, U. (1975): Intrauterine death and circulating anticoagulant 'antithromboplastin'. *Acta Med. Scand.* **197**, 153–159.

Nimpf, J., Bevers, E.M., Bomans, P.H.H. et al. (1986): Prothrombinase activity of human platelets is inhibited by β2-glycoprotein I. *Biochim. Biophys. Acta* **884**, 142–149.

Nimpf, J., Wurm, H. & Kostner, G.M. (1987): β2-glycoprotein I (apoH) inhibits the release reaction of human platelets during ADP-induced aggregation. *Atherosclerosis* **63**, 109–114.

Olee, T., Pierangeli, S.S., Hadley, H.H., Le, D.T., Wei, X., Lai, C.J., En, J., Novotny, W., Harris, E.N., Woods, V.L. & Chen, P.P. (1996): A monoclonal IgG anticardiolipin antibody from a patient with the antiphospholipid syndrome is thrombogenic in mice. *Proc. Natl. Acad. Sci. USA* **93**, 8606–8611.

Oosting, J.D. et al. (1991): *In vitro* studies of antiphospholipid antibodies and its cofactor, beta 2 glycoprotein I, show negligible effects on endothelial cell mediated protein C activation. *Thromb. Haemost.* **66**, 666–671.

Oosting, J.D. et al. (1993): Antiphospholipid antibodies directed against a combination of phospholipid with prothrombin, protein C or protein S: an explanation for their pathogenic mechanism? *Blood* **81**, 2618–2625.

Pangborn, M.C. (1942): Isolation and purification of a serologically active phospholipid from beef heart. *J. Biol. Chem.* **143**, 247–256.

Pierangeli, S.S. & Harris, E.N. (1993): Induction of phospholipid-binding antibodies in mice and rabbits by immunization with human β2-glycoprotein I or anticardiolipin antibodies alone. *Clin. Exp. Immunol.* **93**, 269–272.

Pierangeli, S.S. & Harris, E.N. (1994): Antiphospholipid antibodies in an *in vivo* thrombosis model mice. *Lupus* **3**, 247–251.

Pierangeli, S.S., Liu, X.W., Barker, J.H., Anderson, G. & Harris, E.N. (1995): Induction of thrombosis in a mouse model by IgG, IgM and IgA immunoglobulins from patients with the antiphospholipid syndrome. *Thromb. Haemost.* **74**, 1361–1367.

Pierangeli, A.A. *et al.* (1999): Antiphospholipid antibodies from antiphospholipid syndrome patients activate ECs *in vitro* and *in vivo*. *Circulation* **99**, 1997–2000.

Piona, A., La Rosa, L., Tincani, A., Magno, G., Graso, S., Nicoletti, F., Balestrieri, G. & Meroni, P.L. (1995): Effect of passive transfer of anticardiolipin antibodies on pregnancy outcome in BALB/c mice. *Scand. J. Immunol.* **42**, 27–32.

Radic, M.Z., Ibrahim, S.M., Rauch, J., Camper, S.A. & Weigert, M. (1995): Constitutive secretion of transgene-encoded IgG2b autoantibodies leads to symptoms of autoimmune disease. *J. Immunol.* **155**, 3213–3222.

Rand J.H. (1999): 'Annexinopathies' – A new class of diseases. *N. Engl. J. Med.* **340**, 1035–1036.

Rand, J.H. *et al.* (1994): Reduction of annexin-V (placental anticoagulant protein-I) on placental villi of women with antiphospholipid antibodies and recurrent spontaneous abortion. *Am. J. Obstet. Gynecol.* **171**, 1566–1572.

Rand, J.H. *et al.* (1997): Pregnancy loss in the antiphospholipid-antibody syndrome – A possible thrombogenic mechanism. *N. Engl. J. Med.* **337**, 154–160.

Reutelingsperger, C.P. *et al.* (1988): Purification and characterization of a novel protein from bovine aorta that inhibits coagulation. *Eur. J. Biochem.* **173**, 171–178.

Reverter, J.C., Tassies, D., Font, J. *et al.* (1996): Hypercoagulable state in patients with antiphospholipid syndrome is related to high induced tissue factor expression on monocytes and to low free protein S. *Arterioscler. Thromb. Vasc. Biol.* **16**, 1319–1326.

Roubey, R.A.S. (1997): Antiphospholipid antibody syndrome. In: *Arthritis and allied conditions: a textbook of rheumatology* (13th edn.), W.J. Koopman (ed.), pp. 1393–1406. Philadelphia: Lippincott, Williams & Wilkins.

Roubey, R.A.S., Pratt, C.W., Buyon, J.P. *et al.* (1992): Lupus anticoagulant activity of autoimmune antiphospholipid antibodies is dependent upon β2-glycoprotein I. *J. Clin. Invest.* **90**, 1100–1104.

Shi, W. *et al.* (1993): Anticardiolipin antibodies block the inhibition of β2-glycoprotein I of the factor Xa generating activity of platelets. *Thromb. Haemost.* **70**, 342–345.

Shibata, S. *et al.* (1994): Autoantibodies to heparin from patients with antiphospholipid antibodies syndrome inhibit formation of antithrombin III-thrombin complexes. *Blood* **83**, 2532–2540.

Schorer, A.E. (1997): Discordant effects on eicosanoids and fibrin degradation products in two murine models of antiphospholipid antibody. *Thromb. Res.* **85** (4), 295–304.

Schousboe, I. (1985): β2-glycoprotein I: a plasma inhibitor of the contact activation of the intrinsic blood coagulation pathway. *Blood* **66**, 1086–1091.

Schultze, H.E., Heide, H. & Haupt, H. (1961): Über ein bisher unbekanntes neidemoleculares β2 Globulin des Humanserum. *Naturwissenschaften* **48**, 719–724.

Shu, F. *et al.* (2000): Immunohistochemical study of annexin-V expression in placentae of preeclampsia. *Gynecol. Obstet. Invest.* **49**, 17–23.

Simantov, E. *et al.* (1995): Activation of cultured vascular endothelial cells by antiphospholipid antibodies. *J. Clin. Invest.* **96**, 2211–2219.

Soulier, J.P. & Boffa, M.C. (1980): Avortements à repetition, thromboses et anticoagulant circulant antithromboplastine. *Nouv. Presse Med.* **9**, 859–864.

Tait, J.F. *et al.* (1988): Placental anticoagulant proteins: isolation and comparative characterization of four members of the lipocortin family. *Biochemistry* **27**, 6268–6276.

Thiagarjan, P., Shapiro, S.S. & De Marco, L. (1980): Monoclonal immunoglobulin M lambda coagulation inhibitor with phospholipid specificity. Mechanism of lupus anticoagulant. *J. Clin. Invest.* **66**, 397–405.

Tincani, A., Spatola, L., Prati, E., Allegri, F., Ferremi, P., Cattaneo, R., Meroni, P.L. & Balestrieri, G. (1996): The anti-beta 2-glycoprotein I activity in human antiphospholipid syndrome sera is due to monoreactive low affinity autoantibodies directed to epitopes located on native beta 2-glycoprotein I and preserved during species' evolution. *J. Immunol.* **157,** 5732–5738.

Tincani, A., Balestrieri, G., Spatola, L., Cinquini, M., Meroni, P.L. & Roubey, R.A.S. (1998a): Anticardiolipin and anti-β2 glycoprotein I immunoassay in the diagnosis of antiphospholipid syndrome. *Clin. Exp. Rheumatol.* **16,** 396–402.

Tincani, A., Beltrami, B., Meroni, P.L., Allegri, F., Spatola, L., Cinquini, M., Shoenfeld, Y. & Balestrieri, G. (1998b): Immunization of naive BALB/c mice with human beta 2-glycoprotein I breaks tolerance against the murine molecule. Abstract 8th International Symposium on Antiphospholipid Antibodies, Sapporo, Japan, 1998.

Voges, D. *et al.* (1994): Three-dimensional structure of membrane-bound annexin-V. *J. Mol. Biol.* **238,** 199–213.

Vogt, E., Ah-Kau, N.G. & Rote, N.S. (1996): A model for the antiphospholipid antibody syndrome: monoclonal antiphosphatidylserine antibody induces intrauterine growth restriction in mice. *Am. J. Obstet. Gynecol.* **174,** 700–707.

Vogt, E. *et al.* (1997): Antiphosphatidylserine antibody removes annexin-V and facilitates the binding of prothrombin at the surface of a choriocarcinoma model of trophoblast differentiation. *Am. J. Obstet. Gynecol.* **177,** 964–972.

Wang, X. *et al.* (1999): Annexin-V is critical in the maintenance of murine placental integrity. *Am. J. Obstet. Gynecol.* **180,** 1008–1016.

Willems, G.M. *et al.* (1996): Role of divalency in the high affinity binding of anticardiolipin antibody-β2-glycoprotein-I complexes to lipid membranes. *Biochemistry* **35,** 13833–13842.

Wurm, H. (1984): β-glycoprotein I (apolipoprotein H) interaction with phospholipid vesicles. *Int. J. Biochem.* **16,** 511–515.

Ziporen, L., Shoenfeld, Y., Levy, Y. & Korczyn, A.D. (1997): Neurological dysfunction and hyperactive behavior associated with antiphospholipid antibodies: a mouse model. *J. Clin. Invest.* **100,** 613–619.

Chapter 14

The antiphospholipid syndrome in paediatrics: clinical aspects

Angelo Ravelli

University Department of Paediatric Sciences, IRCCS San Matteo, Piazzale Golgi 2, 27100 Pavia, Italy

Summary

The antiphospholipid syndrome (APS) is characterized by the association between recurrent arterial or venous thrombosis and the presence of circulating antiphospholipid antibodies (aPL). This clinical syndrome is mainly observed in patients with systemic lupus erythematosus, but may occur in other autoimmune or non-autoimmune disorders or even in subjects who do not present any evidence of well-defined systemic disease (so-called 'primary' APS). In recent years, the clinical manifestations of the APS have been increasingly recognized in the paediatric age. In the venous circulation, thrombosis of the deep veins of the lower limbs has been reported more frequently, whereas cerebral arteries are the most common site of arterial occlusion. Since other risk factors pertaining to thrombosis commonly found in adults are not applicable in the paediatric age, the risk of thrombosis and of its recurrences as well as the optimal intensity of oral anticoagulation may be different from those in adults. Because childhood thrombosis is rare, the need for multicentre, controlled, prospective studies is stated to establish the natural history as well as the optimal management of aPL-related thrombosis in paediatric patients.

Introduction

The antiphospholipid syndrome (APS) is defined as the association between recurrent arterial or venous thrombosis and/or recurrent pregnancy loss and circulating antiphospholipid antibodies (aPL), detected as anticardiolipin antibodies (aCL) and/or lupus anticoagulant (LA). This clinical syndrome is mainly observed in patients with systemic lupus erythematosus (SLE), but may occur in a variety of autoimmune or non-autoimmune disorders or even in subjects who do not have any features of a well-defined systemic disease (so-called 'primary' APS). The earliest descriptions of the association between a circulating anticoagulant and vascular thrombosis in the paediatric age were those of Olive *et al.* (1979) and St Clair *et al.* (1981). In the last decade, the features of the APS have been increasingly recognized in children and a growing number of studies have provided information on the clinical significance of aPL in childhood disorders (Ravelli *et al.*, 1994b).

Clinical manifestations of the APS in childhood

Most of the instances of APS in the paediatric age have been described as isolated case reports or small patient series. We have recently identified a total of 50 patients aged less than 16 years in whom detailed clinical and laboratory information was available (Table 1) (Ravelli & Martini, 1997). Of note, arterial thrombosis was more frequent in children aged less than 10 years than in the older age group (62 per cent vs. 28 per cent). The vessels involved and the main clinical manifestations observed in these patients are summarized in Table 2.

Table 1. Clinical characteristics of 50 children with APS reported in the literature (Ravelli & Martini, 1997)

Males/females		31/19
Age at first APS symptom		8 months–16 years (mean: 10.2 years)
Thrombosis		
	Venous	35 patients
	Arterial	22 patients
	Venous + arterial	7 patients
Family history of APS		3 patients

Table 2. Sites of thrombosis and clinical manifestations in 50 children with APS

Vessel involved		Clinical manifestations
VEINS		
Limbs		Deep or superficial vein thrombosis
Large veins		Superior or inferior vena cava thrombosis
Lungs		Pulmonary thromboembolism Pulmonary hypertension
Skin		Livedo reticularis
Brain		Cerebral sinus thrombosis
Adrenal glands		Addison's disease
Liver		
	Large vessels	Budd-Chiari syndrome
	Small vessels	Hepatomegaly, enzyme elevation
Eyes		Retinal vein thrombosis
ARTERIES		
Brain		Stroke, transient ischaemic attacks
Kidney		
	Large vessels	Renal artery thrombosis
	Small vessels	Renal thrombotic microangiopathy
Limbs		Ischaemia, gangrene
Heart		Myocardial infarction
Liver		Hepatic infarction
Gut		Mesenteric artery thrombosis
Spinal cord		Transverse myelopathy

Adapted from Ravelli & Martini, 1997.

Venous thrombosis

As in adults, the deep veins of the lower limbs are the most common site of venous thrombosis at paediatric age. Pulmonary embolism appears to occur less frequently in children than in adults with APS, where it is encountered in approximately one-third of patients with deep vein thrombosis (Cervera et al., 1995). In aPL-positive children with SLE who present with cough, dyspnea, and pleuritic pain, the differential diagnosis with pleurisy is necessary. Thromboembolic pulmonary hypertension is another complication associated with aPL (Asherson & Cervera, 1995). Like pulmonary embolism, thromboembolic pulmonary hypertension seems to be less common in children than in adults, possibly due to a lower tendency toward recurrent thrombosis in the paediatric age. APS is recognized to be a common cause of Budd-Chiari syndrome, with nine of the 11 patients recently reviewed being examples of primary APS (Asherson et al., 1991). Another aPL-associated hepatic manifestation is the so-called 'hepatic veno-occlusive disease', which is clinically similar to the Budd-Chiari syndrome but is caused by occlusion of the central or sublobular veins (Asherson et al., 1991). Hypoadrenalism or Addison's disease have both been linked to aPL (Asherson & Hughes, 1991). Adrenal infarction and haemorrhage are both possible pathogenetic mechanisms. The occurrence of abdominal pain in association with clinical and laboratory signs, suggesting adrenal insufficiency in patients with circulating aPL or APS, should alert the physician to the occurrence of adrenal haemorrhage/infarction. Thrombosis of the cerebral sinuses is another possible complication (Falcini et al., 1991; Uziel et al., 1995). Since early diagnosis is difficult, it has been indicated that severe, unremitting headache, unresponsive to analgesic drugs, in patients with SLE should be considered as a sign of possible intracranial sinus thrombosis and lead to perform appropriate investigations. Livedo reticularis is characterized by a violaceous coloration of the skin in a reticular pattern that is caused by stagnation of blood in dilated superficial capillaries and venules and mainly affects the skin of the thighs, shins and forearms. Areas of normal skin are clearly demarcated from affected areas. It is a common finding in connective tissue diseases, particularly in SLE. The clinical triad of livedo reticularis, cerebrovascular disease and hypertension, known as 'Sneddon's syndrome', was first described in 1965 but linked to APS only in the 1980s (Cervera et al., 1995). This syndrome has rarely been reported in children (Baxter et al., 1993; Tucker, 1994).

Arterial thrombosis

Cerebral ischaemia is the most common neurological manifestation associated with aPL (Brey et al., 1993). In children with arterial thrombosis, cerebral arteries are more commonly affected, with the majority of them presenting with stroke or transient ischaemic attacks. Similarly to what has been observed in adults (Cervera et al., 1995), strokes occur more often in the territory supplied by the middle cerebral artery. We found a high prevalence (76 per cent) of aPL, detected as LA and/or aCL, in 13 unselected children with idiopathic cerebral ischaemia (Angelini et al., 1994). To be defined as aPL-positive, patients had to have circulating LA and/or moderate/high level of aCL on two separate occasions more than two weeks apart; five of the 10 (50 per cent) aPL-positive children had a history of multiple ischaemic events. A high prevalence of aPL, ranging from 57 to 70 per cent, in children with idiopathic cerebral ischaemia has been confirmed by several other groups (Baca et al., 1996; Schoning et al., 1994; Takanashi et al., 1995). These data suggest that aPL must be determined in all children with unexplained cerebral ischaemia. Myocardial infarction due to aPL-related thrombosis represents therefore an additional mechanism, beside vasculitis, for coronary artery disease in children

(Falcini et al., 1991; Miller et al., 1995). Renal complications caused by occlusive arterial disease associated with the presence of aPL include renal artery thrombosis, renal infarction and renal thrombotic microangiopathy (Asherson & Kant, 1993). Jouquan et al. (1986) reported a LA-positive 14-year-old girl with SLE who was admitted with hypertensive encephalopathy. Renal biopsy showed no histological features of proliferative glomerulopathy, but ischaemic changes with shrinkage in almost all glomerular tufts. The authors referred to these changes as 'nephroangiosclerosis' and speculated whether intravascular microthrombosis could have been responsible for this disorder.

'Catastrophic' APS

aPL-positive patients rarely may develop acute medical collapse with severe thrombocytopenia, adult respiratory distress syndrome, and multiorgan failure, often associated with hypertension and/or histopathological evidence of multiple (large/small) vessel occlusion. This frequently fatal condition, which has been linked to widespread and rapid thrombotic events occurring over days to weeks, has been termed 'catastrophic' APS (Asherson, 1998). The differential diagnosis in these patients is often difficult and includes severe lupus vasculitis, thrombotic thrombo-cytopenic purpura and disseminated intravascular coagulation. Two paediatric patients with this syndrome were included in a recent review of 10 patients (Asherson, 1998). The 13-year-old girl described by Ostuni et al. (1990) developed bilateral renal artery thrombosis leading to malignant hypertension and oliguria, probable stenosis of the superior mesenteric artery and a cerebrovascular accident. Inam et al. (1991) reported a 10-year-old boy who developed severe hypertension, hepatomegaly, haematuria and adrenal insufficiency. A liver biopsy showed zonal necrosis and haemorrhage with fibrin thrombi in sinusoid and portal vessels. Renal biopsy revealed a segmental mesangioproliferative glomerulonephritis associated with fibrin thrombi in glomerular capillaries. Three years later, he again had severe hypertension (170/150 mm Hg) with cardiomegaly. Magnetic resonance imaging showed complete adrenal atrophy and repeated renal biopsy revealed glomerulosclerosis. Echocardiogram disclosed mitral regurgitation. These reports show that children with APS can have a clinical course as severe as adults with this syndrome. Prompt recognition of these conditions is important because treatment must be aggressive.

Other aPL-associated clinical manifestations

Autoimmune thrombocytopenia occurs frequently in children with APS and is usually mild (platelet count between 50–150 x 10^9 L). However, platelet-specific antibodies, instead of aPL, appear to be responsible for the pathogenesis of thrombocytopenia in the APS (Galli et al., 1996). Chorea has been observed in adults and children with aPL, either with or without SLE (Asherson et al., 1987). Thrombosis of the small vessels supplying the basal ganglia or binding of aPL to phospholipid in basal ganglia are among the possible pathogenetic mechanisms. The awareness of a possible association of chorea with aPL may help in the differential diagnosis of other, clinically similar, types of chorea, such as Sydenham's chorea. Recently, aPL were detected in a significant proportion of children with migraine, benign intracranial hypertension or unilateral movement disorders (Angelini et al., 1996). Aortic or mitral valve insufficiency attributable to exuberant Libman-Sacks-type vegetations (Asherson & Lubbe, 1988) have been observed in patients with both secondary and primary APS. Additional clinical conditions related to the aPL in the paediatric age include avascular necrosis of the femoral epiphysis (Perthes' disease) (Ura et al., 1992), serous retinal detachment (Ravelli et al., 1993), and Tourette syndrome (Toren et al., 1993).

Antiphospholipid antibodies and juvenile SLE

A large number of the reported children with APS do not fulfil the American College of Rheumatology (ACR) revised 1982 criteria for the classification of SLE (Tan et al., 1982). These patients were generally classified as primary APS. However, many of them had one or more features of SLE, generally low-titre antinuclear antibodies, but also arthritis, alopecia, rheumatoid factor, hypocomplementaemia, proteinuria and even low-titre anti-DNA antibodies. Anti-histone antibodies were detected in four children with primary APS (Massa et al., 1993).

Only few data are available on the frequency and clinical significance of aPL in juvenile SLE (Ravelli & Martini, 1997). The prevalence of aCL and LA ranges from 30 to 87 per cent and from 10 to 42 per cent, respectively. A similar discrepancy in the frequency of aPL has been reported also in adult SLE, with aCL ranging from 17 to 61 per cent and LA from 6 to 65 per cent (Petri, 1994). These disparity may reflect either a different sensitivity and specificity of the assays employed for the detection of aPL or a diversity in the clinical features of the patient populations. The wide variation in the prevalence of aPL noted in the paediatric cohorts may depend at least in part on differences in the disease activity, because some investigators have observed a relationship between the presence and titre of these antibodies and clinical indicators of lupus activity (Ravelli et al., 1994a; Shergy et al., 1988), whereas the lowest prevalence was observed in samples obtained during periods of clinical remission (Molta et al., 1993). Some investigators have found that high levels of aCL are often associated with neurological involvement (Ravelli et al., 1994a; Shergy et al., 1988), whereas others did not observe any association with neuropsychiatric manifestations (Seaman et al., 1995). The frequency of vascular thrombosis ranges from 0 to 24 per cent.

Antiphospholipid antibodies and other systemic disorders

The presence of aPL has been investigated in other chronic rheumatic diseases of children. A prevalence of aCL ranging from 7.9 per cent to 53 per cent has been reported in juvenile idiopathic arthritis (JIA) (Ravelli & Martini, 1997). Leak (1987) found aCL in 10 (29 per cent) of 34 children with ANA-positive JIA and in five (13 per cent) of the 37 patients in the 'other JIA' group (systemic, seropositive and seronegative polyarticular). In the cohort with positive ANA, the presence of aCL was associated with more severe arthritis, younger onset age, and greater number of active joints. No patient had experienced features of the APS. In a similar study of 70 children with JIA, the presence and titre of aCL was not found to be associated with clinical and laboratory variables; no patient had had acute thrombotic events or cytopenia despite a prevalence of aCL of 53 per cent (Caporali et al., 1991). There is one report of aPL-associated thrombosis in a patient with systemic JIA who was exposed to another thrombophilic factor, that was represented by a prolonged plaster immobilization for a healing fracture (Caporali et al., 1992). However, thrombotic complications are rare in JIA despite a high prevalence of aCL. This suggests that aPL may have different pathogenetic potential and, possibly, antigen specificity in different autoimmune disorders. We found a positive aCL test in three out of 14 (21 per cent) children with juvenile dermatomyositis (Montecucco et al., 1990).

Investigation of aPL in rheumatic fever has provided conflicting results. Figueroa et al. (1992) reported 80 per cent aCL positivity in 35 patients with rheumatic fever during the acute attack vs. 40 per cent in the remission stage. The frequency and titre of aCL did not differ between patients with and without Sydenham chorea, but a significant association was found between

IgM aCL and carditis. Reyes et al. (1994) reported 16 per cent aCL in 48 patients with rheumatic heart disease, most with inactive disease, as compared to 0 per cent in congenital heart disease. However, other investigators did not found any aPL-positive cases among patients with rheumatic fever, some of whom with Sydenham chorea (Asherson et al., 1988; Diniz et al., 1994), nor did they detect significant differences in aCL levels between patients with rheumatic fever, chronic rheumatic heart disease or *Streptococcal pharyngitis*, and healthy children (Narin et al., 1996).

Acquired coagulation factor inhibitors and APL

Although the presence of circulating LA corresponds to an increased risk of thrombosis, a positive LA test has been occasionally associated with a bleeding tendency both in adults and in children (Bajaj et al., 1983; Bernini et al., 1993). This condition, named 'acquired hypoprothrombinaemia-lupus anticoagulant syndrome', is characterized by severe haemorrhages, profound acquired hypoprothrombinaemia, and the presence of circulating, high-affinity antibodies that bind prothrombin without neutralizing its coagulant activity; hypoprothrombinaemia is thought to result from a rapid clearance of prothrombin antigen-antibody complexes (Bajaj et al., 1983). The significance of the association between the acquired hypoprothrombinaemia and the LA is unclear; of note, Bajaj et al. (1983) identified both higher- and lower-affinity antibodies to prothrombin. Awareness of this syndrome is important because corticosteroid treatment is effective.

Another condition in which aPL are associated with the presence of acquired coagulation factor inhibitors is a syndrome occasionally observed in children during recovery from chickenpox. It is characterized by multiple thromboses, with or without disseminated intravascular coagulation, that result from an acquired, transient isolated deficiency of protein S due to the presence of a circulating autoantibody to protein S (D'Angelo et al., 1993; Manco-Johnson et al., 1996). This antibody has no direct inhibitory effect on the activity of protein S; the decrease in protein S antigen levels presumably results from rapid clearance of the circulating immune complex.

Neonatal thrombosis

A few cases of thrombosis in neonates born from aPL-positive mothers have been reported (Ravelli & Martini, 1997). In some instances aPL were not detected or tested in the neonate, whereas in others aPL have been found in both the mother and the baby. Teyssier et al. (1995) reported a neonate with cerebral ischaemia, bilateral adrenal haemorrhage and circulating aCL detected during the neonatal period and at 7 months of age; aCL were also found in the mother 5 and 15 weeks after delivery. Contractor et al. (1992) reported a neonate born from a mother with a history of probable SLE who developed left renal vein and inferior vena cava thrombosis; aCL of the IgG class were positive in both the mother and the baby. Four months after delivery aCL had disappeared in the baby whereas they persisted in the mother. The above reports suggest that aPL acquired transplacentally have a pathogenic role in the development of neonatal thrombosis.

Treatment guidelines

Asymptomatic aPL-positive children

In spite of the established association between aPL and thrombosis, most patients who have circulating aPL do not develop thrombosis. To give an example, aCL are positive in low-titre in about 2 per cent of the healthy obstetric population, but this finding has not been associated with major complications (Harris & Spinnato, 1991). Considerable controversy exists concerning whether prophylactic treatment is indicated for individuals with persistently positive aPL who have no history of thrombosis. Several studies have shown that LA is more closely associated with thrombotic events than aCL (Abu-Shakra et al., 1995; Ginsberg et al., 1995), whereas the presence of IgM or low-titre IgG does not seem to confer a significant risk for thrombosis. Nevertheless, the thrombotic risk in asymptomatic aPL-positive patients is yet unknown. At present, these patients generally are given no treatment or just prophylactic low-dose aspirin, although there is no evidence to support the usefulness of the latter (Hunt & Khamashta, 1996). Since children are less exposed than adults to other more general prothrombotic factors, the thrombotic risk in asymptomatic aPL-positive children is likely to be lower than in adults. Nevertheless, prophylaxis of venous thrombosis with subcutaneous heparin can be advised when patients with persistent high levels of IgG aCL or LA activity are exposed to another thrombophilic factor such as prolonged immobilization (Caporali et al., 1992) or surgery (Hunt & Khamashta, 1996). In the adolescent age, other risk factors that might predispose to thrombosis, such as smoking and oral contraceptives that contain estrogens, must be avoided.

aPL-positive children with thrombosis

The management of thrombosis in the acute phase does not differ from that of thrombosis of other cause. Treatment with high-dose corticosteroids, cyclophosphamide or plasmapheresis, aimed at reducing the levels of circulating aPL, is advised, together with adequate anticoagulation, only in life-threatening situations such as catastrophic APS (Asherson, 1998). Otherwise, immunosuppressive therapy, unless required for other accompanying conditions, is not recommended because antibodies rapidly return to previous level after discontinuation of therapy.

Retrospective studies in adults have shown that aPL-associated thromboses tend to recur (Khamashta et al., 1995; Rosove & Brewer, 1992). There is therefore a general agreement on the advisability of treating patients who developed an aPL-related thrombosis to prevent recurrences (Hunt & Khamashta, 1996). However, the duration and dosages of anti-thrombotic therapy are not yet established. Some authors have suggested that it must be continued as long as aPL are detectable, whereas others believe that life-long administration is needed (Lockshin, 1993). Rosove & Brewer (1992) indicated that intermediate- (INR from 2.0 to 2.9) to high-intensity (INR $\geq$ 3) warfarin therapy may confer better anti-thrombotic protection than low- (INR $\geq$ 1.9) to intermediate-intensity warfarin or aspirin therapy. In a large retrospective study, Khamashata et al. (1995) showed that treatment with high-intensity warfarin (producing an INR $\geq$ 3), with or without low-dose aspirin (75 mg/day), was significantly more effective than treatment with low-intensity warfarin, with or without aspirin, or aspirin alone. However, 29 of the 81 patients with INR $\geq$ 3 had significant haemorrhagic complications, which were severe in seven. A very high incidence of recurrence of thrombosis (1.30 per patient/year) was observed during the first six months after the cessation of warfarin administration, which suggests that, once instituted, warfarin therapy should be long-term. These data should be confirmed in prospective, controlled trials.

No data are available on the recurrence rate of thrombosis or on the optimal anticoagulation regimen in children. The whole frequency of vascular thrombosis is much lower in children than in adults and, as previously mentioned, thrombosis appears to be less common in paediatric than in adult SLE. Moreover, warfarin therapy is age- and weight-dependent and requires close monitoring because of evolving requirements (Andrew et al., 1994) and because long-term administration of warfarin at high therapeutic levels raises some concern given the risk of haemorrhage during play and sports. Based on these considerations and in the absence of controlled trials in children, we currently administer intermediate-intensity anticoagulation therapy in association with aspirin to children who have an aPL-related thrombotic event. A similar approach has been proposed by Silverman (1996), who suggested treatment of children with aPL-related thrombosis with heparin followed by warfarin for 6 months to maintain an INR at ≈ 2.5; then, long-term (indefinite) low-dose warfarin should be given to maintain the INR at 1.5–2.0. In Silverman's experience, this therapeutic protocol was not associated with bleeding nor with recurrence of thrombosis.

Thrombocytopenia

Thrombocytopenia in the APS is usually mild and does not require therapy. In the more severe instances, the treatment of choice is represented by corticosteroids. Improvement of corticosteroid-resistant thrombocytopenia with danazol, chloroquine, dapsone, warfarin and low-dose aspirin has been shown in anedoctal reports (Hunt & Khamashta, 1996). Aspirin administration, however, is dangerous in patients with very low platelet counts. Splenectomy is not recommended because the postsplenectomy thrombocytosis may theoretically increase the thrombotic risk; furthermore, in some cases splenectomy has been ineffective (Hunt & Khamashta, 1996). Intravenous gammaglobulin can be useful to temporarily increase the platelet count before surgery.

References

Abu-Shakra, M., Gladman, D.D., Urowitz, M.B. & Farewell, V. (1995): Anticardiolipin antibodies in systemic lupus erythematosus: clinical and laboratory correlations. *Am. J. Med.* **99**, 624–628.

Andrew, M., Marzinotto, V., Brooker, L.A., Adams, M., Ginsberg, J., Freedom, R. & Williams, W. (1994): Oral anticoagulation therapy in pediatric patients: a prospective study. *Thromb. Haemost.* **71**, 265–269.

Angelini, L., Ravelli, A., Caporali, R., Rumi, V., Nardocci, N. & Martini, A. (1994): High prevalence of antiphospholipid antibodies in children with idiopathic cerebral ischemia. *Pediatrics* **94**, 500–503.

Angelini, L., Zibordi, F., Zorzi, G., Nardocci, N., Caporali, R., Ravelli, A. & Martini, A. (1996): Neurological disorders, other than stroke, associated with antiphospholipid antibodies in childhood. *Neuropediatrics* **27**, 149–153.

Asherson, R.A. (1998): The catastrophic antiphospholipid syndrome. A review of the clinical features, possible pathogenesis and treatment. *Lupus* **7** (Suppl. 2), 55–62.

Asherson, R.A. & Cervera, R. (1995): Review: antiphospholipid antibodies and the lung. *J. Rheumatol.* **22**, 62–66.

Asherson, R.A. & Hughes, G.R.V. (1991): Hypoadrenalism, Addison's disease and antiphospholipid antibodies. *J. Rheumatol.* **18**, 1–3.

Asherson, R.A. & Kant, K.S. (1993): Antiphospholipid antibodies and the kidney. *J. Rheumatol.* **20**, 1268–1272.

Asherson, R.A. & Lubbe, W.F. (1988): Cerebral and valve lesions in SLE: association with antiphospholipid antibodies. *J. Rheumatol.* **15**, 539–543.

Asherson, R.A., Derksen, R.H.W.M., Harris, E.N., Bouma, B.N., Gharavi, A.E., Kater, L. & Hughes, G.R.V. (1987): Chorea in systemic lupus erythematosus and 'lupus-like' disease: association with antiphospholipid antibodies. *Semin. Arthritis Rheum.* **16**, 253–259.

Asherson, R.A., Hughes, G.R.V., Gledhill, R. & Quinn, N.P. (1988): Absence of antibodies to cardiolipin in patients with Huntington's chorea, Sydenham's chorea and acute rheumatic fever. *J. Neurol. Neurosurg. Psychiatry* **51**, 1458.

Asherson, R.A., Khamashta, M.A. & Hughes, G.R.V. (1991): The hepatic complications of the antiphospholipid syndrome. *Clin. Exp. Rheumatol.* **9** 341–344.

Baca, V., Garcia-Ramirez, R., Ramirez-Lacayo, M., Marquez-Enriquez, L., Martinez, I. & Lavalle, C. (1996): Cerebral infarction and antiphospholipid syndrome in children. *J. Rheumatol.* **23** 1428–1431.

Bajaj, S.P., Rapaport, S.I., Fierer, D.S., Herbst, K.D. & Schwartz, D.B. (1983): A mechanism for the hypoprothrombinemia of the acquired hypoprothrombinemia-lupus anticoagulant syndrome. *Blood* **61,** 684–692.

Baxter, P., Gardner-Medwin, D., Green, S.H. & Moss, C. (1993): Congenital livedo reticularis and recurrent stroke-like episodes. *Devel. Med. Child. Neurol.* **35,** 917–926.

Bernini, J.C., Buchanan, G.R. & Ashcraft, J. (1993): Hypoprothrombinemia and severe hemorrhage associated with a lupus anticoagulant. *J. Pediatr.* **123,** 937–939.

Brey, R.L., Azzudin, E., Gharavi, A.E. & Lockshin, M.D. (1993): Neurologic complications of antiphospholipid antibodies. *Rheum. Dis. Clin. N. Am.* **19,** 833–850.

Caporali, R., Ravelli, A., De Gennaro, F., Neirotti, G., Montecucco, C. & Martini, A. (1991): Prevalence of anticardiolipin antibodies in juvenile chronic arthritis. *Ann. Rheum. Dis.* **50,** 599–601.

Caporali, R., Ravelli, A., Ramenghi, B., Montecucco, C. & Martini, A. (1992): Antiphospholipid antibody-associated thrombosis in juvenile chronic arthritis. *Arch. Dis. Child.* **67,** 1384–1385.

Cervera, R., Asherson, R.A. & Lie, J.T. (1995): Clinicopathologic correlations of the antiphospholipid syndrome. *Semin. Arthritis Rheum.* **24,** 262–272.

Contractor, S., Hiatt, M., Kosmin, M. & Kim, H.C. (1992): Neonatal thrombosis with anticardiolipin antibody in baby and mother. *Am. J. Perinatol.* **9,** 409–410.

D'Angelo, A., Della Valle, P., Crippa, L., Pattarini, E., Grimaldi, L.M.E. & Viganò D'Angelo, S. (1993): Brief report: autoimmune protein S deficiency in a boy with severe thromboembolic disease. *N. Engl. J. Med.* **328,** 1753–1757.

Diniz, R.E.A.S., Goldenberg, J., Andrade, L.E.C, Leser, P.G., Silva, N.P., Roizenblatt, S. & Hilario, M.O.E. (1994): Antiphospholipid antibodies in rheumatic fever chorea. *J. Rheumatol.* **21,** 1367.

Falcini, F., Taccetti, G., Trapani, S., Tafi, L., Petralli, S. & Matucci-Cerinic, M. (1991): Primary antiphospholipid syndrome: a report of two pediatric cases. *J. Rheumatol.* **18,** 1085–1087.

Figueroa, F., Berrios, X., Gutierrez, M., Carrion, F., Goycolea, J.P., Riedel, I. & Jacobelli, S. (1992): Anticardiolipin antibodies in acute rheumatic fever. *J. Rheumatol.* **19** 1175–1180.

Galli, M., Finazzi, G. & Barbui, T. (1996): Thrombocytopenia in the antiphospholipid syndrome. *Br. J. Rheumatol.* **93** 1–5.

Ginsberg, J.S., Wells, P.S., Brill-Edwards, P., Donovan, D., Moffatt, K., Johnston, M., Stevens, P. & Hirsh, J. (1995): Antiphospholipid antibodies and venous thromboembolism. *Blood* **86,** 3685–3691.

Harris, E.N. & Spinnato, J.A. (1991): Should anticardiolipin tests be performed in otherwise healthy pregnant women? *Am. J. Obstet. Gynecol.* **165,** 1272–1277.

Hunt, B.J. & Khamashta, M.A. (1996): Management of the Hughes syndrome. *Clin. Exp. Rheumatol.* **14,** 115–117.

Inam, S., Sidki, K., Al-Marshedy, A.R. & Judzewitsch, R. (1991): Addison's disease, hypertension, renal and hepatic microthrombosis in 'primary' antiphospholipid syndrome. *Postgrad. Med. J.* **67,** 385–388.

Jouquan, J., Pennec, Y., Mottier, D., Youinou, P., Cledes, J., Leroy, J.P. & Le Menn, G. (1986): Accelerated hypertension associated with lupus anticoagulant and false-positive VDRL in systemic lupus erythematosus. *Arthritis Rheum.* **29,**147.

Khamashta, M.A., Cuadrado, M.J., Mujic, F., Taub, N.A., Hunt, B.J. & Hughes, G.R.V. (1995): The management of thrombosis in the antiphospholipid-antibody syndrome. *N. Engl. J. Med.* **332,** 993–997.

Leak, A.M. (1988): Autoantibody profile in juvenile chronic arthritis. *Ann. Rheum. Dis.* **47,** 178–182.

Lockshin, M.D. (1993): Which patients with antiphospholipid antibody should be treated and how? *Rheum. Dis. Clin. N. Am.* **19,** 235–247.

Manco-Johnson, M.J., Nuss, R., Key, N., Moertel, C., Jacobson, L., Meech, S., Weinberg, A. & Lefkowitz, J. (1996): Lupus anticoagulant and protein S deficiency in children with postvaricella purpura fulminans or thrombosis. *J. Pediatr.* **128,** 319–323.

Massa, M., De Benedetti, F., Ravelli, A. & Martini, A. (1993): Anti-DNA antibodies in the primary antiphospholipid syndrome. *Br. J. Rheumatol.* **32,** 1028.

Miller, D.J., Maisch, S.A., Perez, M.D., Kearney, D.L. & Feltes, T.F. (1995): Fatal myocardial infarction in an 8-year-old girl with systemic lupus erythematosus, Raynaud's phenomenon, and secondary antiphospholipid antibody syndrome. *J. Rheumatol.* **22,** 768–773.

Molta, C., Meyer, O., Dosquet, C., Montes de Oca, M., Babron, M.C., Danon, F., Kaplan, C., Clemenceau, S., Castellano, F. & Levy, M. (1993): Childhood-onset systemic lupus erythematosus: antiphospholipid antibodies in 37 patients and their first-degree relatives. *Pediatrics* **92,** 849–853.

Montecucco, C., Ravelli, A., Caporali, R., Viola, S., De Gennaro, F., Albani, S. & Martini, A. (1990): Autoantibodies in juvenile dermatomyositis. *Clin. Exp. Rheumatol.* **8,** 193–196.

Narin, N., Kutukculer, N., Narin, F., Keser, G. & Doganavsargil, E. *et al.* (1996): Anticardiolipin antibodies in acute rheumatic fever and chronic rheumatic heart disease: is there a significant association? *Clin. Exp. Rheumatol.* **14,** 567–569.

Olive, D., André, E., Brocard, O., Labrude, P. & Alexandre, P. (1979): Lupus érythémateux disséminé révélé par des thrombophlébites des membres inférieurs. *Arch. Fr. Pediatr.* **36,** 807–811.

Ostuni, P.A., Lazzarin, P., Pengo, V., Ruffati, A., Schiavon, F. & Gambari, P. (1990): Renal artery thrombosis and hypertension in a 13-year-old girl with antiphospholipid syndrome. *Ann. Rheum. Dis.* **49,** 184–187.

Petri, M. (1994): Diagnosis of antiphospholipid antibodies. *Rheum. Dis. Clin. N. Am.* **20,** 443–469.

Ravelli, A., Di Fuccia, G., Caporali, R., Malvezzi, F., Montecucco, C. & Martini, A. (1993): Severe retinopathy in systemic lupus erythematosus associated with Ig anticardiolipin antibodies. *Acta Paediatr.* **82,** 624–626.

Ravelli, A., Caporali, R., Di Fuccia, G., Zonta, L., Montecucco, C. & Martini, A. (1994a): Anticardiolipin antibodies in pediatric systemic lupus erythematosus. *Arch. Pediatr. Adolesc. Med.* **148,** 398–402.

Ravelli, A., Martini, A. & Burgio, G.R. (1994b): Antiphospholipid antibodies in paediatrics. *Eur. J. Pediatr.* **153,** 472–479.

Ravelli, A. & Martini, A. (1997): Antiphospholipid antibody syndrome in pediatric patients. *Rheum. Dis. Clin. N. Am.* **23,** 657–676.

Reyes, P.A., Amigo, M.C., Banales, J.L. & Nava, A. (1994): Anticardiolipin antibodies, rheumatic fever and rheumatic heart disease. *J. Rheumatol.* **21,** 2389.

Rosove, M.H. & Brewer, P.M. (1992): Antiphospholipid thrombosis: clinical course after the first thrombotic event in 70 patients. *Ann. Intern. Med.* **117,** 303–308.

Schoning, M., Klein, R., Krageloh-Mann, I., Falck, M., Bien, S., Berg, P.A. & Michaelis R. (1993): Antiphospholipid antibodies in cerebrovascular ischemia and stroke in childhood. *Neuropediatrics* **25,** 8–14.

Seaman, D.E., Londino, A.V., Kwoh, C.K., Medsger, T.A. & Manzi, S. (1995): Antiphospholipid antibodies in pediatric systemic lupus erythematosus. *Pediatrics* **96,** 1040–1045.

Shergy, W.J., Kredich, D.W. & Pisetsky, D.S. (1988): The relationship of anticardiolipin antibodies to disease manifestations in pediatric systemic lupus erythematosus. *J. Rheumatol.* **15,** 1389–1394.

Silverman, E. (1996): What's new in the treatment of pediatric SLE? *J. Rheumatol.* **23,** 1657–1660.

St Clair, W., Jones, B., Rogers, J.S., Crouch, M. & Hrabovsky, E. (1981): Deep venous thrombosis and a circulating anticoagulant in systemic lupus erythematosus. *Am. J. Dis. Child.* **135,** 230–232.

Takanashi, J., Sugita, K., Miyazato, S., Sakao, E., Miyamoto, H. & Niimi, H. (1995): Antiphospholipid antibody syndrome in childhood strokes. *Pediatr. Neurol.* **13,** 323–326.

Tan, E.M., Cohen, A.S., Fries, J.F., Masi, A.T., McShane, D.J., Rothfield, N.F., Green Schaller, J., Talal, N. & Winchester, R.J. (1982): The 1982 revised criteria for the classification of systemic lupus erythematosus. *Arthritis Rheum.* **25,** 1271–1277.

Teyssier, G., Gautheron, V., Absi, L., Galambrun, C., Ravni, C. & Lepetit, J.C. (1995): Anticorps anticardiolipine, ischémie cérébrale et hémorragie surrénalienne chez un nouveau-né. *Arch. Pédiatr.* **2,** 1086–1088.

Toren, A., Toren, P., Many, A., Mandel, M., Mester, R., Neumann, Y., Kende, G., Moses, T., Gitel, S. & Levanon, M. (1993): Spectrum of clinical manifestations of antiphospholipid antibodies in childhood and adolescence. *Pediatr. Hematol. Oncol.* **10,** 311–315.

Tucker, L.B. (1994): Antiphospholipid syndrome in childhood: the great unknown. *Lupus* **3,** 367–369.

Ura, Y., Hara, T., Mori, Y., Matsuo, M., Fujioka, Y., Kuno, T., Okue, A. & Miyazaki, S. (1992): Development of Perthes' disease in a 3-year-old boy with idiopathic thrombocytopenic purpura and antiphospholipid antibodies. *Pediatr. Hematol. Oncol.* **9,** 77–80.

Uziel, Y., Laxer, R.M., Blaser, S., Andrew, M., Schneider, R. & Silverman, E.D. (1995): Cerebral vein thrombosis in childhood systemic lupus erythematosus. *J. Pediatr.* **126,** 722–727.

Chapter 15

Neurologic disorders associated with antiphospholipid antibodies

Federica Zibordi and Lucia Angelini

Department of Child Neurology, Istituto Nazionale Neurologico 'C. Besta', via Celoria 11, 20133 Milan, Italy

Summary

Different neurologic conditions associated with antiphospholipid antibodies have recently been described in children. Stroke is the prominent neurologic manifestation. Disorders other than stroke such as chorea, migraine, partial epilepsy, transverse myelitis, benign intracranial hypertension have also been reported. The presumed pathophysiologic mechanism underlying these manifestations is thought to be a cerebral ischaemia in some, but not all, cases. A direct reaction against neuronal membrane components rather than antiphospholipid-associated thrombosis seems to be an alternative pathogenetic mechanism.

We report the prevalence of antiphospholipid antibodies in a group of children with idiopathic cerebral ischaemia and with non-stroke neurological disease including migraine, benign intracranial hypertension, unilateral movement disorders and cryptogenetic partial seizures. The strongest association appears to be with ischaemic cerebrovascular disease and the contribution of antiphospholipid antibodies to cerebral ischaemia may be particularly relevant in childhood, where other stroke risk factors are not present. The association between antiphospholipid antibodies and neurological conditions other than stroke may suggest a possible pathogenetic mechanism of disorders usually regarded as cryptogenetic.

Introduction

The antiphospholipid syndrome (APS) has been detected in a significant number of children with cerebrovascular ischaemic events, but its significance is variably appreciated. Recent reports have drawn attention to a variety of neurologic conditions associated with the presence of antiphospholipid antibodies (aPL) (Brey & Escalante, 1998). This association may be due to systemic lupus erithematosus (SLE) or lupus-like disease, but may also occur without any of the clinical or serological features of SLE in the so-called primary antiphospholipid antibodies syndrome (PAPS). This syndrome is defined as a combination of vascular occlusion and thrombocytopenia, with a persistent increase of anticardiolipin antibodies (aCL) and/or the presence of lupus anticoagulant (LA) (Harris *et al.*, 1998).

The neurologic conditions associated with aPL may be grouped, in accordance with the literature, into cerebrovascular disease and neurological disorders other than stroke (Asherson & Cervera, 1993).

Cerebral infarction, and related conditions such as TIA, stroke and ocular ischaemia are the prominent neurological manifestations, well known in adults and very recently also recognized in children.

The second group of neurologic disorders includes chorea and other movement disorders, migraine, epilepsy, transverse myelitis and pseudotumour cerebri.

Pathogenetic remarks

While thrombosis of large vessels is responsible for the clinical manifestations as in other organs and/or systems (Ravelli and colleagues), ischaemic events may be insufficient to explain other aPL-associated disorders.

Imaging studies of subjects with aPL and neurological disease have given no conclusive results, revealing either cerebral infarction due to demonstrable arterial occlusion or multiple white matter and cortical grey matter abnormalities scattered in non-specific patterns for a vascular injury (Provenzale et al., 1994).

Furthermore experimental data have provided evidence suggesting thrombotic pathogenesis (Tincani et al., 1998) but also the occurrence of non-occlusive mechanisms.

Two possible mechanisms triggered by aPL have been proposed: occlusive vascular events involving small vessels or, alternatively, a direct reaction against neuronal membrane components (Asherson & Cervera, 1993; Mc Neil et al., 1991).

MRL/lpr mice, which spontaneously develop SLE and elevated titres of aCL and MRL/++ mice, which produce aCL after immunization with β2-glycoprotein I (GPI), may both manifest neurologic diseases. Clinicopathological studies in neurologically affected animals failed to reveal thrombosis or cerebral infarction, suggesting pathogenetic mechanisms based on a direct reaction between aPL and CNS tissue. This process first requires either intratechal antibody production or blood-brain barrier compromise to allow access of serum aPL to the CNS. It also requires that aPL bind to tissues in the CNS and that binding alter the function of the tissue, resulting in aPL-related symptoms. The site and effect of the bound between aPL and neural tissue has yet to be established (Kent et al., 1997).

A few studies, however, have suggested that aPL may have direct reactivity with the CNS. Interestingly, according to Miyazawa (1992), monoclonal aPL may directly react with neurons in developing rat cerebellum.

Furthermore purified pooled polyclonal aCL, from patients with SLE, have been shown by Sun et al. (1992), to have inhibitory effects on cultured murine brain astrocytes proliferation. In this experiment, normal rat astrocytes were used as target cells: micelle purified aCL in serum samples from patients with SLE were proven to exert suppressive effects on these cells in a dose-dependent manner. The astrocytes became spherical and their membranes depolarized. It appears that aCL derange the structure and function of the blood-brain barrier, probably through their membrane effect, with the entrance of noxious substances, including cytotoxic antibodies.

Even if aPL react with CNS tissue, they must first reach the CNS. aCL have been found simultaneously in the liquor and serum of patients with SLE, suggesting that aCL had crossed the blood-brain barrier from the serum (Lolli et al., 1991). However, local production of aCL has also been observed within the CNS in several patients with multiple sclerosis, AIDS and Guillain-Barré syndrome (Brey et al., 1991).

The hypotheses of CNS injury resulting from thrombosis or from direct binding to neural tissues are not mutually exclusive. Tight junctions (between endothelial cells of blood vessels and epithelial cells of the choroid plexus of the CNS) are believed to be responsible for blood-brain barrier function. If aPL alter endothelial cell functions, with or without thrombosis, the barrier may be compromised, allowing aPL access to the CNS (Kent et al., 1997).

Neurologic disorders mediated by aPL may be the result of a combination of events.

To support the notion that aPL are involved in the pathophisiology of neurologic symptoms associated with APS in a mouse model Ziporen et al. (1997), using active immunization of a monoclonal aCL, produced neurologic behavioural abnormalities consisting in hyperreactivity and reduced motor coordination with diminished performance of reflex activities. The iperkinetic movements observed in APS mice are reminiscent of chorea reported in several patients in association with elevated aPL. This may point to a defect in the functioning of basal ganglia in APS mice. The movement disorder observed probably derives from the combination of different autoimmune pathways in which aPL or anti-β2GPI are involved, affecting the dopaminergic system either by occlusion of microvessels within the basal ganglia, or by direct binding of autoantibodies to the neurons (Ziporen et al., 1997)

The effective role of the aPL still remains unclear. Whether these antibodies are epiphenomenal markers of the disease or participant in pathogenesis has yet to be determined.

Case studies

The series consisted of children referred in the last decade to the Department of Neuropaediatrics of the National Neurological Institute of Milan. The neurologic conditions of these children, in accordance with the literature, were grouped into cerebrovascular diseases (stroke, transient ischaemic attacks, ocular ischaemia) and neurological disorders other than stroke (migraine, pseudotumour cerebri, unilateral movement disorders and partial seizures).

Cerebrovascular disease

As previously reported (Angelini et al., 1994) a high prevalence of aPL in children with idiopathic cerebral ischaemia was observed. The clinical data are shown in Table 1. Ten of 13 (76 per cent) patients were positive, according to the proposed APS criteria, for either LA or aCL. Stroke had occurred in five patients. Three patients had transient ischaemic attacks (TIA), which represented the first episode in one and a recurrence in two. Two patients had ocular ischaemia. Six (46 per cent) of the 13 patients had a history of multiple ischaemic events.

Several studies have shown that aPL are positive in 7–9 per cent of patients of all ages with TIA or stroke, whereas unselected young adults with cerebral ischaemia have a prevalence of circulating aPL ranging from 18 to 46 per cent. These findings, together with the high frequency (76 per cent) of aPL observed in the reported study in children, show that the prevalence of aPL in idiopathic cerebral ischaemia is inversely related to age (Angelini et al., 1994; Levine et al., 1995).

Neurologic diseases other than stroke

In a systematic study on the association of aPL with cryptogenetic neurological disease other than stroke, positive aPL were found in six out of 17 patients suffering from migraine, in three out of the four children with benign intracranial hypertension (including both pseudotumour cerebri and communicating hydrocephalus) and in all of the five patients affected by acute or subacute unilateral movement disorder (hemidystonia in three cases and chorea in two) (Angelini et al., 1996). The clinical data are reported in Table 2.

Table. 1. Main demographic data, ischaemic events and results of LA and aCL determination in 13 children with cerebral ischaemia

Patient no.	Age (years)	Sex	Ischaemic event	First determination			Second determination		
				IgG aCL	IgM aCL	LA	IgG aCL	IgM aCL	LA
1	14	M	Stroke	–	–	+	25	–	+
2	5	M	Stroke	32	–	–	32	–	–
3	4	M	Stroke	21	–	–	15	6	–
4	12	F	Stroke	50	–	–	>100	–	–
5	16	M	Stroke	22	–	–	15	7	–
6	12	M	TIA	23	–	–	20	–	–
7	14	M	TIA	9	17	–	–	15	–
8	5	M	TIA	20	8	–	22	–	–
9	7	F	OI	–	–	+	27	–	–
10	10	F	OI	15	–	–	17	–	–
11	7	F	Stroke	–	–	–	8	–	–
12	12	F	Stroke	–	–	–	11	–	–
13	14	F	Stroke	–	–	–	–	–	–

TIA = transient ischaemic attack; OI = ocular ischaemia.

Table. 2. Main demographic data results of LAC and aCL determination in 14 aPL-positive children

Patient no.	Age (years)	Sex	Ischaemic event	First determination			Second determination		
				IgG aCL	IgM aCL	LA	IgG aCL	IgM aCL	LA
1	7	F	Migraine	25	–	–	–	15	+
2	13	M	Migraine	44	–	–	24	11	–
3	10	F	Migraine	>100	–	–	23	–	–
4	13	M	Migraine	27	–	–	–	16	–
5	16	F	Migraine	31	–	–	22	–	–
6	17	F	Migraine	46	28	–	20	–	–
7	4	F	BIH	24	–	–	19	–	–
8	12	M	BIH	27	–	–	15	–	–
9	6	M	BIH	10	–	+	–	–	+
10	17	F	Chorea	–	–	+	19	5	+
11	7	M	Chorea	22	–	–	16	–	–
12	12	M	Dystonia	6	18	–	29	33	–
13	7	F	Dystonia	27	–	–	25	–	–
14	5	F	Dystonia	21	29	+	6	35	+

BIH= Benign intracranial hypertension.

Migraine

Though the association between migraine and aPL in adults has been described in several reports, even if with debatable results, no similar data for childhood population are available in the literature. The prevalence of aPL in patients with migraine does not appear to be increased, even in an SLE population in whom the prevalence of both migraine and aPL are increased over the general population. The largest case-control study to date has failed to demonstrate an association of aCL immunoreactivity in patients under 60 years of age with migraine with or without aura compared to controls (Tjetjen et al., 1998) These data highlight the importance of considering the presence of aPL in migrainous stroke; however, there is insufficient evidence to support a need to evaluate all migraine patients for aPL (Brey & Escalante, 1998).

Benign intracranial hypertension

Benign intracranial hypertension (BIH) associated with aPL has been sporadically described in SLE and was reported in one child who presented deep thrombosis and cranial sinuses occlusion in the absence of serological evidence of underlying systemic disease.

Movement disorders

Hemidystonia is usually symptomatic of basal ganglia damage, often of vascular origin, but in the five children here reported neuroimaging failed to demonstrate any alteration in these structures.

Chorea is a well-known manifestation of SLE. Only a few reports of chorea associated with APS exist. Cervera et al. (1997) have reviewed cases found in the literature on neuroimaging in chorea and aPL: in the majority of patients, CT or MRI scans were normal. MRI revealed caudate nuclei involvement in two out of seven patients with PAPS. The main hypothesis on the mechanism of chorea in aPL is a vascular disorder involving the small vessels of the basal ganglia (Brey et al., 1993). Another hypothesis is that chorea in patients with reversible iperkinesia may be caused by striatal dysfunction induced by the binding of aPL to phospholipid-rich regions of the basal ganglia (Asherson & Hughes, 1988). This hypothesis is supported by several recent case reports describing transient hypermetabolism in basal ganglia in patients with aPL-associated chorea studied using positron emission tomography (Furie et al., 1994; Sunden-Culberg et al., 1998).

Epilepsy

Lastly, aPL positivity in three out of a series of 23 consecutive children presenting partial epileptic seizures was reported (Angelini et al., 1998) All three presented clinical ictal phenomena suggesting frontal lobe epilepsy. The clinical data are showed in Table 3. aPL have been reported with increased frequency in SLE patients with epilepsy, where the aetiology consisted in cerebral infarction, while in these reported patients imaging of the brain showed no evidence of vascular lesions, ruling out an ischaemic aetiology for the partial seizures. Seizures have been described in patients with cerebrovascular disesase and aPL, but only in two reports (Inzelberg & Korczyn, 1989; Spreafico et al., 1994) seizures associated with APS were not related to ischaemic events. Although a pathogenetic role for occult occlusive micrangiopathy can not be excluded, the normal imaging findings suggest that a cross-reaction between aPL and neurones is more likely.

None of the patients included in this series developed any clinical or serologic features of SLE or other connective tissue disease and were diagnosed as affected by PAPS during follow-up. No differences were found between aPL-positive and aPL-negative patients with respect to clinical manifestations or radiological features.

Table 3. Results of LA and aCL determination in three aPL-positive children

Patient no.	Sex	First determination			Second determination		
		IgG aCL	IgM aCL	LA	IgG aCL	IgM aCL	LA
1	F	2	14	+	6	11	+
2	M	–	30	–	8	>100	–
3	F	12	29	–	1	18	–

Conclusions

The consensus is that aPL play a pathogenetic role in ischaemic disease. Cumulative evidence from a number of recent studies has suggested an association between increased aPL levels and cerebrovascular disease in individuals without SLE.

The age at occurrence of the first ischaemic cerebrovascular event is younger in patients with elevated aPL levels than in general population with strokes.

Seizures, chorea and other movement disorders as well as transverse myelitis all appear to be associated with antiphospholipid antibodies and for these diseases an interaction between aPL and CNS rather than aPL-associated thrombosis seems to be a more plausible mechanism. Migraine, on the other hand, does not appear to be associated with aPL in SLE or non-SLE patients.

On the basis of these findings, a systematic screening for aPL has been recommended in patients with transient or permanent ischaemic cerebrovascular events, recurrent thromboses or other clinical features suggesting antiphospholipid antibody syndrome, like chorea, partial seizures, Guillain-Barré and pseudotumour cerebri of no recognizable aetiology.

References

Angelini, L., Ravelli, A., Caporali, R., Rumi, V., Nardocci, N. & Martini, A. (1994): High prevalence of antiphospholipid antibodies in children with idiopathic cerebral ischemia. *Pediatrics* **94**, 500–503.

Angelini, L., Zibordi, F., Zorzi, G., Nardocci, N., Caporali, R., Ravelli, A. & Martini, A. (1996): Neurological disorders, other than stroke, associated with antiphospholipid antibodies in childhood. *Neuropediatrics* **27**, 1–5.

Angelini, L., Granata, T., Zibordi, F., Binelli, S., Zorzi, G. & Besana, C. (1998): Partial seizures associated with antiphospholipid antibodies in childhood. *Neuropediatrics* **29**, 1–5.

Asherson, R. & Cervera, R. (1993): Antiphospholipid syndrome. *J. Invest. Dermatol.* **100**, 21S–27S.

Asherson, R.A. & Hughes, G.R.V. (1988): Antiphospholipid and chorea. *J. Rheumatol.* **15**. 377–379

Brey, R.L. & Escalante, A. (1998): Neurological manifestations of antiphospholipid antibodies syndrome. *Lupus* **7**, S67–S74.

Brey, R. L., Arroyo, R. & Boswell, R.N. (1991): Cerebrospinal fluid anticardiolipin antibodies in patients with HIV-1 infection. *J. Acquir. Immuno. Def. Syndr.* **4**, 435–441.

Brey, R.L., Gharavi, A.E., Lockshin, M.D. (1993): Neurologic complications of antiphospholipid antibodies. *Rheum. Dis. Clin. North. Am.* **19**, 833–850.

Cervera, R., Asherson, R.A., Font, J., Tikly, M., Pallares, L., Chamorro, A. & Ingelmo, M. (1997): Chorea in the antiphospholipid syndrome. *Medicine* **76**, 203–212.

Furie, R., Ishikawa, T., Dhawan, V. & Eidelberg, D. (1994): Alternating hemichorea in PAPS: evidence for contralateral striatal metabolism. *Neurology* **44**, 2197–2199.

Harris, E.N. Pierangeli, S.S., Gharavi, A.E. (1998): Diagnosis of the antiphospholipid syndrome: a proposal of use of laboratory tests. *Lupus* **7,** S144–S148.

Inzelberg, R. & Korczyn, A.D. (1989): Lupus anticoagulant and late-onset seizures. *Acta. Neurol. Scand.* **79,** 114–118.

Kent, M., Alvarez, F., Vogt, E., Fyffe, R., Ng, A.-K. & Rot, N. (1997): Monoclonal antiphosphatidylserine antibodies react directly with feline and murine central nervous system. *J. Rheumatol.* **24,** 1725–1733.

Levine, S.R., Brey, R.L., Sawayak, J., Salowich-Palm, L., Kokkinos, J., Kostrema, B., Perru, M., Havstad, S. & Carey, J. (1995): Recurrent stroke and thrombo-occlusive events in the antiphospholipid syndrome. *Ann. Neurol.* **38,** 119–134.

Lolli, F., Mata, S., Baruffi, M.C. & Amaducci, L. (1991): Cerebrospinal fluid anticardiolipin antibodies in neurological diseases. *Clin. Immunol. Immunopathol.* **59,** 314–321.

Mc Neil, H.P., Chesterman, C.N. & Krilis, S.A. (1991): Immunology and clinical importance of antiphospholipid antibodies. *Adv. Immunol.* **49,** 193–280.

Miyazawa, A., Inoue, H. & Yoshioka, T. (1992): Monoclonal antibody analysis of phosphatidylserine and protein kinase C localisation in developing rat cerebellum. *J. Neurochem.* **59,** 1547–1554.

Provenzale, J.M., Heinzer, E.R., Ortel, T.L., Macik, G.B., Charles, L.A. & Alberts, M.J. (1994): Antiphospholipid antibodies in patients without systemic lupus erythematosus: neuroradiologic findings. *Radiology* **192,** 531–537.

Spreafico, R., Binelli, S., Bruzzone, M.G., Croci, D., Rumi, V. & Angelini, A. (1994): Primary antiphospholipid antibodies syndrome (PAPS) and isolated partial seizures. A case report. *Ital. J. Neurol. Sci.* **15,** 297–301.

Sun, K., Liu, W., Tsai, C., Lin, W. & Yu, C. (1992): Inhibition of astrocyte proliferation and binding to brain tissue of anticardiolipin antibodies purified from lupus serum. *Ann. Rheum. Dis.* **51,** 707–712.

Sunden-Culberg, J., Tedroff, J. & Aquilonius, S.-M. (1998): Reversible chorea in PAPS. *Mov. Dis.* **13,** 147–149.

Tjetjen, G.E., Day, M., Norris, L., Aurora, S., Halvorsen, A., Schultz, L.R. & Levine, S.R. (1998): Role of anticardiolipin antibodies in young persons with migraine and transient focal neurologic events. *Neurology* **50,** 1433–1440.

Tincani, A., Spatola, L., Cinquini, M., Meroni, P., Balestrieri, G. & Shoenfeld, Y. (1998): Animal models of antiphospolipid syndrome. *Rev. Rhum. Engl. Ed.* **65,** 614–618.

Ziporen, L., Shoenfeld, Y., Levy, Y. & Korczyn, A.D. (1997): Neurological dysfunction and hyperactive behavior associated with antiphospholipid antibodies. *J. Clin. Invest.* **100,** 613–619.

Chapter 16

Endothelial cell role in the pathogenesis of the antiphospholipid syndrome

Cristina Luzzana, Elena Raschi, Luca Catelli, Paola Panzeri,
Monica Riboni, Cinzia Testoni, Maria Orietta Borghi, Nicoletta Del Papa*
and Pier Luigi Meroni

*Clinical Immunology Unit, IRCCS Istituto Auxologico Italiano, University of Milan, via L. Ariosto 13, 20145 Milan, Italy; *IRCCS Policlinico, Milan, Italy*

Summary

The antiphospholipid syndrome (APS) is a multisystem disease with predominant clinical features of a thrombophilic disorder (arterial and venous thrombosis), foetal loss, thrombocytopoenia and antiphospholipid antibodies (aPL). An important and serious characteristic of APS is the involvement of the central nervous system (CNS) by cerebral thrombosis that results in several clinical manifestations: cerebrovascular accidents, epilepsy (or abnormal EEG), chorea and migraine.

Despite a large number of studies, a clear mechanism of aPL-associated thrombosis has not yet been demonstrated. Nevertheless, there is now sound evidence that endothelial cells (EC) do play a role in the induction of the pro-thrombotic diathesis of the syndrome. The reactivity of aPL with endothelial membranes appears to be the necessary prerequisite; actually, such an event seems to be strictly related to the involvement of plasma cofactors, especially beta 2-glycoprotein I (β2GPI).

Endothelial cells obtained from brain tissue specimens do bind β2GPI that can be recognized by β2GPI-dependent aPL or by anti-β2GPI antibodies. The antibody binding is followed by the appearance of a pro-inflammatory phenotype. Interestingly, β2GPI seems to display a higher binding to brain EC in comparison to EC from venous macro-vessels. These findings could represent the biological basis to explain the frequent involvement of CNS vessels in the syndrome.

Endothelial cells

Endothelial cells (EC) form a multifunctional cell lining that covers all of the inner surface of blood vessels and regulates several important physiological and pathological reactions. These include also inflammation-immune reactions, blood vessel tone and haemostasis-thrombosis functions. Particularly, EC produce cytokines that regulate the haematopoietic system (G-CSF and GM-CSF), the proliferation and differentiation of T- and B-cells and the recruitment of leukocytes at sites of inflammation by expression of adhesive structures on their membrane. In resting condition, EC express two integral membrane proteins denominated 'intercellular adhesion molecules' (ICAM-1 and ICAM-2). When EC are activated by the inflammatory mediators (IL-1 and TNF), the expression of ICAM-1 is up-regulated and two novel adhesion structures are induced (ELAM-1 and VCAM) (Dejana et al., 1991).

The prototypes of cytokines which induce proinflammatory-protrombotic changes in EC are IL-1 and TNF. These cytokines promote activation of the coagulation system by induction of thrombomodulin-protein C pathway (Nawrot et al., 1986), and moreover induce production of 'platelet activating factor' (PAF) (Bussolino et al., 1986) and increase the secretion of a plasminogen activator inhibitor, thus impairing the cell ability to dissolve a fibrin clot (Gramse et al., 1986).

Thus, EC possess a main role in the regulation of haemostasis and contribute to maintain blood fluidity. Their anti-thrombogenic functions, in unperturbed conditions, include the production of thrombomodulin (TM) as well as prostacyclin (PGI_2), nitric oxide (NO), heparan sulphate proteoglycans, protein S and plasminogen activator. NO and PGI_2 are responsible for blood dilatation and inhibit platelet functions (Furchgott & Zawadski, 1980; Weksler et al., 1977). The secretion of tissue plasminogen activator enhances fibrinolysis by activation of plasminogen to plasmin (Plow et al., 1995). Heparan sulphate proteoglycans activate antithrombin III that in turn inhibits activation of factor Xa and thrombin (Hatton et al., 1978). TM is an endothelial natural anticoagulant factor and plays an important role by the conversion of thrombin from a procoagulant to an anticoagulant protease (Esmon, 1989; 1995). TM acts as an endothelial cofactor for the activation of protein C by thrombin. In the presence of protein S, calcium and membrane phospholipids activated protein C degrades factor Va and VIIIa, preventing the formation of new thrombin molecules that, also, become unable to act on their procoagulant substrates (fibrinogen and factor V) or to aggregate platelets (Fig. 1). On the contrary, when these delicate mechanisms are perturbed, the effective natural antithrombotic and haemostatic mechanism may lead to intravascular coagulation and thrombus formation. Actually, EC produce tissue factor, plasminogen-activation inhibitors and specific binding sites for several coagulation factors involved in the coagulation cascade (Cines et al., 1998).

Endothelial cells and antiphospholipid antibodies

There is a close association between circulating antiphospholipid antibodies (aPL) and a thrombophilic diathesis (Hughes, 1998). The mechanisms by which aPL might cause the thrombi formation is yet unclear; actually a great deal of attention has been paid to the relationship between aPL, platelets and endothelial cells involved in the coagulation cascade (Roubey, 1998).

Recently, different in vitro studies demonstrated that aPL induce functional modification on EC by the expression of pro-adhesive and pro-inflammatory phenotype. It has been shown that aPL IgG (both polyclonal and monoclonal anti-β2GPI antibodies) bind the EC and induce a phenotypic change: cells were shown to express E-selectin, ICAM-1 and VCAM-1 and to increase the secretion of pro-inflammatory cytokines such as IL-1β and IL-6 (Del Papa et al., 1995, 1997; Simantov et al., 1995; George et al., 1998). It should be pointed out that vascular cell activation has been reported as associated with the appearance of a pro-coagulant state (Nawrot & Stern, 1987). Moreover, mononuclear leukocytes, adhering to activated endothelium, can be

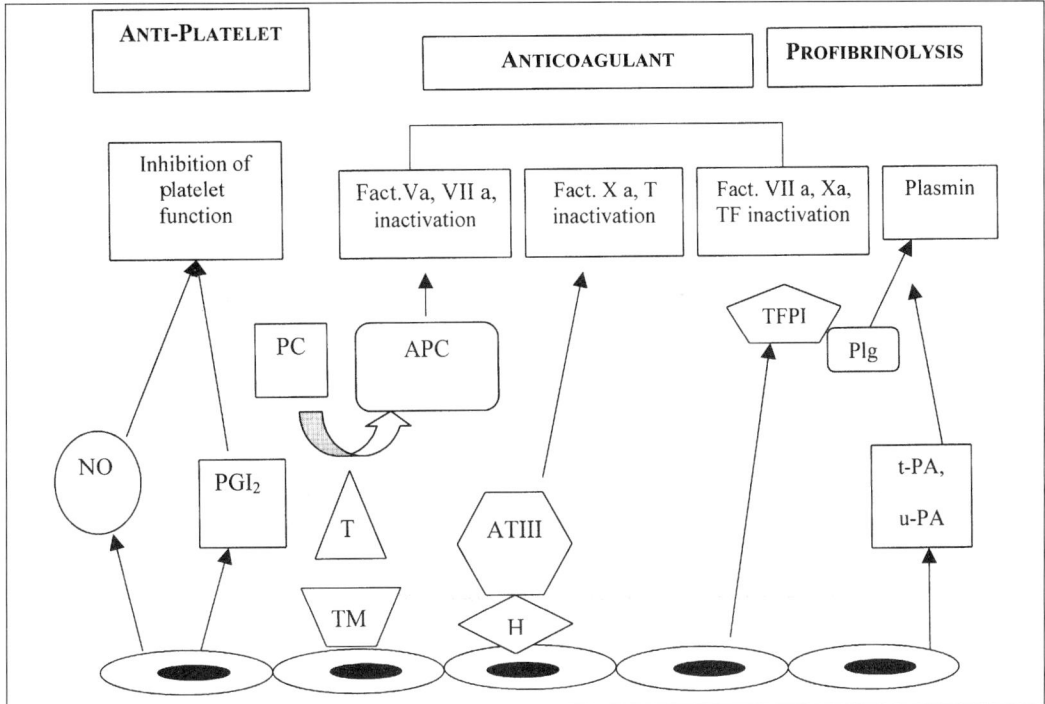

Fig. 1. Endothelial cells: anti-thrombogenic function.
NO, nitric oxide; PGI_2, prostacyclin; T, thrombin; TM, thrombomodulin; PC, protein C; APC, activate protein C; H, heparin; ATIII, antithrombin III; TFPI, tissue factor pathway inhibitor; Plg, plasminogen; t-PA, tissue type Plg activator; u-PA, urokinase type Plg activator.

activated by endothelial inflammatory cytokines and induced to display a procoagulant phenotype, further contributing to the thrombophilic state in APS (Nawrot & Stern, 1987). It is reasonable to presume that such a series of events might occur not only *in vitro* but *in vivo* too. This hypothesis is also supported by the demonstration that plasma levels of soluble VCAM-1 are increased in patients with primary APS (Kaplanski, 1996). Actually, adhesion molecules, once upregulated on cell membranes, are shed into the circulation as soluble forms (Carlos & Harlam, 1994). Pierangeli *et al.* (1998) described an *in vivo* model of pinch-induced thrombosis that supports the hypothesis that aPL can exert their thrombogenicity, at least in part, via EC activation. In this *in vivo* model the passive transfer of aPL was shown to increase the size of the thrombus and to slow its resolution after a mechanical trauma on the venous vessel wall. The authors also described a locally increased endothelial leukocyte adhesion and enhanced adhesion molecule expression (Pierangeli *et al.*, 1998).

The first hypothesis that aPL-positive sera or plasma might induce the conversion of EC from anti-thrombotic to procoagulant state, was supposed by Carreras & Vermylen (1982). The authors, in studies with lupus anticoagulant (LA) positive plasmas, suggested that aPL were able to suppress prostacyclin (PGI_2) production by vascular bovine endothelium. Because PGI_2 is known to be a potent inhibitor of platelet aggregation, it was suggested that this mechanism could be involved in the *in vivo* thrombotic diathesis (Carreras *et al.*, 1982). Different groups, in subsequent studies, did not confirm a clear cross-reactivity between aPL and EC. The suppressing effect of LA was observed only in a minority of instances. Different sources of EC and aPL (whole sera or plasmas, different Ig fractions, etc.) and differences in techniques have been regarded as the most likely reasons to explain the discrepancies (Carreras & Martinuzzo, 1993; Carreras et al., 1996). In order to reduce the technical variables linked to the use of whole plasmas or sera or polyclonal IgG fractions, we evaluated the effect of human anti-β2GPI mAbs on the production of 6-keto-PGF$_{1\alpha}$ – the main product of arachidonic acid metabolism – by HUVEC monolayers. The authors found that the monoclonal antibodies induced a dose-dependent increase of 6-keto-PGF$_{1\alpha}$ that correlated with other parameters of EC activation, such as adhesion molecule up-regulation and cytokine secretion (Del Papa et al., 1997).

It has been reported that HUVEC incubated in the presence of IgG from four APS patients displayed an increase of the inducible cycloxygenase (COX-2). These patients showed also a high urinary excretion of 11-dehydrothromboxane B2, an indirect parameter for *in vivo* platelet activation (Habib et al., 1995). These data might sustain the hypothesis that an antibody-mediated increase in enzyme availability could be responsible for the enhanced metabolic degradation of PGI$_2$. However, the same authors did not find any effect on 6-keto-PGF$_{1\alpha}$ production unless APS IgG were incubated in the presence of thrombin (Habib et al., 1995).

Moreover, Lellouche et al., in an *ex-vivo* study, showed an increase in urinary excretion of thromboxane A (TXA)-platelet-derived metabolites and a smaller increase in 6-keto-PGF$_{1\alpha}$ in APS patients (Lellouche et al., 1991). These results underline, once again, the difficulty to extrapolate from *in vitro* studies data that can be applied to *in vivo* situations in which several variables are present. These data might support the hypothesis that the TXA$_2$/PGI$_2$ imbalance is apparently more linked to an enhanced TXA$_2$ secretion than to the involvement of vascular PGI$_2$ as predisposing state for thrombosis.

Do aPL recognize EC?

To sustain the hypothesis that aPL-positive samples were able to induce thrombophilic diathesis, it was necessary to accept that the autoantibodies can recognize phospholipid determinants on endothelial surfaces. Different groups independently reported a higher prevalence of anti-endothelial binding activity in sera from both primary and secondary APS in comparison with sera from aPL-negative patients; nevertheless, a direct reactivity of purified aPL with EC membranes was not clearly demonstrated (Vismara et al., 1988; Hasselaar et al., 1990; Del Papa et al., 1992, 1993; Le Roux et al., 1986; Rosenbaum et al., 1988; McCrae et al., 1991). Absorption studies with cardiolipin liposome suspensions showed that aPL reactivity was completely inhibited, but endothelial binding was affected in a minority of sera and only partially (Vismara et al., 1988; Hasselaar et al., 1990; McCrae et al., 1991; Cervera et al., 1991). Altogether these findings were quite in line with the fact that EC surface membranes in the resting state do not expose negatively charged phospholipids on the outer leaflet but only on the inner one, as in the majority of cell types. Moreover, it has been demonstrated that, differently from platelets (Khamashta et al., 1988), endothelial activation following several stimuli (such as cytokines, phorbol esters or LPS) did not affect at all the anti-endothelial binding of aPL-positive sera. This evidence once again disproves the hypothesis that epitopes specific for aPL could be at least available on the surface of activated human EC (Del Papa et al., 1992). In addition our own group has been also unable to demonstrate any binding of a human monoclonal antibody (mAb) reactive with anionic phospholipids in a β2-glycoprotein I (β2GPI)-independent manner to both resting- or cytokine-activated human umbilical vein endothelial cells (HUVEC) (Meroni, personal communication).

At last two groups, by using an immunoprecipitation assay with radiolabelled HUVEC surface proteins, independently demonstrated that aPL-positive sera reacted with a heterogeneous family of membrane structures (proteins with a molecular weight ranging from 200 to 24 kD) (McCrae et al., 1991; Del Papa et al., 1994). These latter findings suggested the existence of autoantibodies directed against endothelial constitutive membrane proteins unrelated to the known phospholipid epitopes (McCrae et al., 1991; Del Papa et al., 1994), but did not explain the close association between anti-endothelial cell antibodies (AECA) and aPL. In APS both aPL and AECA could occur as separate antibody populations.

EC and the plasma cofactor β2GPI

Another possible mechanism to explain the close association between anti-endothelial activity and aPL has been suggested by our own group and by Le Tonquèze et al. (Del Papa et al., 1995; Le Tonquèze et al., 1995). The authors reported that affinity-purified anti-cardiolipin antibodies (aCL) from sera positive for both AECA and aCL did react with a human endothelioma cell line (EAhy926) only when the IgG fractions were co-eluted with β2GPI, the major plasma cofactor for aPL. Moreover, the demonstration that addition of exogenous β2GPI allowed the endothelial binding of affinity-purified aCL IgG, further underlined the role of β2GPI in the reaction of aCL with EC (Le Tonquèze et al., 1995). The previously reported ability of β2GPI to bind human EC in vitro (Del Papa et al., 1993) and the in vivo immunohistological demonstration of its binding to endothelial membranes in trophoblast vessel walls (McIntyre, 1992; La Rosa et al., 1994) were in agreement with these data.

In 1995, for the first time, we confirmed that β2GPI is able to mediate the binding of aPL to EC surfaces (Del Papa et al., 1995). Actually, whole sera positive for AECA, aCL and anti-β2GPI antibodies were analysed for their binding activity to EC cultured in the presence or in the absence of foetal calf serum; we found that the incubation of EC in serum-free medium significantly reduced the anti-endothelial activity, which was restored by the addition of exogenous purified human β2GPI in a dose-dependent manner. These findings strongly supported the hypothesis that foetal calf serum in the cell-culturing media could represent a source of β2GPI taking into account the close homology between bovine and human β2GPI (Kandhia & Krilis, 1994). In agreement, affinity-purified anti-β2GPI IgG fractions reacted with EC cultured in the presence of the cofactor but not with cells in serum-free medium. The addition of purified β2GPI to the cultures restored the binding once again. Human IgM mAbs – previously characterized as antibodies recognizing β2GPI – showed comparable EC binding (Del Papa et al., 1997). Altogether these findings suggest that endothelial β2GPI adherence offers suitable epitopes for anti-β2GPI antibodies either by making available high-density immunogenic epitopes or by displaying new cryptic epitopes comparable to those detectable on γ-irradiated type C plates utilized for anti-β2GPI detection. It has been in fact demonstrated that a highly positively charged aminoacid sequence, located in the fifth domain of β2GPI, is the phospholipid-binding site involved in the binding to CL-coated plates (Hunt et al., 1993; Hunt & Krilis, 1994, Sheng et al., 1996). A single aminoacid substitution from Lys^{286} to Glu (mutant 1k) decreased the binding of β2GPI to CL in a significant manner; further substitutions (mutant 2k, 2ka, 3k) completely abolished the ability of β2GPI to bind to CL-coated plates (Sheng et al., 1996). We found that, while the synthetic wild-type molecule was able to bind to EC, mutant 1k binding declined; in contrast, no binding at all was detected with 2k, 2ka and 3k mutants. Altogether, these data suggest that β2GPI binds to human endothelium by the major phospholipid-binding aminoacid sequence in the fifth domain. This observation was further supported by the reactivity of anti-β2GPI mAbs with EC incubated in the presence of the synthetic P1 peptide, spanning the aminoacid sequence of the phospholipid-binding activity. On the contrary, another peptide (P8), identical to P1 but not displaying any phospholipid-binding activity (because of the substitution of Cys^{281} and Cys^{288} with serine residues) did not bind to EC. Furthermore, polyclonal anti-β2GPI IgG fractions from patients with APS were also shown to recognize P1 adhered to endothelial monolayers (Del Papa et al., 1998).

Although the above-mentioned findings do support the adhesion of β2GPI to EC membranes, it is still not clear to which structures β2GPI binds. Since heparan sulphate (HS) – the major proteoglycan of the vascular endothelium – constitutes the majority of the endothelial anionic sites, we investigated whether HS could be involved in the binding of cationic β2GPI to HUVEC. Actually HUVEC monolayers pre-treated with heparitinase I, an enzyme able to cleave specifically the α-N-acetyl-D-glycosaminidic linkage in HS, significantly down-regulates their ability to bind β2GPI (Del Papa et al., unpublished data). It should be pointed out that the effect of heparitinase I on β2GPI binding was dose-dependent and that the highest enzyme concentrations produced an inhibition of up to 65 per cent. Taken together, these findings suggest that if it is true that HS is involved in β2GPI binding, endothelial structures other than HS might be also responsible for the cofactor adhesion.

Brain endothelium

The most common aPL-associated thromboocclusive event occurs in the central nervous system (CNS) (Coull et al., 1992) suggesting a selective susceptibility of CNS vascular endothelium to aPL. There is increasing evidence that EC are heterogeneous (Fajardo, 1989) and differ from organ to organ in their antigenic characteristics, secretion of prostaglandins, expression of adhesion molecules, and their thrombogenicity (Page et al., 1992). Hess et al. (1993) showed that sera from patients with stroke and aPL had increased IgG binding to cultured human microvascular brain endothelial cells (BEC) compared with healthy controls and a group of stroke patients without aPL (Hess et al., 1993). However the same authors could not find any difference in the binding activity to HUVEC or to BEC when sera from aPL-positive patients with cerebral vascular accidents (CVA) were compared with sera from aPL-positive patients without CVAs (Hess et al., 1993). Our own group recently observed the ability of human polyclonal and monoclonal anti-β2GPI antibodies to recognize the cofactor adhered to BEC and to induce a pro-adhesive and a pro-inflammatory cell phenotype (Del Papa, personal communication). Altogether these data demonstrate that: (i) β2GPI adhesion to cell membranes is a phenomenon common to both macro- and microvascular EC, and (ii) the binding of antibodies to the adhered cofactor is also able to activate EC from the microvasculature.

Interestingly, anti-β2GPI mAbs showed a significantly increased binding activity to BEC in comparison to HUVEC, suggesting a higher β2GPI adherence. In addition, at variance with HUVEC, the antibody cell-reactivity decreased but did not decline to background levels when BEC were cultured in serum-free medium (Del Papa et al., personal communication).

APL and vessel tone regulation

Antiphospholipid antibodies also appear to play a role in vessel tone regulation. In fact, recently, Atsumi et al. raised another interesting hypothesis that might support once again the disregulation of EC function (Atsumi et al., 1998). Actually, it has been demonstrated that plasma levels of endothelin-1 (ET-1) peptide, the most potent endothelium-derived contracting factor, correlated significantly with the history of arterial thrombosis in APS patients. In addition, the authors showed, in an in vitro study, that the treatment of EC monolayers with anti-β2GPI monoclonal antibodies induced the expression of ET-1 mRNA. These data suggest that the aPL-induced endothelial dysfunction might also be related to alterations of the vessel tone (especially in the arterial tree).

APL and endothelial apoptosis

It has been demonstrated that antiphospholipid antibodies bind to apoptotic cells, including EC (Goldman *et al.*, 1995). The exposure of plasma membrane phosphatidylserine (PS) on the cells undergoing apoptosis and the binding of antiphospholipid antibodies might be related (Fadok *et al.*, 1992). Moreover, several groups reported β2GPI binding to apoptotic cells (Casciola-Rosen *et al.*, 1996; Manfredi *et al.*, 1998a, b; Rouch *et al.*, 1998). Endothelial membrane-bound β2GPI, either by exposing cryptic epitopes after the formation of a complex with PS or by displaying high antigen density, would satisfy the requisites for the binding of β2GPI-dependent aPL or of antibodies specifically reacting with β2GPI. Conversely, it has been showed that aPL themselves were able to induce EC apoptosis (Nakamura *et al.*, 1994). Bordron *et al.* recently demonstrated that some but not all AECA can be responsible for PS exposure, using hypoploid cell enumeration, DNA fragmentation, optical and ultrastructural analyses to confirm EC apoptosis. Such data suggest a possible role for AECA to induce endothelial programmed cell death (Bordron *et al.*, 1998). In conclusion the authors hypothesized that the AECA-induced EC apoptosis could explain, at least in part, the association between AECA and aPL, since the latter could be produced after the exposure of PS (or PS/phospholipid-binding protein complexes) on apoptotic EC. However, only a minority of sera from APS patients were found to display such an activity in *in vitro* studies.

Annexin-V and aPL interactions

Recently, attention has been focussed on the interactions between aPL antibodies and annexin-V, a protein found in different tissues and also in blood, which displays a potent anti-coagulant activity based on its high affinity for anionic phospholipids. It has been shown, by Rand *et al.* (1997), that aPL IgG affect the *in vitro* binding of annexin-V both on cultured trophoblasts and on HUVEC, thus increasing the procoagulant activity of these cells (Rand *et al.*, 1997). In their study the authors showed a decrease in levels of annexin-V on the surface of vascular EC after exposure to aPL IgG. This reduction was followed by a shortening of plasma coagulation time. So, they suggested that when aPL are absent, a 'shield' of annexin-V can cover the negatively charged structures on the EC membranes (and trophoblast cells), thus inhibiting coagulation. Deposition of aPL or aPL/phospholipid-binding protein complexes on the cell membranes would displace such a shield, allowing negatively charged molecules to activate the coagulation cascade. Since β2GPI has been suggested to play a pivotal role in these events, these data further stress the importance of the binding of this 'phospholipid-cofactor' to cell membranes.

References

Atsumi, T., Khamashta, M.A., Haworth, R.S., Brooks, G., Amengual, O., Ichikawa, K., Koike, T. & Hughes, G.R.V. (1998): Arterial disease and thrombosis in the antiphospholipid syndrome: a pathogenic role for endothelin 1. *Arthritis Rheum.* **41,** 800–807.

Bordron, A., Dueymes, M., Levy, Y., Jamin, C., Ziporen, L., Piette, J.C., Shoenfeld, Y. & Youinou, P. (1998): Anti-endothelial cell antibody binding makes negatively charged phospholipids accessible to antiphospholipid antibodies. *Arthritis Rheum.* **41,** 1738–1747.

Bussolino, F., Breviario, F., Tetta, C., Aglietta, M., Mantovani, A. & Dejana, E. (1986): Interleukin-1 stimulates platelet-activating factor production in cultured human endothelial cells. *J. Clin. Invest.* **77,** 2027–2033.

Carlos, T.M. & Harlam, J.M. (1994): Leukocyte-endothelial adhesion molecule. *Blood* **84**, 2068–2101.

Carreras, L.O. & Martinuzzo, M.O. (1993): The lupus anticoagulant and eicosanoids. *Prostaglandins leukotrienes and essential fatty acids* **49**, 483–488.

Carreras, L.O., Defreyn, G. & Machin, S.J. (1981): Arterial thrombosis intrauterine death and 'lupus' anticoagulant. Detection of immunoglobulin interfering with prostacyclin formation. *Lancet* **i**, 244–246.

Carreras, L.O. & Vermylen, J.G. (1982): Lupus anticoagulant and thrombosis: possible role of inhibition of prostacyclin formation. *Thromb. Haemost.* **48**, 38–40.

Carreras, L.O., Martinuzzo, M.O. & Maclouf, J. (1996): Antiphospholipid antibodies, eicosanoids and expression of endothelial cyclooxygenase-2. *Lupus* **5** (Suppl.), 494–497.

Casciola-Rosen, L., Rosen, A., Petri, M. & Schlissel, M. (1996): Surface blebs on apoptotic cells are sites of enhanced pro-coagulant activity implications for coagulation events and antigenic spread in SLE. *Proc. Natl. Acad. Sci. USA* **93**, 1624–1629.

Cervera, R., Khamashta, M.A., Font, J., Ramirez, J., D'Cruz, D., Montalban, J., Lopez-Soto, A., Asherson, R.A., Ingelmo, M. & Hughes, G.R.V. (1991): Anti-endothelial cell antibodies in patients with the antiphospholipid syndrome. *Autoimmunity* **11**, 1–6.

Cines, D., Pollak, E., Buck, C. *et al.* (1998): Endothelial cells in physiology and in the pathophysiology of vascular disorders. *Blood* **91**, 3527–3561.

Coull, B.M., Levine, S.R. & Brey, R.L. (1992): The role of antiphospholipid antibodies and stroke. *Neurol. Clin.* **10**, 125–143.

Del Papa, N., Meroni, P.L., Tincani, A., Harris, E.N., Pierangeli, S.S., Barcellini, W., Borghi, M.O., Balestrieri, G. & Zanussi, C. (1992): Relationship between antiphospholipid and antiendothelial antibodies: further characterization of the reactivity on resting and cytokine-activated endothelial cells. *Clin. Exp. Rheum.* **10**, 37–42.

Del Papa, N., Conforti, G., Gambini, D., Barcellini, W., Borghi, M.O., Fain, C., Tincani, A., Balestrieri, G., Tedesco, F. & Meroni, P.L. (1993): Characterization of anti-endothelial cell antibodies in antiphospholipid syndrome. In: *Molecular bases of human diseases*, ed. E.E. Polli, pp. 67–74. Amsterdam: Excerpta Medica.

Del Papa, N., Conforti, G., Gambini, D., La Rosa, L., Tincani, A., D'Cruz, D., Khamashta, M., Hughes, G.R.V., Balestrieri, G. & Meroni, P.L. (1994): Characterization of the endothelial surface proteins recognized by anti-endothelial antibodies in primary and secondary autoimmune vasculitis. *Clin. Immunol. Immunopathol.* **70**, 211–216.

Del Papa, N., Guidali, L., Spatola, L., Bonara, P., Borghi, M.O., Tincani, A., Balestrieri, G. & Meroni, P.L. (1995): Relationship between antiphospholipid and anti-endothelial antibodies III: β2-glycoprotein I mediates the antibody binding to endothelial membranes and induces the expression of adhesion molecules. *Clin. Exp. Rheumatol.* **13**, 179–186.

Del Papa, N., Guidali, L., Sala, A., Buccellati, C., Khamashta, M.A., Ichikawa, K., Koike, T., Balestrieri, G., Tincani, A., Hughes, G.R.V. & Meroni, P.L. (1997): Endothelial cell as target for antiphospholipid antibodies. *Arthritis. Rheum.* **40**, 551–561.

Del Papa, N., Sheng, Y.H., Raschi, E., Kandiah, D.A., Tincani, A., Khamashta, M.A., Atsumi, T., Hughes, G.R.V., Ichikawa, K., Koike, T., Balestrieri, G., Krilis, S.A. & Meroni, P.L. (1998): Human β2-glycoprotein I binds to endothelial cells through a cluster of lysine residues that are critical for anionic phospholipid binding and offers epitopes for anti-β2-glycoprotein I antibodies. *J. Immunol.* 160: 5572–5578.

Dejana, E., Bazzoni, G., Martin-Padura, I., Walter, S. & Mantovani, A. (1991): Endothelial cells as targets for and producers of cytokines. In: *Vascular endothelium. Physiological basis of clinical problems*. New York and London: Plenum Press.

Esmon, C.T. (1989): The role of protein C and thrombomodulin in the regulation of blood coagulation. *J. Biol. Chem.* **264**, 4743–4746.

Esmon, C.T. (1995): Thrombomodulin as a model of molecular mechanisms that modulate protease specificy and function at the vessel surface. *FASEB J.* **9**, 946–955.

Fadok, V.A., Voelker, D.R., Campbell, P.A., Cohen, J.J., Bratton, D.L. & Henson, P.M. (1992): Exposure of phosphatidylserine on the surface of apoptotic lymphocytes triggers specific recognition and removal by macrophages. *J. Immunol.* **148,** 2207–2215.

Fajardo, L.F. (1989): The complexity of endothelial cells. *Am. J. Pathol.* **92,** 241–250.

Furchgott, R.F. & Zawadzki, J.V. (1980): The obligatory role of endothelial cells in the relaxation of arterial smooth muscle by acetylcholine. *Nature* **228,** 373–376.

George, J., Blank, M., Levy, Y., Meroni, P.L., Damianovich, M., Tincani, A. & Shoenfeld, Y. (1998): Differential effects of anti-beta 2 glycoprotein I antibodies on endothelial cells and on the manifestations of experimental antiphospholipid syndrome. *Circulation* **97,** 900–906.

Goldman, D., Philips, G., Back, K. & Petri, M. (1995): Binding of SLE antibodies on apoptotic cells. *Arthritis Rheum.* **38** (Suppl.), S214 (Abstract).

Gramse, M., Breviario, F., Pintucci, G., Millet, I. & Dejana, E. (1986): Enhancement by interleukin-1 (IL-1) of plasminogen activator inhibitor (PA-I) activity in cultured human endothelial cells. *Biochem. Biophys. Res. Commun.* **139,** 720–727.

Habib, A., Martinuzzo, M., Carreras, L.O., Levy-Toledano, S. & Maclouf, J. (1995): Increased expression of inducible cyclooxygenase-2 in human endothelial cells by antiphospholipid antibodies. *Thrombosis Haemost.* **74,** 770–777.

Hasselaar, P., Derksen, R.H.W., Blokzjil, L. & De Groot, P.G. (1990): Cross-reactivity of antibodies directed against cardiolipin, DNA, endothelial cells and blood platelets. *Thromb. Haemost.* **63,** 169–173.

Hatton, M.W.C., Berry, L.R. & Regoeczi, E. (1978): Inhibition of thrombin by antithrombin III in presence of certain glycosaminoglycans found in the mammalian aorta. *Thomb. Res.* **13,** 655–670.

Hess, D.C., Shepard, J.C. & Adams, R.J. (1993): Increased immunoglobulin binding to cerebral endothelium in patients with aPL. *Stroke* **24,** 994–999.

Hughes, G.R.V. (1998): Hughes' syndrome: The antiphospholipid syndrome. A historical view. *Lupus* **7** (Suppl), S1–4.

Hunt, J.E. & Krilis, S.A. (1994): The fifth domain of β2-glycoprotein I contains a phospholipid binding site (Cys ^{281}-Cys ^{288}) and a region recognized by anti-cardiolipin antibodies. *J. Immunol.* **152,** 653–661.

Hunt, J.E., Simpson, R.J. & Krilis, S.A. (1993): Identification of a region of β2-glycoprotein I critical for lipid binding and anti-cardiolipin antibody cofactor activity. *Proc. Natl. Acad. Sci. USA* **90,** 2141–2149.

Kandhia, D.A. & Krilis, S.A. (1994): Beta 2-glycoprotein. *Lupus* **3** (Suppl.), 207–212.

Kaplanski, G. (1996): Increased serum soluble VCAM-1 in the antiphospholipid syndrome. *Lupus* **5** (Suppl.), S548 (Abstract).

Khamashta, M.A., Harris, E.N., Gharavi, A.E., Derue, G., Gil, A., Vasquez, J.J. & Hughes, G.R.V. (1988): Immune-mediated mechanisms for thrombosis: antiphospholipid antibody binding to platelet membranes. *Ann. Rheum. Dis.* **47,** 849–852.

La Rosa, L., Meroni, P.L., Tincani, A., Balestrieri, G., Faden, A., Lojacono, A., Morassi, L., Brocchi, E., Del Papa, N., Gharavi, A.E., Sammaritano, L. & Lockshin, M.D. (1994): β2-glycoprotein I and placental anti-coagulant protein I in placentae from patients with antiphospholipid syndrome *J. Rheumatol.* **21,** 1684–1698.

Le Roux, G., Wautier, M.P., Guillevin, L. & Wautier, J.L. (1986): IgG binding to endothelial cells in systemic lupus erythematosus. *Thromb. Haemost.* **56,** 144–146.

Le Tonqueze, M., Salozhin, K., Dueymes, M., Piette, J.C., Lovalev, V., Shoenfeld, Y., Nassonov, E. & Youinou, P. (1995): Role of β2-glycoprotein I in the antiphospholipid antibody binding to endothelial cells. *Lupus* **4,** 179–186.

Lellouche, F., Martinuzzo, M.E., Said, P., Maclouf, J. & Carreras, L.O. (1991): Imbalance of thromboxane/prostacyclin biosynthesis in patients with lupus anticoagulant. *Blood* **78,** 2894–2899.

Manfredi, A.A., Rovere, P. Galati, G., Heltai, S., Bozzolo, E., Soldini, L., Davoust, J., Balestrieri, G., Tincani, A. & Sabbadini, M.G. (1998a): Apoptotic cell clearance in systemic lupus erythematosus. I. Opsonization by antiphospholipid antibodies. *Arthritis Rheum.* **40**, 205–214.

Manfredi AA, Rovere P, Heltai S, Galati G, Nebbia G, Tincani A, Balestrieri G, Sabbadini MG (1998b): Apoptotic cell clearance in systemic lupus erythematosus. II. Role of β2-glycoprotein I. *Arthritis. Rheum.* **40** (2), 215–222.

McCrae, K.R., De Michele, A., Samuels, P., Roth, D., Kuo, A., Meg, Q.H., Rauch, J. & Cines, D.A. (1991): Detection of endothelial cell reactive immunoglobulin in patients with antiphospholipid antibodies. *Br. J. Haematol.* **79**, 595–605.

McIntyre, J.A. (1992): Immune recognition at the maternal-fetal interface: overview. *Am. J. Reprod. Immunol.* **28**, 127–131.

Nakamura, N., Shidara, Y., Kawaguchi, N., Azuma, C., Mitsuda, N., Onishi, S., Yamaji, K., Wada, Y. (1994): Lupus anticoagulant autoantibody induces apoptosis in HUVEC: involvement of annexin-V. *Biochem. Byophys. Res. Commun.* **205**, 1488–1493.

Nawrot, P. & Stern, D. (1987): Endothelial cell procoagulant properties and the host response. *Semin. Thromb. Hemost.* **13**, 391–398.

Nawrot, P.P., Handley, D.A., Esmond, C.T. & Stern, D.M. (1986): Interleukin-1 induces endothelial cells procoagulant while suppressing cell-surface anticoagulant activity. *Proc. Natl. Acad. Sci. USA* **83**, 4360–4364.

Page, C., Rose, M., Yacoub, M. & Pigott, R. (1992): Antigenic heterogeneity of vascular endothelium. *Am. J. Pathol.* **14**, 673–683.

Pierangeli, S., Colden-Stanfield, M., Liu, X. & Harris, E.N. (1998): Antiphospholipid antibodies activate endothelial cells *in vitro* and *in vivo*. *Lupus* **7** (Suppl.), S179 (Abstract).

Plow, E.F. *et al.* (1995): The biology of the plasminogen system. *FASEB J.* **9**, 939–945.

Rand, J.H., Wu, X.X., Andree, H.A.M., Lockwood, C.J., Guller, S., Scher, J. & Harpel, P.C. (1997): Pregnancy loss in the antiphospholipid-antibody syndrome – a possible thrombogenic mechanism. *N. Engl. J. Med.* **337**, 154–160.

Rosenbaum, J., Pottinger, B.E., Woo, P., Black, C.M., Louzou, S., Byron, M.A. & Pearson, J.D. (1988): Measurement and characterization of circulating anti-endothelial cell IgG in connective tissue diseases. *Clin. Exp. Immunol.* **72**, 450–456.

Roubey, R.A.S. (1998): Mechanisms of autoantibody-mediated thrombosis. *Lupus* **7** (Suppl.), S114–119.

Rouch, J., Subang, R., Koh, J.S. & Levine, J.S. (1998): Induction of antiphospholipid antibodies by β2-glycoprotein I bound to apoptotic thymocytes. *Lupus* **7** (Suppl.), 66.

Sheng, Y., Sali, A., Herzog, H., Lahnstein, J. & Krilis, S. (1996): Site-directed mutagenesis of recombinant human β2-glycoprotein I identifies a cluster of lysine residues that are critical for phospholipid binding and anti-cardiolipin antibody activity. *J. Immunol.* **157**, 3744–3751.

Simantov, R., LaSala, J.M., Lo, S.K., Gharavi, A.E., Sammaritano, L.R., Salmon, J.E. & Silverstein, R.L. (1995): Activation of cultured vascular endothelial cells by antiphospholipid antibodies. *J. Clin. Invest.* **96**, 2211–2219.

Vismara, A., Meroni, P.L., Tincani, A., Harris, E.N., Barcellini, W., Brucato, A., Khamashta, M.A., Hughes, G.R.V., Zanussi, C. & Balestrieri, G. (1988): Antiphospholipid antibodies and endothelial cells. *Clin. Exp. Immunol.* **74**, 247–253.

Weksler, B.B., Marcus, A.S. & Jaffe, E.A. (1977): Synthesis of prostaglandin I_2 (prostacyclin) by a cultured human and bovine endothelial cells. *Proc. Natl. Acad. Sci. USA* **74**, 3922–3926.

Chapter 17

Central nervous system vasculitis

Maurizia Rasura, Alexia Anzini and Cesare Fieschi

First Neurological Clinic, Department of Neurosciences, University of Rome 'La Sapienza', viale dell'Università 30, 00185 Rome, Italy

Summary

Vasculitis is a clinicopathologic descriptive term for a heterogeneous group of relatively rare diseases characterized by various types of inflammation and necrosis of vessel walls leading to ischaemic and thrombotic events – or to rupture of aneurysm formation, resulting in haemorrhage. Vasculitis may be a primary, independent inflammation of blood vessels, or a component of a systemic condition, such as an infectious disease. Virtually any type of blood vessel anywhere in the body may be affected. The specific vasculitic manifestations and complications in a given case depend on whether the disease pattern is slow or fulminant, local or general; on the number of organ systems involved; on the size of most of the vessels involved; and on the predominant cell type in the inflammatory process. In many respects vasculitic syndromes are among the most variable and complex of inflammatory diseases. For years this diversity has caused difficulties in classifying and standardizing the vasculitides. One approach to classifying nonfectious vasculitides categorizes them, in part, on the basis of the predominant type of vessel affected. There is, however, substantial overlap among different vasculitides, and the type of vessel involved is merely one of many features that must be determined before a diagnosis can be reached.

The usual symptoms are mental confusion, delirium and seizures rather than the more focal symptoms that usually characterize stroke due to infarction or haemorrhage. Arteriograms are often normal, since in many cases involved arteries are too small to be imaged by conventional angiography. When the vessels seen on angiogram are involved, the multiple successive stenoses ('beading') consistent with arteritis are not specific for the diagnosis. In the end, brain biopsy to examine the meningeal and cortical vessels may be the key to diagnosis.

Treatment of vasculitides is generally with variable doses of corticosteroids and immunosuppressants. Prednisone (oral) and methylprednisolone (usually intravenous) are the most commonly used corticosteroids. Cyclophosphamide is one of the most potent drugs available to treat severe, life-threatening vasculitis. It is administered as oral or intravenous single daily dose regimen or as intravenous pulse therapy. Although general treatment guidelines can be suggested, treatment should be individualized for each vasculitic syndrome.

Vasculitides are a very heterogeneous group of multisystem disorders characterized by an immunomediated pathologic process involving blood vessel walls with inflammation and necrosis and, ultimately, with stenosis of the lumen and ischaemia of perfused tissues. Vessels of any type in any organ can be affected, a fact that results in a wide variety of signs and symptoms. Clinical expression depends on the site, type and size of involved vessels, and the severity of the associated inflammatory features. These protean clinical manifestations, combined with the aetiologic non-specificity of the histologic lesions, complicate the diagnosis of specific forms of vasculitis. This is problematic because different vasculitides with indistinguishable clinical presentations have very different prognoses and treatments.

Within the spectrum of vascular inflammatory diseases, vasculitis affecting the central nervous system (CNS) is traditionally viewed as one of the most challenging clinical problems. The reasons for this include: lack of specificity of associated signs and symptoms, inaccessibility of the end organ tissues for pathologic examination, lack of efficient noninvasive diagnostic tests and the relative rarity of the disorders (Fieschi et al., 1998).

The cerebral vasculature has unique characteristics that serve to protect the internal milieu of the CNS. The physical characteristics of the CNS vessels depend upon two functionally different systems: the blood-brain barrier and the blood-cerebrospinal fluid barrier. The natural and experimental acute inflammatory response in many types of injury to the brain differs from that of other tissues. Rapid recruitment of neutrophils to the site of injury is almost absent and monocytic response is delayed by several days. Furthermore, leukocyte adhesion to vessel walls and migration into the parenchyma are decreased in the CNS compared with other tissues.

It is widely believed that several CNS vasculitides are explained by one of three possible basic immune mechanisms. First, immune complexes may form at the arterial wall, activating complement components with accumulation of polymorphonuclear leukocytes, whose enzymes damage the vessel wall. Alternatively, circulating immune complexes may be deposited in vessel walls. Second, a direct attack on the vessel wall may occur from antibodies, but this possibility is still unproven. Third, cell-mediated immune reactions may be present in many of the primary vasculitides, in which endothelial cells act as antigen-presenting cells with a response of T-cells. Current hypotheses also include a possible role of perivascular microglial cells and smooth muscle cells in immune interactions bearing on the vessel wall. The histologic structure of granulomas also suggests a participation of monocytes and macrophages. Antiphospholipid antibodies, such as lupus anticoagulant and anticardiolipin antibodies, although associated with a thrombotic tendency, may be markers for vasculitis.

Vasculitides can be primary (a major manifestation of a disease process) or secondary (associated with an infection or a connective tissue disease). Primary vasculitides, without identifiable underlying pathogenesis, are further divided on the basis of the distribution of clinical features and the pattern of histologic abnormalities. Involvement can be widespread, involving multiple organ systems. Neurological involvement may include both the peripheral nervous system (PNS) and the CNS. CNS complications of vasculitis are not uncommon and carry with them significant morbidity and mortality if not recognized early and treated aggressively.

Nearly all vasculitides can entail significant CNS involvement, but this is most common in isolated angiitis of the CNS (IACNS) and Takayasu's arteritis (Cohen Tervaert & Kallenberg, 1993). In both of these disorders the CNS is affected early and, especially in IACNS, is typically the only organ affected. In the remaining disorders, CNS involvement is more variable and tends not to be present at the onset of the illness. CNS involvement is rarely the only site affected in these other diseases and the PNS is more often affected (Moore & Cupps, 1983; Moore & Fauci, 1981).

In recent years there has been substantial progress in identifying the attributes of specific types of vasculitis that allow accurate diagnosis. One approach to classifying non-infectious vasculitides categorizes them, in part, on the basis of the predominant type of vessel affected (Table 1) (Jennette et al., 1994; Jennette & Falk, 1997). There is, however, substantial overlap among different vasculitides, and the type of vessel involved is merely one of many features that must be determined before a diagnosis can be obtained.

Table 1. Major categories of non-infectious vasculitis

Large-vessel vasculitis

Giant-cell arteritis
Takayasu's arteritis

Medium-sized-vessel vasculitis

Polyarteritis nodosa
Kawasaki's disease
Primary granulomatous central nervous system vasculitis

Small-vessel vasculitis

ANCA-associated small-vessel vasculitis
    Microscopic polyangiitis
    Wegener's granulomatosis
    Churg-Strauss syndrome
    Drug-induced ANCA-associated vasculitis

Immune complex small-vessel vasculitis
    Henoch-Schonlein purpura
    Cryoglobulinaemic vasculitis
    Lupus vasculitis
    Rheumatoid vasculitis
    Sjogren's syndrome vasculitis
    Hypocomplementaemic urticarial vasculitis
    Behçet's disease
    Goodpasture's syndrome
    Serum-sickness vasculitis
    Drug-induced immune-complex vasculitis
    Infection-induced immune-complex vasculitis

Paraneoplastic small-vessel vasculitis
    Lymphoproliferative neoplasm-induced vasculitis
    Myeloproliferative neoplasm-induced vasculitis
    Carcinoma induced vasculitis

Inflammatory bowel disease vasculitis

The diagnostic approach is defined by three salient clinical features: (1) many but not all of the disorders are serious; (2) many imply an extensive differential diagnosis that includes equally serious and potentially treatable alternative disorders; (3) treatment has a major impact on outcome but involves long-term administration of drugs with serious risks and side effects. Consequently, it is important to make a definitive diagnosis which depends on a combination of clinical, radiographic, and pathologic features; the gold standard is confirmation of vasculitis in a biopsy specimen. Treatment is always far more effective when initiated early in the disease course. Thus, definitive diagnostic evaluation should be obtained as quickly as possible.

CNS manifestations of vasculitis may be acute, subacute or insidious, and are frequently non-specific. The symptoms of CNS involvement may include: recurrent headache, transient visual loss, transient or progressive weakness, cranial neuropathy, dementia; patients may present either diffuse or focal/multifocal cortical dysfunction. Diffuse dysfunction manifests as subacute memory loss, acute encephalopathy, behavioural changes or seizures; focal disturbances may occur anywhere along the neuraxis and may affect both grey and white matter structures.

All patients with suspected CNS vasculitis should undergo neuroimaging, cerebrospinal fluid (CSF) analysis and, if necessary, brain biopsy. CSF analysis may be normal or demonstrate elevations in the protein and/or the cell count. In general, if the cell count is elevated this is predominantly due to increases in lymphocytes. Further studies such as viral, bacterial, fungal and mycobacterial cultures, as well as cytology, may need to be performed if infection or neoplasm is suspected. Although brain biopsy remains the 'gold standard', a presumptive diagnosis of cerebral vasculitis can be made using neuroimaging studies. Besides, because involvement is frequently diffuse, the presence of a negative biopsy result does not entirely exclude the diagnosis of vasculitis.

Cerebral angiography provides useful and supportive, but not diagnostic evidence of CNS vasculitis. Angiography does not distinguish among several types of vasculopathy. In addition, vasculitis may not be identified in an angiogram particularly when only small vessels are affected, and so it is also for magnetic resonance angiography. However, characteristic abnormalities include segmental narrowing, dilatation, occlusions, collateral formation, microaneurysms and vascular beading (multiple successive stenoses corresponding to focal or segmental lesions of arteritis); but these are all non-specific findings indistinguishable from non-vasculitic intracranial atherosclerosis, vasospasm, mycotic aneurysms, emboli, or tumour. Serial cerebral angiography can be used however to monitor disease progression before and after therapy. Cranial MRI and CT adequately delineate tissue damage secondary to vasculitis but they do not detect early vasculitis, predict histologic features, or distinguish underlying causes; MRI findings suggestive of vasculitis are generally multifocal, bilateral, and involve grey and white matter.

Giant-cell arteritis

Also known as temporal arteritis, cranial arteritis, or Horton's disease, is an inflammatory disease that affects the medium- and large-sized arteries throughout the body, including the aorta and most of its major branches, and sparing the capillaries and veins; this is a systemic form of necrotizing vasculitis histologically characterized by the formation of giant cells. The pattern of pathologic involvement is usually patchy, so that severe arteritis and normal vessel wall may be found side by side in a single biopsy specimen. Generally, different stages of the vasculitic process are found in the same patient, ranging from inflammatory infiltrates in the media with mononuclear cells, fragmentation of the internal elastic lamina, and necrosis of the total vessel wall due to aneurysm formation or narrowing due to fibrosis and proliferation. The disease could be rightly termed extracranial, as intracranial lesions are exceptional once the arteries have pierced the dura. Perhaps the paucity of elastic tissue in the intracranial arteries is the explanation.

Giant-cell arteritis is not a rare disease, the incidence ranging between 0.35 and 21.5 per 100,000 inhabitants per year. The seventh and eighth decades are the most common age for this disease; before the age of 50 years, temporal arteritis is very uncommon. There is a dramatic increase in incidence with age. Women are affected two to three times as often as men.

The presenting symptoms of temporal arteritis are: headache, jaw claudication, polymyalgia rheumatica (a syndrome of limb girdle muscle pain and stiffness); despite its name, it is a systemic disease and consequently, even when not associated with polymyalgia (as it is in 50 per cent of cases), cranial manifestations are typically accompanied by systemic symptoms including malaise, fever, anorexia, weight loss, arthralgias, myalgias, depression, or even flu-like symptoms. Most patients with giant-cell arteritis have symptoms of polymyalgia rheumatica for weeks to months before developing headache, jaw claudication, or visual loss (Ostberg, 1973). On clinical examination, patients may show a thickened, swollen, nodular and tender superficial temporal artery. Involvement of other larger vessels may be identifiable by bruits or pulse and blood pressure differences. Claudication of the tongue and/or pharyngeal muscles and necrosis of the scalp or the tongue may also occur. The headache of temporal arteritis reflects persistent ischaemia of pain-sensitive structures; consequently, it tends to be persistent, asymmetric if not unilateral, especially common at night and interfering with sleep. It is located predominantly in the temporal area, but may radiate to the scalp, face, jaw or occiput (Hamilton et al., 1971). The symptom most likely to bring the patient into a neurological emergency ward is amaurosis fugax; it reflects retinal or choroidal ischaemia and imminent and almost irreversible loss of vision in one or both eyes. This is an emergency situation requiring prompt diagnostic and therapeutic action. Frequently, the disease affects both eyes and therapeutic intervention is directed at saving the remaining eye. Ophthalmoscopic signs of anterior ischaemic optic neuropathy may precede visual loss by 1 or 2 days. Therapy must be started when the diagnosis is suspected and must not be delayed pending the results of the biopsy.

The patients with giant-cell arteritis may be at higher risk for stroke during the active phase of their disease and it may occur as the first indication of the disease. In a brief report of a necropsy series, Missen (1972) noted that obstruction of the arterial lumen due to giant-cell arteritis was 'three times as frequent in the vertebral arteries as in the internal carotids' and that 'infarction was found more often in the hind-brain than in the forebrain'.

Diagnosis of vasculitis depends on a combination of clinical, radiographic and pathologic features. The gold standard in diagnosis is confirmation of vasculitis in a biopsy specimen. Biopsy of the superficial temporal artery or less commonly the occipital artery is the most helpful diagnostic procedure and may be performed after starting steroid therapy, but it plays a minimal role in patients with clinically likely disease; its major value is in patients in whom temporal arteritis enters into the differential diagnosis but is thought unlikely on clinical grounds. Due to the segmental nature of the inflammatory foci (skip lesions) the biopsy should be generous and multiple histopathological sections should be examined because a normal temporal artery biopsy does not exclude the diagnosis of giant-cell arteritis; abnormalities of the superficial temporal artery are common in the elderly; therefore, a biopsy should be considered diagnostic only if there is evidence of a chronic granulomatous infiltrate. Doppler sonography of branches of the superficial temporal artery may disclose segmental stenosis and help to find the artery in severe stenosis and thus may be useful for selecting the site for biopsy.

For diagnosis the most common laboratory abnormality in patients with giant-cell arteritis is a markedly elevated erythrocyte sedimentation rate (ESR), reflecting the systemic nature of the disease. However, a normal ESR does not exclude the diagnosis (Wong & Korn, 1986). Most patients have a mild to moderate normochromic or slightly hypochromic anaemia. White blood cell counts are normal or moderately elevated.

Angiographic signs are infrequently present. The superficial temporal arteriogram may demonstrate areas of dilatation and constriction along the length of the artery. Changes may also be seen in the internal carotid artery siphon segments.

Ideally, the therapy of each vasculitis should focus on the specific immunologic mechanism causing the disease. Such specific interventions are not yet available. In general the agents currently available induce global immunosuppression.

Once the diagnosis of giant-cell arteritis is suspected, the patient should be started on steroids, the treatment of choice. An initial dose of 40 to 60 mg/day of prednisone is recommended for the first month, or until symptoms of the disease are controlled (Huston & Hunder, 1980). Symptoms usually respond promptly to steroids, although visual loss and stroke may occur after the beginning of treatment. Steroids may be tapered while monitoring symptoms and the ESR. There is controversy over the duration of therapy but normally the treatment must be continued for at least 12 months and maintenance with low steroid dosage (5–10 mg prednisone per day) is recommended for 18–24 months. Given the side effects of corticosteroids, physicians and patients wish to use them for the shortest necessary period of time, but rapid tapering is thought to lead to relapse more often than very slow tapering. Usually it is possible to reduce the corticosteroid dose to about 20–40 mg daily over a period of 8–12 weeks. Recurrence of symptoms or elevation of the ESR after initial control of the disease indicates relapse and should prompt resumption of higher doses of steroids. The relapse rates after withdrawal of steroid therapy bore little relationship to the duration of treatment (Andersson *et al.*, 1986). Alternate-day treatment regimens are felt to be less effective than daily administration of steroids, and carry not only the risk of relapses but also of blindness in the other eye.

Takayasu's arteritis

Takayasu's arteritis (pulseless disease, idiopathic aortitis) is a large-vessel granulomatous chronic arteritis that affects the aorta, its main branches, and occasionally the pulmonary artery. Most cases have been reported from Asia, but the disease is found world-wide. It generally occurs in young female patients who initially present with a fever and non-specific systemic complaints. In fact it is characterized by an initial inflammatory stage associated with systemic symptoms that overlap to one degree or another with a later obliterative phase defined by manifestations of ischaemia. Over weeks to months, this pre-pulseless phase ends and the effect of the vasculitis becomes apparent with the pulseless phase of the illness. Claudication and other symptoms/signs of large artery insufficiency develop, such as hypertension secondary to renal artery stenosis or stroke with CNS involvement (Nasu, 1975). Ischaemic symptoms are produced through stenosis rather than thrombosis and embolism and the patients more often present with orthostatic syncope or presyncope, occasionally with ischaemic retinopathy (Hall *et al.*, 1985). Brachial pressures and pulses are frequently asymmetric, and there may be asymmetry between pressures in the arms and legs.

The early inflammatory phase of the disease may be characterized by a mild normochromic, normocytic anaemia, modest leukocytosis, elevated ESR, and hypergammaglobulinaemia. Aortic arteriography is the definitive diagnostic procedure. It may need to be repeated later to monitor the progress of the disease and the need for continued treatment. Ultrasonography, MR imaging and MR angiography (MRA) provide useful noninvasive means of monitoring disease progress (Sun *et al.*, 1996). Characteristic angiographic abnormalities include irregular vessel walls, stenoses or occlusions, poststenotic dilatation, aneurysm formation, and evidence of increased collateral circulation, often with pronounced neovascularization.

Treatment is most beneficial during the early, inflammatory phase of the illness and usually consists of high dose daily oral corticosteroids which can be tapered over months to years. Other immunosuppressive agents (cyclophosphamide) have been used in combination with and to spare steroids, which are then tapered gradually over several months to years after signs of inflammation have resolved. Relapses are common and require retreatment also with a combination of these modalities (Shelhamer *et al.*, 1985). Regression of carotid stenosis has been reported after administration of corticosteroids (Ishikawa & Yonekawa, 1987). A variety of surgical reconstructive and bypass procedures have been employed, including extracranial-intracranial bypass with saphenous vein grafts and femoral artery to internal carotid artery bypass using synthetic grafts (Yamamoto *et al.*, 1984).

Primary angiitis of the central nervous system

Primary CNS vasculitis was first described by Harbitz (1922). The terms non-infectious granulomatous angiitis involving the CNS, granulomatous angiitis of the brain (GAB), granulomatous angiitis of the nervous system (GANS), giant-cell arteritis involving small meningeal and intracerebral vessels, isolated angiitis of the CNS (IACNS), and primary angiitis of the CNS (PACNS), have all been used interchangeably in the past.

It is by definition an idiopathic recurrent inflammatory disease of the small-and medium-sized vessels, confined to the brain and the spinal cord circulation. Mononuclear infiltrates with some accompanying polymorphonuclear cells are usually to be found. Different stages of the vasculitis with and without infiltrates and necrosis may be seen in the same patient at the time of examination, supporting the view that IACNS is a recurrent and progressive vasculitis. Because of the variability in the pathology, the presentation is protean and often presents a major diagnostic challenge.

The disease affects both sexes at all ages, with a peak incidence in the 40- to 60-year range. Persisting headaches and the signs and symptoms of encephalopathy with personality changes, cognitive disorders, and memory disturbances are the most frequent presenting symptoms of the disease and follow a more insidious course, with relapses and slowly progressive cognitive disorder. Confusional states, drowsiness, stupour, seizures, focal deficits resulting from recurrent cerebral ischaemia and cranial nerve involvement (e.g. hemiplegia, aphasia, hemianopia), elevated intracranial pressure with papilloedema, and myelopathy are possible. Systemic manifestations, such as arthralgias, myalgias or fever are usually absent, but if present are mild.

None of the standard laboratory tests are diagnostic for granulomatous angiitis, and normal findings do not exclude the diagnosis. There are no consistent haematologic or serologic abnormalities, no inflammatory signs; the ESR is normal. There are no detectable immunocomplexes, autoantibodies, or antibodies against bacteria, fungi, or viruses. The CSF usually shows increased protein content, and a lymphocytic pleocytosis occurs. Despite the frequent CSF findings, the examination can be normal. Imaging studies in early stages of the disease may be normal. Most imaging studies reveal focal abnormalities of gray or white matter, usually with a regional preponderance and asymmetric distribution within the brain. There may be diffuse lobar or hemispheric oedema, a poorly defined tumour-like mass, contrast enhancement of lesions, and focal or multifocal haemorrhage.

Cerebral angiography demonstrates vascular abnormalities only when there is macrovascular involvement, approximately 40 per cent of cases. MRA provides a useful noninvasive screening tool, but usually the greater resolution of conventional angiography is required. Angiographic abnormalities typically consist of fairly abrupt irregularities and segmental constrictions and ectasia (beading) in major vessels or their branches. This pattern is a non-specific sign that may be seen in a variety of vasculitides and other conditions; in fact, similar abnormalities are consistently seen in reversible cerebral vasospasm and provide the basis for the misdiagnosis of vasculitis in these patients. Furthermore, the clinical context and the typically more disseminated arteriographic abnormalities of reversible cerebral vasospasm help to distinguish it.

Because of the size of the differential diagnosis of PACNS (Table 2), the existence of many alternative disorders with specific treatments, and the usually non-diagnostic results of conventional neurodiagnostic studies, brain biopsy should be viewed as mandatory. One major problem with brain biopsy is that almost certainly there are a number of undefined inflammatory disorders mimicking PACNS.

Table 2. Differential diagnosis of central nervous system vasculitis

Vasculitis: idiopathic	
	Systemic vasculitis (polyarteritis nodosa, Churg-Strauss syndrome, Wegener's granulomatosis)
	Behçet's disease
	Isolated angiitis of the central nervous system
Vasculitis: secondary	
	Infections (fungi, viral, bacterial, treponemal, mycobacterial)
	Neoplasia (Hodgkin's lymphoma, paraneoplastic)
	Toxins (amphetamines, cocaine)
	Collagen vascular disease (systemic lupus erythematosus, Sjogren's syndrome, rheumatoid arthritis)
Vasculopathy	
	Amyloidosis
	Postirradiation
	Fibromuscular dysplasia
	Neoplasia (lymphoma)
	Degenerative (systemic lupus erythematosus)
Coagulopathy	
	Thrombotic thrombocytopenic purpura (TTP)
	Hyperviscosity
	Antiphospholipid/cardiolipin antibody (systemic lupus erythematosus)
	Anti factor VII antibody
	Paraproteinaemia
	Sickle cell disease

There is no standard treatment. Progression of the disease and death have frequently occurred despite treatment. Until recently, therapy for patients with PACNS has been a combination of corticosteroids and cyclophosphamide but the recognition of clinical heterogeneity among patients with PACNS suggests that not all patients with PACNS should be treated in the same manner. It is possible to gauge therapy based upon the clinical picture. For patients with a histologically based diagnosis of chronic progressive inflammatory disease, we advocate combined therapy using corticosteroids and cyclophosphamide, which is continued for at least 6 to 12 months after the patient is in remission.

In conclusion, the treatment of most forms of systemic vasculitis can be divided into three phases.

The *acute phase* of therapy refers to the brief time during the initial attempt to control the disease, where the highest level of immunosuppression is needed. But the treatment requires consideration of both disease-specific and patient-specific factors. Diseases that are limited in their severity and activity may require little or no therapy at all. Alternatively, life-threatening or rapidly progressive vasculitic disease, particularly involving the renal, cardiovascular, pulmonary, or CNS, generally requires high-dose glucocorticoids (GC). The decision to administer GC by a single daily dose, split, or pulse therapy with or without combination cytotoxic therapy depends on the individual situation. In rapidly progressive diseases, therapy should be initiated with intravenous pulse GC therapy, consisting of three daily infusions of 1000 mg of methylprednisone. In hyperacute and immediately life-threatening disease both GC and cytotoxic drugs should be administered intravenously to avoid the uncertainty of bioavailability. During the *subacute phase* there is tapering of the intense phase of immunosuppressive therapy while attempting to limit treatment- and disease-associated comorbidity. During the *consolidation phase* of therapy, efforts are aimed at minimizing long-term treatment-related toxicity and ultimately the discontinuation of immunosuppressive therapy.

Finally, one of the greatest pitfalls in the long-term management of any form of vasculitis is the failure to recognize when the disease becomes inactive. Patients with vasculitis involving the central or peripheral nervous systems are particularly challenging because of the limited capacity of these end-organs to regenerate. Every effort should therefore be made to find reliable surrogate markers of disease activity, but this task is also often frustrating.

References

Andersson, R., Malmvall, B.E. & Bengtsson, B.A. (1986): Long-term corticosteroid treatment in giant-cell arteritis. *Acta Med. Scand.* **220,** 465.

Cohen Tervaert, J.W. & Kallenberg, C. (1993): Neurologic manifestations of systemic vasculitides. *Rheum. Dis. Clin. North Am.* **19,** 913–40.

Fieschi, C., Rasura, M., Anzini, A. & Beccia, M. (1998): Central nervous system vasculitis. *J. Neurol. Sciences* **153,** 159–171.

Hall, S., Barr, W., Lie, J.T., Stanson, A.W., Kazmier, F.J. & Hunder, G.G. (1985): Takayasu's arteritis: a study of 32 North American patients. *Medicine (Baltimore)* **64,** 89.

Hamilton, C.R., Shelley, W.M. & Tumulty, P.A. (1971): Giant-cell arteritis: including temporal arteritis and polymyalgia rheumatica. *Medicine (Baltimore)* **50,** 1.

Harbitz, F. (1922): Unknown forms of arteritis with special reference to their relation to syphilitic arteritis and periarteritis nodosa. *Am. J. Med. Sci.* **163,** 250.

Huston, K.A. & Hunder, G.G. (1980): Giant-cell (cranial) arteritis: a clinical review. *Am. Heart J.* **100,** 99.

Ishikawa, K. & Yonekawa, Y. (1987): Regression of carotid stenoses after corticosteroid therapy in occlusive thromboaortopathy (Takayasu's disease). *Stroke* **18,** 677.

Jennette, J.C. & Falk, R.J. (1997): Small-vessel vasculitis. *New Engl. J. Med.* **337,** 1512–1523.

Jennette, J.C., Falk, R.J., Andrassy, K., Bacon, P.A., Churg, J., Gross, W.L., Hagen, E.C., Hoffman, G.S., Hunder, G.G. & Kallenberg, C.G. (1994): Nomenclature of systemic vasculitides: proposal of an international consensus conference. *Arthritis Rheum.* **37,** 187–92.

Missen, G.A. (1972): Involvement of the vertebrocarotid arterial system in giant-cell arteritis. *J. Pathol.* **106,** ii.

Moore, P.M. & Cupps, T.R. (1983): Neurologic complications of vasculitis. *Ann. Neurol.* **14,** 155–167.

Moore, P.M. & Fauci, A.S. (1981): Neurological manifestations of systemic vasculitis: a retrospective and prospective study of the clinicopathologic features and responses to therapy in 25 patients. *Am. J. Med.* **71,** 517–524.

Nasu, T. (1975): Takayasu's truncoarteritis in Japan: a statistical observation of 76 autopsy cases. *Pathol. Microbiol.* **43,** 140.

Ostberg, G. (1973): On arteritis with special reference to polymyalgia arteritica. *Acta Pathol. Microbiol. Scand.* **237** (Suppl. A), 1.

Shelhamer, J.H., Volkman, D.J., Parrillo, J.E., Lawley, T.J., Johnston, M.R. & Fauci, A.S. (1985): Takayasu's arteritis and its therapy. *Ann. Intern. Med.* **103,** 121.

Sun, Y., Yip, P., Jeng, J., Hwang, B. & Lin, W. (1996): Ultrasonographic study and long-term follow-up of Takayasu's arteritis. *Stroke* **27,** 2178–2182.

Wong, R.L. & Korn, J.H. (1986): Temporal arteritis without an elevated erythrocyte sedimentation rate: case report and review of the literature. *Am. J. Med.* **80,** 959.

Yamamoto, S., Nozawa, T., Aoki, H. & Isobe, Y. (1984): Femoro-internal carotid artery bypass for cerebral ischemia in Takayasu's arteritis. *Arch. Surg.* **119,** 1426.

Chapter 18

Neurological impairment in systemic vasculitides

Marina Cao, Marco Ferrari, Mario Beccia and Cesare Fieschi

Department of Neurological Sciences, University of Rome 'La Sapienza', viale dell'Università 30, 00185 Rome, Italy

Summary

Vasculitides are still a debated entity and their central nervous system and peripheral nervous system involvement needs further investigation. Neurological manifestations are common in medical practice. In this paper the authors describe the clinical and diagnostic characteristics of primary and secondary vasculitides, as well as therapeutic approaches. Clinical aspects rather than morphological features of the vessels involved are discussed to identify neurological and systemic signs and humoral patterns which may lead to diagnosis. According to the Villringer and Moore classification, vasculitides are divided in two groups: primary vasculitides which include several diseases characterized by the lack of any pathological process thought to be responsible for the development of vasculitides; and secondary vasculitides, associated with collagen vascular diseases, infections, toxins and neoplasms, whose relation to the disease is well known. Pharmacological approaches, mainly steroids and immunosuppressors, are described, as well as new therapeutic trends.

Finally, the authors describe differential diagnosis with other neurological conditions (multiple sclerosis, stroke due to causes other than vasculitis and non-atherosclerotic vasculopathies). The main differential diagnostic criteria which may be useful in clinical practice are indicated.

Introduction

In recent years much progress has been made regarding the diagnosis, pathogenesis and treatment of vasculitides. These are systemic diseases which may commonly involve the central nervous system (CNS) (Calabrese, 1995) and peripheral nervous system (PNS) (Nadeau, 1997). Therefore, the role of the neurologist is to identify the disease thought to be responsible for the neurological disease. This review describes the most common neurological signs associated with vasculitides, as well as diagnostic criteria and therapeutic approaches.

Neurological involvement in vasculitides

Numerous vasculitis classifications are now available (Fieschi *et al.*, 1998; Ostrov & Barron, 1995; Jennette *et al.*, 1994; Lie, 1990); but for the neurologist a classification which relates vasculitis development and nervous system impairment may be more useful, such as that described by Villringer & Moore (1996) (Table 1). As shown in Table 1, vasculitides are divided in primitive and secondary; the first group includes, in addition to isolated CNS vasculitides, described by other authors, the following diseases: panarteritis nodosa, Wegener's granulomatosis, Churg-Strauss syndrome, lymphomatoid granulomatosis, hypersensitivity vasculitides, giant-cell vasculitides; the latter group includes vasculitides which occur during autoimmune diseases, infections and neoplasms.

Table 1. Vasculitis classification

Primary vasculitides
Polyarteritis nodosa
Churg-Strauss syndrome
Wegener's granulomatosis
Isolated angiitis of CNS
Giant-cell arteritis
Takayasu's arteritis
Temporal arteritis
Hypersensitivity vasculitis
Secondary vasculitides
Associated with:
Collagen vascular diseases
Infections
Toxins
Neoplasms

Villringer & Moore (1996), modified.

Polyarteritis nodosa (PAN)

This is a necrotizing vasculitis involving small- and medium-size vessels. It is a well studied pathology; the annual prevalence is 5/100,000 and it accounts for 15 per cent of all vasculitides. Males are more frequently affected than females (2.5/1). One clinical characteristic is the lack of spleen and lung involvement (Baranger et al., 1995). Data regarding the organs involved are shown in Table 2.

PNS is frequently impaired: multiple and peripheral neuropathies are common features and can be the onset symptoms. Signs can be represented by neuropathy in the legs with painful disaesthesia followed by hypoaesthesia and anaesthesia. A common feature is cranial nerve involvement. CNS can be affected by brain ischaemia and/or haemorrhage.

Diagnosis is based on the clinical features, weight loss, inflammatory signs, and sometimes by the occurrence of seric HbsAg (Gocke et al., 1970). Some authors have reported the presence of p-ANCA; this finding, however, has not been confirmed in other studies (Baranger et al., 1995; Moore & Calabrese, 1994).

Treatment is based on steroids (prednisone-PDN at the dosage of 60 mg/day) combined with cyclophosphamide.

Table 2. Percentage of involved organs in systemic vasculitides

Organ	Polyarteritis nodosa	Wegener's granulomatosis	Churg-Strauss syndrome	Lymphomatoid granulomatosis
Kidney	85	83	40	uncommon
Liver	62	uncommon	uncommon	12
Spleen	0	uncommon	uncommon	18
Lung	0	100	100**	97
Upper respiratory tract	uncommon	100	100**	0
Skin	51	46*	70	39
Gastrointestinal	51	uncommon	40	uncommon
Lymphoadenopathy	uncommon	uncommon	uncommon	8
Eye	uncommon	41	uncommon	uncommon
Middle ear	uncommon	39	uncommon	uncommon
Heart or Pericardium	76	28	85	uncommon
Muscle	uncommon	46*	23	uncommon
Joints	uncommon	39	uncommon	uncommon
CNS	uncommon	7	62	19
PNS	67	23	65	18

*Skin and muscles; **Lung and upper respiratory tract.

Churg-Strauss syndrome (Chumbley et al., 1977)

This is a small- and medium-size vasculitis characterized by allergic diathesis, lung involvement and peripheral eosinophilia. There are no absolute data on incidence and prevalence. Males are more often affected than females (1.4/1) (Villringer & Moore, 1996). Data regarding the organs involved are shown in Table 2. CNS and PNS are involved in 60 per cent of cases, with a slight prevalence of PNS, and the clinical manifestations are the same as those of *polyarteritis nodosa*.

Clinical diagnosis is based on eosinophilia with history of asthma, bronchitis, pneumonia, fever, and is confirmed by angiography of the organs involved and biopsy. In 60–80 per cent of cases p-ANCA is positive (Moore & Calabrese, 1994; Reinhold-Keller et al., 1995; Schmitt & Gross, 1998). Treatment is based on a combination of steroids and immunosuppressors. Some authors report plasmapheresis as an important element in the treatment (Fregoni et al., 1995).

Wegener's granulomatosis (Fauci et al., 1973)

This is a necrotizing granulomatous vasculitis that involves the upper and lower respiratory tracts and kidney. There are no absolute epidemiological data; it can occur at any age, with a mean age at onset of 51.6 years. One characteristic is the abundance of granulomatous lesions in the upper and lower respiratory tracts, focal segmental glomerulitis and necrotizing vasculitides.

CNS and PNS involvement is common after upper respiratory tract involvement and is due both to local extension of the granulomas from the upper respiratory tract to the brain and to vasculitis itself which leads to tissue ischaemia (Nishino et al., 1993). Polyneuropathy is a common sign; seizures, related to cerebral ischaemia, can also occur: brain granulomatosis is, however, a characteristic pattern (Villiringer & Moore, 1996).

Diagnosis is based on the occurrence of granulomatosis in the upper respiratory tract, epistaxis, haemoptysis and deafness. In addition, mild fever, anaemia, leucocytosis, thrombocytosis and an elevated blood sedimentation rate are usual.

The mainstay of diagnosis is histology. Theoretically, any tissue involved may show the typical findings; however, nasal biopsies and needle biopsies of the respiratory tract may be non-specific. Renal lesions are often revelatory. The most conclusive procedure may be open lung biopsy. In most, but not all patients, c-ANCA is positive. However, there are many controversies on the role of c-ANCA as a marker of the disease (Reinhold-Keller *et al.*, 1995; Schmitt & Gross, 1998).

In addition to the combination of steroids with cyclophosphamide, some authors proposed the association between co-trimoxazole and methotrexate (Villringer & Moore, 1996).

Lymphomatoid granulomatosis

This can be considered as a premalignant or ever angiocentric, angiodestructive T-cell lymphoma. The walls of the vessels are infiltrated, which leads to narrowing and occlusion of the lumen. It is a very rare illness which can occur at any age.

The respiratory tract is usually involved, but not its upper tract; this finding is mandatory for diagnosis, as are the lack of systemic symptoms and/or elevated blood sedimentation rate.

CNS involvement is uncommon: injury is due to meningeal and brain damage; cranial neuropathy may also be present. Nystagmus, ataxia, seizures as well as blindness are common symptoms.

The prognosis of the disease, if untreated, is poor: about half the patients develop lymphoma. Mortality was 63.5 per cent in Katzenstein's series of 157 patients with a median survival of 14 months (Katzanstein *et al.*, 1979). With early treatment, the prognosis improves; however, the mortality rate remains nearly 50 per cent. Therapy is based on the use of steroids and immunosuppressors. In addition, some authors report that cranial irradiation may be beneficial (Villringer & Moore, 1996).

Hypersensitivity vasculitides

This is a heterogeneous group which includes (Table 3): (a) hypersensitivity vasculitis of Zeek (Zeek *et al.*, 1948); (b) drug-induced vasculitis; (c) serum sickness; (d) hypersensitivity vasculitis associated with infection, malignancy, connective tissue disease; (e) Schönlein-Henoch purpura; (f) hypocomplementaemic vasculitis; (g) cryoglobulinaemia; (h) cutaneous vasculitis.

Table 3. Hypersensitivity vasculitides

Vasculitis of Zeek
Drug-induced vasculitis
Serum sickness
Associated with: malignancy
infections
connective tissue diseases
Schönlein-Henoch purpura
Hypocomplementaemic vasculitis
Cryoglobulinaemia
Cutaneous vasculitis

There are few data on the incidence of this group of vasculitides. According to Hunder, hypersensitivity vasculitis represents 22 per cent of vasculitides (Hunder *et al.*, 1990).

Vasculitis of Zeek (Angiitis) is a multisystemic disease with skin (100 per cent), pulmonary, myocardial, gastrointestinal, renal, musculoskeletal involvement. The nervous system is involved in 20 per cent of cases: polyneuropathy, myositis, seizures, and stroke are usual findings (Villringer & Moore, 1996). Diagnosis is based on the absence of other clinical characteristics which assign the illness to a specific subgroup.

Drug-induced vasculitis: these patients have a history of drug exposure 3–21 days before illness onset. The clinical features are similar to Zeek vasculitis, combined with eosinophilia.

Serum sickness: patients have a history of exposure to heterologous serum 7–10 days before symptoms, as well as some drugs, particularly penicillin. In addition to lymphoadenopathy, which is the most prominent sign, there is arthralgia, fever and urticaria, while involvement of other organs is less frequent. Typical neurological signs are headache and drowsiness.

Hypersensitivity vasculitis associated with infection, malignancy, connective tissue disease: many types of infection produce immune complexes which can lead to glomerulonephritis and neurological impairment. A similar feature may occur in connective tissue diseases – systemic lupus erythematosus (SLE) and rheumatoid arthritis (RA). Polyneuropathy is the most common sign; CNS may be involved though its frequency is unknown.

Schönlein-Henoch purpura: this occurs mainly in children and is characterized by non-thrombocytopoenic purpura, arthralgia and abdominal pain. Headache is common; seizures, subdural and cortical haemorrhage, stroke have also been described (Szer, 1994). The skin lesions are characterized by 2–5 mm, purpuric lesions over extensor surfaces of lower extremities and buttocks. Diagnosis is based on a history of food allergies; IgA seems to play an important pathogenetic role. The prognosis is good: the process is self-limited in nearly all cases.

Hypocomplementaemic vasculitis: this is defined by episodic or persistent generalized urticaria and migratory arthralgias with depressed complement levels. It occurs in women between 30–60 years with a history of asthma and rhinitis. Papillo-oedema, myositis, carpal tunnel syndrome and mononeuritis have been reported.

Cryoglobulinaemia: cryoglobulins are seric proteins able to precipitate reversibly below 37 °C inducing occlusion of vessels by gelatinous material, bland thrombosis of small arteries, endothelial proliferation and basement membrane thickening and hypersensitivity vasculitis. This pathology is associated with viral, fungal, bacterial infections and autoimmune disease, lymphoproliferative disease, renal and liver disease, breast and esophagous malignancy, heroin use, as well as a familial and essential form. Dominant signs are: dermatitis, arthralgia and cold sensitivity; the most common neurological symptom is a sensorimotor neuropathy (7–15 per cent) due to vasculitis. CNS manifestations are rare.

Cutaneous vasculitis is a pure cutaneous form without any neurological manifestation. An inflammatory pattern, with an elevated blood sedimentary rate, is common (Villringer & Moore, 1996).

Secondary vasculitides

These are a heterogeneous group of diseases, characterized by a pathogenetic noxa thought to be able to start the process. Some of them have been revisited and defined as hypersensitivity vasculitides. Vasculitides secondary to autoimmune disease are common: SLE, RA and other systemic illness are correlated with vasculitis development.

Secondary vasculitides related to infection are thought to be caused by organisms which can directly damage the brain. While there is extensive evidence of the role of *Herpes zoster* in the development of CNS damage, there are few data on the role of hepatitis B virus, if we exclude its role in PAN, which has been well studied.

HIV is related to a systemic syndrome and it is difficult to define the aetiopathogenetic role of the virus in the development of vasculitis. During HIV infection, many other organisms besides neoplasms able to create an autoimmune process may be involved. Mycotic infections, such as mucormycosis and candida, may be responsible for intracranial vasculitis.

Amphetamines, cocaine and other sympathomimetic amines are involved in vasculitis development. This finding is supported by angiographic patterns showing narrowing of the vessels or aneurysms. The CNS is frequently involved with headache, hemiparesis and seizures (Giang, 1994).

Differential diagnosis

Vasculitides can mimic other neurological diseases (Berlit, 1994): multiple sclerosis (MS), for example, is a common disease which involves young adult people, especially women, characterized by CNS demyelination, but it is an autoimmune process involving the CNS whose cause is unknown. The clinical signs which allow a diagnosis to be made are based on Schumacher's criteria (Schumacher et al., 1965). In addition, in MS MRI may show a characteristic demyelination in the white matter of brain and spine. A production of IgG is frequent in cerebrospinal fluid test; in contrast, no serological pattern is unequivocally present (Fieschi et al., 1995).

Stroke in the young adult population is not rare: it is frequently due to cardiac embolic sources, autoimmune disease with vasculitides, artery dissection and metabolic and clotting disorders (Fieschi et al., 1996). Cardiac embolic sources comprise atrial fibrillation, myocardiopathies, myocardial infarction and patent foramen ovale (PFO). This last source is a congenital malformation which leads to an atrial communication with paradoxical emboli. The diagnosis is based on the features of PFO at transesophageal echocardiography.

Hereditary diseases such as CADASIL (Cerebral autosomal dominant arteriopathy with subcortical infarct leukoencephalopathy) and MELAS (mitochondrial myopathy, encephalopathy and stroke-like episodes), a mithocondrial disease, can mimic vasculitis: diagnosis is based on genetic screening and, in the latter, on muscle biopsy.

Some hereditary diseases, such as clotting abnormalities (deficit of V and II factors) can be the cause of stroke in young adult people, and have to be differentiated from vasculitides.

Table 4. Other nonatherosclerotic vasculopathies

Fibromuscular dysplasia
Moya Moya disease
Sneddon's syndrome
Amyloid angiopathy

Finally, some non-atherosclerotic vasculopathies must be differentiated from vasculitis (Table 4): Moya Moya disease occurs mainly in Japanese and Korean populations; its incidence is low and its aetiology is unknown, while its pathogenesis is characterized by the occlusion of proximal arteries compensated by a network of dilated small arteries (Gotoh, 1983). Sneddon's syndrome is a condition which affects mainly young women, characterized by ischaemic stroke and livedo reticularis. Most, but not all patients have high titres of antiphospholipid antibodies (Stockhammer et al., 1993).

Cerebral amyloid angiopathy (CAA) is an important cause of spontaneous intracerebral lobar haemorrhage which occurs in the elderly (Vinters, 1987). TIA have been reported. CAA may be rarely associated with granulomatous or giant-cell vasculitis (Moore & Calabrese, 1994).

Fibromuscular dysplasia involves the cervicocephalic arteries, particularly the extracranial internal carotid artery (Mettinger & Erickson, 1982). Transient cerebral ischaemia may be accompanied by headache, haemorrhage and encephalopathy and can predispose the patient to arterial dissection (Sato & Hata, 1982).

References

Baranger, T.A., Audrain, M.A., Testa, A., Besnier, D., Guillevin, L. & Esnault, V.L. (1995): Anti-neutrophil cytoplasm antibodies in patients with ACR criteria for polyarteritis nodosa: help for systemic vasculitides classification? *Autoimmunity* **20**, 33–37.

Berlit, P. (1994): The spectrum of vasculopathies in the differential diagnosis of vasculitides. *Sem. Neurol.* **14**, 370–379.

Calabrese, L.H. (1995): Vasculitides of the central nervous system. *Rheum. Dis. Clin. North. Am.* **21**, 1059–1076.

Chumbley, L.C., Harrison, E.G. Jr & Deremee, R.A. (1977): Allergic granulomatosis and angiitis (Churg-Strauss syndrome). Report and analysis of 30 cases. *Mayo Clin. Proc.* **52**, 477–484.

Fauci, A.S. & Wolff, S.M. (1973): Wegener's granulomatosis: studies in eighteen patients and a review of the literature. *Medicine (Baltimore)* **52**, 535–561.

Fieschi, C., Gasperini, C., Ristori, G., Bastianello, S., Girmenia, F., Leuzzi, A., Buttinelli, C. & Rasura, M. (1995): Patients with clinically defined abnormalities on MRI and normal CSF. If not multiple sclerosis, what is it? *J. Neurol. Neurosurg. Psychiatry* **59**, 255–256.

Fieschi, C., Rasura, M., Anzini, A., De Castro, S., Di Gianfilippo, G., Valesini, G., Violi, F. & Zanette, E.M. (1996): A diagnostic approach to ischemic stroke in young and middle-aged adults. *Eur. J. Neurol.* **3**, 324–330.

Fieschi, C., Rasura, M., Anzini, A. & Beccia, M (1998): Central nervous system vasculitides. *J. Neurol. Sci.* **153**, 159–171.

Fregoni, V., Perseghin, P., Epis, R., De Fazio, P. & Nalli, G. (1995): Churg-Strauss syndrome with peripheral polyneuropathy refractory to steroideal and immunosuppressive therapy successfully treated with plasma exchange. *Recent Prog. Med.* **86**, 353–354.

Giang, D.W. (1994): Central nervous system vasculitides secondary to infections, toxins and neoplasms. *Semin. Neurol.* 14, 313–319.

Gocke, D.J., Hsu, K., Morgan, C., Bombardieri, S., Lockshin, M. & Christian, C.L. (1970): Association between polyarteritis and Australia antigen. *Lancet* **5**, 1149–1153.

Gotoh, F. (1983): Annual report (1982) of the Research Committee on spontaneous occlusion of the circle of Willis (Moya Moya disease). Ministry of health and welfare, Japan.

Hunder, G.G., Arend, W.P., Bloch, D.A., Calabrese, L.H., Fauci, A.S., Fries, J.F., Leavitt, R.Y., Lie, J.T., Lightfoot, R.W. Jr, Masi, A.T. *et al.* (1990). The American College of Rheumatology 1990 Criteria for the classification of vasculitides. Introduction. *Arthritis Rheum.* **33**, 1065–1067.

Jennette, J.C., Falk, R.J., Andrassy, K., Bacon, P.A., Churg, J., Gross, W.L., Hagen, E.C., Hoffman, G.S., Hunder, G.G., Kallenberg, C.G. *et al.* (1994): Nomenclature of systemic vasculitides: proposal of an international consensus conference. *Arthritis Rheum.* **37**, 187–192.

Katzenstein, A.L., Carrington, C.B. & Liebow, A.A. (1979): Lymphomatoid granulomatosis: a clinicopathologic study of 152 cases. *Cancer* **43**, 360–373.

Lie, J.T. (1990): Diagnostic histopathology of major systemic and pulmonary vasculitic syndromes. *Rheum. Dis. Clin. North. Am.* **16**, 269–292.

Mettinger, K.L. & Erickson, K. (1982): Fibromuscolar dysplasia and the brain: observations on angiographic, clinical and genetic characteristics. *Stroke* **13,** 46–52.

Moore, P.M. & Calabrese, L.H. (1994): Neurologic manifestations of systemic vasculitides. *Semin. Neurol.* **14,** 300–306.

Nadeau, S.E. (1997): Diagnostic approach to central and peripheral nervous system vasculitides. *Neurol. Clin.* **15,** 759–777.

Nishino, H., Rubino, F.A., Deremee, R.A., Swanson, J.W. & Parisi, J.E. (1993): Neurological involvement in Wegener granulomatosis: an analysis of 324 consecutive patients at the Mayo Clinic. *Ann. Neurol.* **33,** 4–9.

Ostrov, B.E. & Barron, T.F. (1995): Cerebral vasculitides: diagnosis and current treatment recommendations. *CNS Drugs* **3,** 115–125.

Reinhold-Keller, E., Tatsis, E. & Gross, W.L. (1995): ANCA-associated vasculitides (Wegener's granulomatosis, Churg-Strauss syndrome, microscopic polyangiitis). 3. Therapeutic procedures. *Z. Rheumatol.* **54** (5), 303–309.

Sato, S. & Hata, J. (1982): Fibromuscolar dysplasia: its occurrence with a dissecting aneurysm of the internal carotid artery. *Arch. Pathol. Lab. Med.* **106,** 332–335.

Schmitt, W.H. & Gross, W.L. (1998): Vasculitides in the seriously ill patient: diagnostic approaches and therapeutic options in ANCA-associated vasculitides. *Kidney Int. Suppl.* **64,** S39–44.

Schumacher, G.A., Beebe, G., Kibler, R.E. et al. (1965): Problems of experimental trials of therapy in multiple sclerosis. *Ann. NY Acad. Sci.* **122,** 552–568.

Stockhammer, G., Felber, S.R., Zelger, B., Sepp, N., Birbamer, G.G., Fritsch, P.O. & Aichner, T. (1993): Sneddon's syndrome: diagnosis by skin biopsy and MRI in 17 patients. *Stroke* **24,** 685.

Szer, I.S. (1994): Henoch-Schonlein purpura. *Curr. Opin. Rheumatol.* **6** (1), 25–31.

Villringer, A. & Moore, P.M. (1996): Vasculitides and other nonatherosclerotic vasculopaties of the nervous system. In: *Neurological disorders: course and treatment*, eds. Brand, Caplan, Dichgans, Diener, Kennard, pp. 305–326. London: Academic Press.

Vinters, H.V. (1987): Cerebral amyloid angiopathy: a critical review. *Stroke* **18,** 311–324.

Zeek, P.M., Smith, C.C. & Weeter, J.C. (1948): Studies on periarteritis nodosa. III. The differentiation between the vascular lesions of periarteritis nodosa and of hypersensitivity. *Am. J. Pathol.* **24,** 889–917.

Chapter 19

Diagnostic and prognostic role of autoantibodies in connective tissue diseases

Fabrizia Corona and Mirella Scarazatti

Paediatric Rheumatology Centre, First Paediatric Clinic, University of Milan, via Commenda 9, 20122 Milan, Italy

Summary

Connective tissue diseases are frequently considered in the differential diagnosis of skin, joint, lung and other disorders. The simplest screening test and practical starting point is the research of antinuclear antibody (ANA) and anti-neutrophil cytoplasmic antibodies (ANCA).

Among the many antibody specificities that have been identified, some of them seem to represent specific markers for a given disease and/or have been correlated with symptoms or with specific organ involvement. The identification of a growing number of new antibody specificities has allowed researchers to establish serological profiles for various morphological entities. In this study, before reporting data concerning our patients, we report the main studies of the literature regarding the most important autoantibodies in childhood connective tissue diseases: ANA and ANCA and their diagnostic and prognostic correlations.

Introduction

The connective tissue diseases include a group of disorders whose clinical manifestations may greatly vary, although the presence of circulating antinuclear antibodies is considered to be one of its major characteristics. Notwithstanding most of the research conducted in the past few years (Fritzler, 1985; Nakamura *et al.*, 1984; Bombardieri *et al.*, 1987), the significance of these autoantibodies and the mechanisms underlying their production and their role in human pathology has not yet been fully understood. The presence in sera of autoantibodies has a different meaning according to whether these autoantibodies are organ-specific or non-organ-specific; the clinical correlation between autoimmune diseases and autoantibodies is particularly interesting for the non-organ-specific autoantibodies. Whereas the correlation between organ-specific autoantibodies and clinical manifestations is clear (for example antibodies against pancreatic insula and insulin-dependent diabetes), it is more difficult to recognize the correlation between non-organ-specific autoantibodies and diseases. Indeed the role of these autoantibodies is not understood and this phenomenon occurs mainly in paediatric connective tissue diseases. In this study we evaluated the most important, common and known autoantibodies in childhood connective tissue diseases: antinuclear antibody and anti-neutrophil cytoplasmic antibodies.

Antinuclear antibody

Antinuclear antibody (ANA) are immunoglobulins directed against different nuclear antigens, which are divided into:

- *ANA directed against not extractable nuclear antigens*: anti-DNA antibody, anti-histone and anti-ribonuclear protein (Nakamura *et al.*, 1984);

- *ANA directed against extractable nuclear antigens*: the most important are anti-RNP antibody, anti-SS-A, anti-SS-B, anti-Scl 70, anti-PCNA, anti-Jo-1, anti-Mi-1 (Nakamura *et al.*, 1984).

Methods of ANA detection

The technique of indirect immunofluorescence (IIF) has been widely used for many years and also now serves as the primary screening test; at present the techniques of double diffusion, counterimmunoelectrophoresis in agarose gels, immunoblotting, immunoprecipitation, enzyme-linked immunosorbent assay (ELISA) and radioimmunoassay (RIA) support the IIF assay (Wilk, 1987; Tan, 1983). Currently, ANA is performed by IIF using an epithelial cell line, Hep-2, as a substrate.

This substrate is far better than mouse kidney or liver as regards sensitivity and ability to distinguish staining patterns of autoantibodies.

The patterns obtained by immunofluorescence provide a clue to autoantibody specificity.

With IIF it is possible to identify different patterns:

- Homogeneous or peripheric: specific for anti-dsDNA antibody, anti-ssDNA and anti-histones;

- Speckled: specific for anti-Sm antibody, anti-RNP, anti-Scl70, anti-SS-A(Ro), anti-SS-B(La);

- Nucleolar: specific for anti-RNA.

However, autoantibody specificities cannot be diagnosed with certainty by the immunofluorescence pattern. Gel precipitation or immunoassay using purified antigens are used for determination of autoantibody specificity; the next step is immunoprecipitation and Western blotting (Jaskovski, 1996).

Clinical correlations

The clinical correlations between ANA and connective tissue diseases are particularly interesting especially in childhood. Among the many antibody specificities that have been identified, some of them seem to represent specific markers for a definite disease and/or have been correlated with symptoms or with specific organ involvement. The identification of a growing number of new antibody specificities has allowed researchers to establish serological profiles for several morphological entities.

Before considering the possible clinical correlations, some points should be established:

- The presence of ANA only does not imply disease;
- The autoantibody titre must be at least 1:40 and persistent in time;
- Autoantibodies can be present in normal, healthy children (up to 7.3 per cent), with a low titre (1:40) and a homogeneous or diffuse pattern and can be found in 3.3 per cent of normal adults also with high titre (1:320);
- Many drugs (procainamide, hydralazine) may help develop a positive ANA;
- Antinuclear antibodies have been associated with chronic infectious diseases (parasitic and bacterial infections, malaria, hepatitis, tuberculosis, leprosy etc.);
- Various malignancies have been reported to be associated with ANA, including lymphomas, leukemias and solid tumours;
- Antinuclear antibodies may be absent at the beginning of the disease and appear only when the symptoms become evident;
- The anticorpal titre varies during the course of the disease.

Clinical data

Before reporting data concerning our patients, we report the main studies about paediatric connective tissue diseases.

Juvenile idiopathic arthritis (JIA): the prevalence of ANA in children affected by JIA varies according to the different subtypes:

- Systemic JIA : 2–17 per cent (Wilk, 1987; Leak, 1998)
- Polyarticular JIA : 10–80 per cent (Wilk, 1987; Leak, 1998)
- Pauciarticular JIA : 30–90 per cent (Wilk, 1987; Leak, 1998)

Considering pauciarticular JIA type I with anterior uveitis, the frequency of ANA positivity is close to 100 per cent (Leak & Woo, 1991). In a recent study Rosenberg *et al.* (1996) found a higher ANA positivity in patients with iridocyclitis compared with the children without iridocyclitis.

The immunofluorescence pattern is largely homogeneous (55–75 per cent of patients), sometimes speckled (25–42 per cent), rarely nucleolar (18 per cent) (Leak, 1998; Rosenberg *et al.* (1996).

Systemic lupus erythematosus (SLE) is the prototype of the autoimmune diseases characterized by the production of ANA directed to various nuclear constituents, in which anti-DNA autoantibodies are the most characteristic. These antibodies are markers of diagnostic and prognostic significance. ANA are detected in nearly 100 per cent of children with SLE; although some ANA are expressed at relatively constant levels during the course of SLE, anti-DNA levels are highly variable and frequently fluctuate with disease activity and appear especially sensitive to the effects of immunomodulatory agents: after corticosteroid therapy, anti-DNA may fall to undetectable levels (Fritzler, 1985). The percentage of positivity is reported: for anti-dsDNA antibody 75–80 per cent, for anti-histones 70 per cent, for anti-Sm 30 per cent, for anti-RNP 30 per cent, for anti-SS-A(Ro) 35 per cent and anti SS-B(La) 15 per cent (Fritzler, 1985; Kohda *et al.*, 1989). The strongest clinical association of anti-DNA is found with nephritis (70–90 per cent). Anti-Sm is detected in 10–30 per cent of patients with SLE; associations with pulmonary fibrosis, pericarditis and nervous system involvement have been reported and it has also been suggested that anti-Sm levels are useful indicators of disease activity (Bombardieri et al., 1987). Other autoantibodies can be present in SLE: anti-histone in drug-induced lupus (between 35 and 95 per cent), anti-SS-A(Ro) in subacute cutaneous lupus erythematosus or in infants with congenital heart block (between 25 and 33 per cent) (Bombardieri et al., 1987). Table 1 reports the clinical meaning and frequency of ANA in SLE.

Table 1. Clinical meaning and frequency of ANA in SLE

ANA	Frequency, %	Clinical meaning
Anti-dsDNA	75–80	Diagnostic, correlation with disease activity and renal involvement
Anti-histone	25–40	Correlation with renal involvement
	100	Drug-induced SLE
Anti-Sm	10–40	Diagnostic
Anti-RNP	30	–
Anti SS-A(Ro)	25–40	Correlation with congenital heart block
Anti SS-B(La)	15	–

Dermatomyositis (DM) is the most common childhood myopathy; ANA may be detected in 10–50 per cent of patients, often in very high titre. However a particular antigenic specificity is found only in a minority of patients and these autoantibodies have been considered as 'myositis-specific-autoantibodies' (MSA) (Pachman, 1995).

The most common MSA is anti-Jo-1, seen in 15–20 per cent of all myositis patients and directed at histidyl-tRNA synthetase (HSR). In patients with lung involvement, anti-Jo-1 is reported to be present in 50–75 per cent of the cases (Montecucco et al., 1990).

Scleroderma: the presence of ANA is a central feature of systemic sclerosis (SSc) and localized scleroderma and has long been reported with a prevalence of 40–90 per cent, with a speckled pattern in 60 per cent of these patients.

The serological subsets tend to be associated with certain patterns of clinical expression and, at present, eight antibody profiles can be used to classify about 85 per cent of scleroderma population.

Thus, antibodies to certain nonhistone proteins associated with the nucleolar organizer region such as topoisomerase 1, RNA polymerases and U3RNA are found in patients with diffuse skin disease and systemic involvement. For example, antibodies to topoisomerase 1 and RNA polymerase are associated respectively with pulmonary and renal involvement.

By contrast, anti-kinetochore antibodies are found in patients with limited skin disease, including up to 90 per cent of those defined as CREST, and may identify patients at risk of severe vascular complications. Yet other antibodies, for example antibodies to the PM-Scl system, are associated with the development of overlap syndromes with prominent myositis (Spencer-Green et al., 1997).

Mixed connective tissue disease (MCTD) is uncommon in children and is characterized by features of more than one of the rheumatic disorders with ANA antibodies in a speckled pattern and with antibodies to nuclear ribonucleoprotein (nRNP) with high titre.

Sjögren syndrome is a rare condition in childhood; anti-SS-A(Ro) and anti-SS-B(La) antibody can be present with a prevalence respectively of 60 and 70 per cent. Table 2 shows ANA frequency in connective tissue disease, obtained from clinical data.

Table 2. Clinical meaning and frequency of ANA in connective tissue disease

Disease	ANA	Frequency, %	Clinical meaning
Systemic JIA		2–17	–
Polyarticular JIA		10–80	–
Pauciarticular JIA		30–90	–
SLE	Anti-dsDNA	75–80	Diagnostic
DM	Anti-Jo 1	15–20	–
Scleroderma	Anti-Scl70	20–50	Diagnostic
MCTD	Anti-RNP	95–100	Diagnostic
	Anti-dsDNA	< 5	–
Sjögren syndrome	Anti-SS-A(Ro)	55	Correlation with xerostomia and xeroftalmia
	Anti-SS-B(La)	40–50	

Table 3. ANA positivity: personal experience

Disease	Antibody	Percentage positivity
JIA		
Systemic (24 patients)	ANA	61
Systemic ev poly (38 patients)	ANA	68
Polyarticular (56 patients)	ANA	55
Pauciarticular (167 patients)	ANA	87
Pauciarticular ext (31 patients)	ANA	87
SLE		
(76 patients)	ANA	94
	Anti-dsDNA	67.1
	Anti-ssDNA	7.9
	Anti-DNP	15.8
	Anti SSA/SS-B	14.5
	Anti-RNP	7.9
	Anti-Sm/RNP	7.9
	Anti-histone	9.2
DM		
(28 patients)	ANA	61
	Anti SS-A/SS-B e Sm/RNP	3.5
	Anti-Jo 1	0
Scleroderma		
(12 patients)	ANA	75
– 6 localized	Anti-Scl 70	0
– 6 systemic sclerosis	ANA	80
	ANA	100
MCTD		
(7 patients)	ANA	100
	RNP	100
Sjögren syndrome		
(1 patient)	Anti SS-A/SS-B	100

Personal experience

In our study, comprehensive of 440 patients affected by connective tissue diseases, we evaluated the diagnostic meaning and the prognostic correlation of ANA.

For the *diagnostic correlation*, we found ANA positivity in 94 per cent of our children affected by SLE, anti-dsDNA positivity in 67.1 per cent, anti-Sm positivity in 7.9 per cent.

In all seven patients with MCTD the determination of anti-RNP autoantibodies tested positive with high titre. In one patient with Sjögren's syndrome, an unusual disease in childhood, anti-SS-A(Ro)/SS-B(La) autoantibodies were positive. We found ANA positivity in 61 per cent of the 28 patients affected by DMT; only one had ENA positivity, none had anti Jo-1.

In localized scleroderma ANA were detected in 80 per cent of patients, while these autoantibodies were found in 100 per cent of patients suffering from systemic sclerosis: none had anti-Scl-70 antibody, usually present in adult with SSc. Table 3 reports ANA positivity in our patients.

In summary, our experience confirms that ANA positivity is diagnostic for a very low number of connective tissue diseases; therefore the mere presence of autoantibodies cannot justify a diagnosis.

In connective tissue disease the *prognosis* is multifactorial and ANA presence is only one of the various aspects.

As far as SLE is concerned, the presence and the increase of anti ds-DNA and anti-Sm titre correlate with nephropathy. Anti-RNP autoantibodies are frequently present in SLE with severe vasculitis, anti-P autoantibodies in SLE with neuropsychiatric, renal and hepatic involvement and anti-SS-A in cutaneous SLE (Table 4).

Table 4. ANA in SLE: prognostic correlation

ANA	Clinical meaning
Anti-dsDNA	Renal involvement
Anti-histone	Renal involvement
Anti-Sm	Renal, neurological involvement
Anti-RNP	Raynaud's phenomenon, nephropathy, hepatopathy
Anti SS-A(Ro)	Cutaneous involvement

In our patients affected by SLE, 26 out of 76 children with renal involvement, at the moment of diagnosis, had respectively ANA positivity of 80 per cent and anti-dsDNA positivity of 62 per cent; when the nephropathy developed, ANA positivity was close to 100 per cent and anti-dsDNA positivity was 80 per cent. Conversely in 15 patients in partial remission the titre was generally very low (Fig. 1).

JIA: as far as prognostic meaning between JIA and ANA titre is concerned, the results of our research confirm the literature data. The prevalence of ANA in children varied according to the different subtypes: pauciarticular JIA 87 per cent, polyarticular JIA 55 per cent and systemic JIA 61 per cent. With IIF we recognized different patterns: homogeneous in pauciarticular JIA, speckled in systemic and polyarticular JIA.

Another important prognostic correlation between ANA titre and flare-up of arthritis in pauciarticular JIA came out of our study: 28 out of 31 patients (90 per cent) that had a flare-up of disease activity showed an increase in ANA titre. In 78 patients in complete remission we

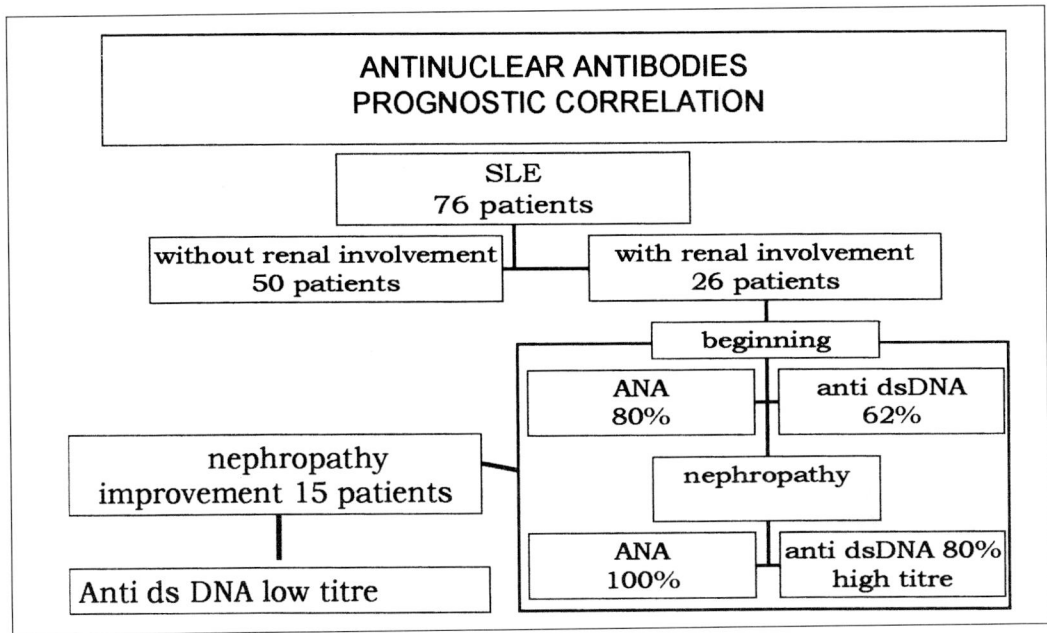

Fig. 1. Antinuclear antibodies prognostic correlation.

observed a decrease of ANA titre only in 55 per cent. In pauciarticular JIA population we observed no difference of ANA positivity between the groups with iridocyclitis (63 patients) and without iridocyclitis (109 patients): 94.5 per cent vs. 83 per cent ($P > 0.05$); on the contrary ANA levels increased in patients who experience iridocyclitis relapse (74 per cent ANA rise in iridocyclitis relapse).

Overall, in JIA the ANA are more frequent in the pauciarticular subtype with a homogeneous pattern and the increase of the titre is a considerable risk factor for relapse.

Antineutrophil cytoplasmic antibodies

Antineutrophil cytoplasmic antibodies (ANCA) are autoantibodies directed against cytoplasmic constituents of neutrophils and monocytes.

Since the first description of ANCA the number of diseases in which ANCA may be discovered has continued to increase. In addition to the systemic vasculitides such as Wegener's granulomatosis (WG), microscopic polyangiitis (MPA), necrotizing glomerulonephritis (GN), polyarteritis nodosa (PAN) and Churg-Strauss syndrome (CCS), the list now includes various rheumatic autoimmune diseases such as juvenile idiopathic arthritis (JIA) and systemic lupus erythematosus (SLE), inflammatory bowel disease (IBD), autoimmune liver disease, infections, malignancies and myelodysplastic process (Hoffman & Specks, 1998).

Methods of ANCA detection

The most common screening method for detection of ANCA is still the indirect immunofluorescence technique (IIF) using ethanol-fixed human granulocytes from normal blood donors as substrate.

Fixation of the cells by ethanol allows discrimination between the two major fluorescence patterns: c-ANCA and p-ANCA. Falk & Jenette (1998) first demonstrated that the p-ANCA pattern is an artifact of alcohol fixation. If fixation is done in formaldeyde it is impossible to discriminate between p-ANCA and c-ANCA, because both exhibit the same cytoplasmic staining pattern.

The current terminology that distinguishes between classic cytoplasmic ANCA (c-ANCA) and perinuclear ANCA (p-ANCA) is based on the fluorescence appearance on ethanol-fixed neutrophil cytospin preparation: c-ANCA indicates cytoplasmic staining and refers to the coarse granular, centrally accentuated, cytoplasmic fluorescence pattern. The characteristic c-ANCA pattern is usually caused by antibodies against proteinase 3 (PR3), a neutral serine protease present in the azurophil granules of neutrophils.

Autoantibodies against other defined and undefined cytoplasmic antigens, including bactericidal/permeability-increasing protein (BPI) and, rarely, myeloperoxidase (MPO), can cause cytoplasmic fluorescence on polymorphonuclear cell slides.

Clearly distinct from the c-ANCA is the p-ANCA (perinuclear) fluorescence pattern on ethanol-fixed neutrophils; the p-ANCA fluorescence pattern represents an artifact of ethanol fixation which allows the rearrangement of positively charged granule constituents around and on the negatively charged membrane (Falk & Jenette, 1998).

In conclusion it is possible to recognize:

- C-ANCA: classic granular cytoplasmic fluorescence with central or interlobular accentuation;

- C-ANCA (atypical): diffuse flat cytoplasmic fluorescence without interlobular accentuation;

- P-ANCA: perinuclear fluorescence, with or without nuclear extension; includes granulocyte-specific ANA;

- Atypical ANCA: includes all other neutrophil-specific or monocyte-specific IFN reactivity, most commonly a combination of cytoplasmic and perinuclear fluorescence.

The original method of ANCA detection is IIF and while it remains the most widely used method, it does not identify the specific antigen for the ANCA responsible for immunofluorerescence. Enzyme-linked immunosorbent assay (ELISA) is used to target antigen-specific ANCA determination. There are other detection methods, such as radioimmunoassay, immunoblotting, or immunoprecipitation techniques, that at present are not practical for routine ANCA testing (Hoffman & Specks, 1998).

Also for ANCA we can acknowledge a diagnostic meaning and a prognostic correlation in systemic vasculitis and in rheumatic autoimmune diseases.

ANCA in systemic vasculitis and in rheumatic autoimmune diseases

The systemic vasculitides are dynamic processes that evolve in variable time frames and patterns in different patients. The early phases of diseases are often associated with non-specific features that are more frequently noted in common illnesses such as infections, atopic disorders, or malignancies.

For the *diagnostic meaning*, the most clear-cut association of a disease with ANCA directed against a specific target antigen remains the association between WG and PR3-ANCA. ANCA occur in at least 80–90 per cent of these patients, almost all of these are c-ANCA (between 80 per cent and 95 per cent) (Cohen Tervaerj et al., 1990). Only an estimated 5–20 per cent of ANCA may be p-ANCA, which are mostly directed against MPO and only rarely directed against other known target antigens such as elastase or even PR3.

C-ANCA induced by PR3-ANCA are highly sensitive and specific (specificity = proportion of patients without WG who have a negative result test; sensitivity = proportion of patients with established disease who have a positive test result) for WG. In experienced laboratories, the specificity of c-ANCA is about 95 per cent, and the sensitivity depends on the activity of the disease: it is about 50 per cent in patients with 'initial phase' WG and close to 100 per cent in patients with active generalized disease characterized by clinical symptoms due to small-vessel vasculitis (Cohen Tervaerj et al., 1990).

The association of MPA with p-ANCA/MPO-ANCA is reported to be in the range of 40–80 per cent. ANCA-positive, anti-MPO-negative patients with MPA most often have antibody specificity for PR3. The reported sensitivity of MPO-ANCA has ranged from 23 per cent to 75 per cent, and the combined sensitivity of c-ANCA/PR3 plus p-ANCA/MPO has been 51–90 per cent (Cohen Tervaerj et al., 1990).

C-ANCA have been detected with variable frequency in patients with CCS (Cohen Tervaerj et al., 1990), and both PR3 and MPO have been described as target antigens; they are not found at all or occur only rarely in other forms of vasculitides such as giant-cell arteritis, Takayasu arteritis, and Behçet's disease (Locke et al., 1997).

In conclusion ANCA pattern type implies a diagnostic meaning. In fact while the fluorescence patterns discovered in systemic vasculitis are usually c-ANCA, in rheumatic autoimmune diseases they are mostly p-ANCA.

P-ANCA have been described in patients with a variety of rheumatic autoimmune diseases, including rheumatoid arthritis (Mulder et al., 1997), systemic lupus erythematosus (Schnabel et al., 1995), Sjögren's syndrome (Falk & Jenette, 1998), polymyositis and dermatomyositis (Falk & Jenette, 1998), juvenile chronic arthritis (Mulder et al., 1997); in these patients, ANCA levels are often low and clinically unclear. In addition to this uncertainty, ANCA in scleroderma are also uncommon (Locke et al., 1997).

In a recent study, Mulder et al. (1997) evaluated the prevalence of ANCA in JIA; ANCA were detected in the sera from 35 per cent of patients with JIA; regarding the onset type of JIA, ANCA were present in 44 per cent of patients with oligoarticular onset, in 36 per cent with polyarticular onset and in 16 per cent with systemic onset. All but one ANCA positive serum samples produced a perinuclear fluorescence pattern on ethanol-fixed granulocytes. However, on neutrophils fixed with paraformaldehyde either a cytoplasmic (14 per cent) or a nuclear (23 per cent) staining pattern was observed, suggesting that both cytoplasmic and nuclear autoantibodies occur in JIA. Further characterization studies showed that ANCA in JIA are not directed against proteinase 3, elastase or myeloperoxidase. On Western blots ANCA in JIA incidentally showed reactivity either to lactoferrin (5 per cent) or polypeptides (Mulder et al., 1997) (Table 6).

The prevalence and antigen specificity of ANCA were studied also in sera from 23 children with active SLE; ANCA were present in 69 per cent of these patients and consisted of IgM and IgG antibodies of variable specificities, but did not correlate with organ involvement or disease activities. It remains unclear whether they have pathogenic significance or they are epiphenomena in B-cell activation process (Schnabel et al., 1995).

Atypical ANCA and sometimes p-ANCA are found in some drug-induced vasculitides but are otherwise of uncertain clinical significance (Falk & Jenette, 1998).

ANCA, particularly perinuclear, have been found more frequently in sera from children with ulcerative colitis (UC) (33 patients with UC) than in sera from Crohn's disease (CD) (64 patients with CD) or unclassified enterocolitis (UE) (five patients with UE); the prevalence was respectively of 80 per cent, 73 per cent and 14 per cent and in this study (Falk & Jenette, 1998) there was no link between ANCA-positive sera and disease activity, so that it cannot be used to monitor medical treatment or surgical indications.

However, concerning the *prognostic meaning*, the most important autoantibodies are c-ANCA.

C-ANCA are not detectable in most patients with MPA and WG in complete remission, and are generally very low in those in partial remission. Persistent or intermittent positivity for c-ANCA in patients entering remission is a considerable risk factor for relapse.

In WG and microscopic polyangiitis, ANCA levels usually decrease with treatment but increase in about 50 per cent of patients who experience a relapse; conversely, about 50 per cent of patients in whom ANCA recur will relapse. Because titre level corresponds to disease activity, serial c-ANCA testing is useful for monitoring patients with WG (Savige *et al.*, 1999).

In Tables 5 and 6 percentage of ANCA positivity is reported.

Table 5. ANCA in systemic vasculitis

	ANCA positivity, %	Target antigen
Wegener's granulomatosis	c-ANCA 80–95%	Proteinase 3 (PR3-ANCA)
	p-ANCA 5–20%	Myeloperoxidase (MPO-ANCA)
Microscopic polyangiitis	c-ANCA 80–85%	Proteinase 3 (PR3-ANCA)
	p-ANCA 80–85%	Myeloperoxidase (MPO-ANCA)
Churg-Strauss syndrome	c-ANCA 50%	Proteinase 3 (PR3-ANCA)
	p-ANCA 50%	Myeloperoxidase (MPO-ANCA)
Polyarteritis nodosa	p-ANCA 80%	Myeloperoxidase (MPO-ANCA)

Table 6. ANCA in rheumatic disorders

	ANCA positivity, %	Target antigen
JIA	GS-ANA/p-ANCA/athipic-ANCA (30%)	Lactoferrin
SLE	p-ANCA < 20%	Lactoferrin elastase
		Myeloperoxidase (MPO-ANCA)

Table 7. ANCA in vasculitis and in connective tissue diseases: personal experience

	Patients	Positivity, %	c-ANCA, %	p-ANCA, %	Atypical, %
JIA	61	28	22	88	0
SLE	26	42	0	91	9
Other CTD	21	48	20	80	0
Vasculitis	13	54	57	43	0

In our study (Table 7) we measured ANCA by indirect immunofluorescence in the serum of 108 children with connective tissue disease (CTD) (61 JIA, 26 SLE, 21 other CTD) and in the serum of 13 patients with vasculitis. ANA were detected in 28 per cent of patients with JIA (88 per cent p-ANCA, 22 per cent c-ANCA), in 42 per cent of children with SLE (91 per cent p-ANCA, 9 per cent atypic pattern), in 54 per cent with systemic vasculitis (43 per cent p-ANCA, 57 per cent c-ANCA) and in 48 per cent of other rheumatic diseases (80 per cent p-ANCA, 20 per cent c-ANCA). ANCA prevalence in CTD is not statistically different from ANCA prevalence in vasculitis patients (39 per cent vs. 54 per cent).

In JIA we observed an association of p-ANCA titre with high Steinbrocker grades (severe and progressive JIA), higher duration of disease activity (92 months vs. 60 months, $P < 0.05$) and lower duration of remission (5.9 months vs. 17 months, $P < 0.003$).

In patients with SLE, persistent high titres or rising titres of ANCA were often associated with severe disease activity or a relapse.

Our preliminary data suggest that ANCA profile could offer a correlation with disease activity even if at the moment the prognostic value of a rise in ANCA is imperfect. Moreover the presence of ANCA in our patients showed a high specificity (95 per cent) for diagnosis of connective tissue disease but a low sensitivity (37 per cent).

P-ANCA patterns had a higher prevalence in systemic CTD compared to vasculitis ($P < 0.02$); c-ANCA are prevalent in patients with vasculitis (specificity 89 per cent).

The establishment of a disease in the human body is very likely the result of a genetically controlled response to various triggered factors (viral infection or toxic agents). This response may take various forms, such as polyclonal activation, direct cytotoxicity, or molecular mimicry.

The study of the fine specificity and the potential mechanism of formation of antinuclear antibodies could help to shed light on the diagnostic picture and the physiopathological mechanisms of systemic autoimmune diseases.

References

Bombardieri, S., Neri, R., Tartarelli, G., D'Ascanio, A. & Giovanelli, L. (1987): The clinical relevance of antinuclear antibodies in connective tissue diseases. *Scand. J. Rheumatol* **66**, S35–45.

Cohen Tervaerj, J.W., Goldschmeding, R., Elema, J.P., Limburg, P.C., van der Gissen, M., Huitema, M.G. et al (1990): Association of autoantibodies to myeloperoxidase with different forms of vasculitis. *Arthritis Rheum.* **33**, 1264–1272.

Falk, R.J. & Jenette, C. (1998): Antineutrophil cytoplasmic antibodies with specificity for myeloperoxidase in patients with systemic vasculitis and idiopathic necrotizing and crescentic glomerulonephritis. *N. Engl. J. Med.* **25**, 1651–1657.

Fritzler, M. (1985): Antinuclear antibodies in the investigation of the rheumatic diseases. *Bull. Rheum. Dis.* **35** (6), 1–10.

Hoffman, G & Specks, U. (1998): Antineutrophil cytoplasmic antibodies. *Arthritis Rheum.* **41** (9), 1521–1537.

Jaskowski, T.D., Schroder, C., Martins, T.B., Mouritsen, C.L., Litwin, C.M. & Hill, H.R. (1996): Screening for antinuclear antibodies by enzyme immunoassay. *Am. J. Clin. Pathol.* **105**, 468–473.

Kohda, S., Kanayama, Y., Okamura, M., Amatju, K., Negoro, N., Takeda, T. & Inoue, T. (1989): Clinical significance of antibodies to histones in systemic lupus erythematosus. *J. Rheumatol.* **16** (1), 24–28.

Leak, A.M (1998): Autoantibody profile in juvenile chronic arthritis. *Annals of the Rheum. Dis.* **47**, 178–182

Leak, A.M. & Woo, P. (1991): Juvenile chronic arthritis, chronic iridocyclitis, and reactivity to histones. *Ann. Rheum. Dis.* **50,** 653–657.

Locke, I.C., Worral, I.G., Leaker, B., Black, C.M. & Cambridge, G. (1997): Autoantibodies to myeloperoxidase in systemic sclerosis. *J. Rheumatol.* **24,** 86–89.

Montecucco, S., Ravelli, A., Caporali, R., Viola, S. & Martini, A. (1990): Autoantibodies in juvenile dermatomyositis. *Clin. Exp. Rheumatol.* **8,** 193–196.

Mulder, L., Horst, G, Kuis, W. *et al.* (1997): Antineutrophil cytoplasmic antibodies in juvenile chronic arthrtitis. *J. Rheumatol.* **24,** 568–575.

Nakamura, R., Peebles, C.L., Molden, D.P. & Tan, E.M. (1984): Advances in laboratory tests for autoantibodies to nuclear antigens in systemic rheumatic diseases. *Lab. Med.* **15** (3), 25–50.

Pachman, L.M. (1995): An update on juvenile dermatomyositis (1995): *Curr. Opinion Rheumatol.* **7** (5), 437–441.

Rosenberg, A.M, Hauta, S.A., Prokopchuk, P.A. & Romanchuk, K.G. (1996): Studies on associations of antinuclear antibodies with antibodies to an uveogenic peptide of retinal S-antigen in children with uveitis. *J. Rheumatol.* **23,** 370–373.

Savige, J., Gillis, D. *et al.* (1999): International consensus statement on testing and reporting of ANCA. *Am. J. Clin. Pathol.* **117,** 507–513.

Schnabel, A., Csernok, E., Jsenberg, D.A., Mrowka, C. & Gross, W.L. (1995): Antineutrophil cytoplasmic antibodies in Systemic lupus erythematosus. *Arthritis Rheum.* **38,** 633–637.

Spencer-Green, G., Alter, D. & Welch, H.G. (1997): Test performance in systemic sclerosis: anti-centromere and anti-Scl 70 antibodies. *Am. J. Med.* **103,** 242–248.

Tan, E.M. (1983): Autoantibodies to nuclear antigens (ANA): their immunobiology and medicine. *Adv. Immunol.* **33,** 167–240.

Wilk, A. (1987): The value of specific ANA determination in rheumatology. *Allergy* **42,** 241–261.

Chapter 20

Immune-mediated disorders of the CNS at paediatric age: neuroradiological findings

Elio Maccagnano and Mario Savoiardo

Department of Neuroradiology, Istituto Nazionale Neurologico 'C. Besta', via Celoria 11, 20133 Milan, Italy

Summary

The neuroradiological findings observed in immune-mediated disorders of the CNS are heterogeneous. Two groups can be identified: disorders that mainly affect the nervous tissue, like multiple sclerosis, acute disseminated encephalomyelitis, Rasmussen's encephalitis, Sydenham's chorea, and disorders that mainly affect the blood vessels, like systemic and primary CNS vasculitides. The pattern of CNS involvement demonstrated by MRI and its evolution may allow the neuroradiologist to suggest the differential diagnosis. Close interaction between the neuroradiologist and the paediatric neurologist is necessary in order to choose the appropriate laboratory tests or plan a biopsy that may lead to definite diagnosis and appropriate treatment.

Introduction

The neuroradiological findings observed in immune-mediated disorders that affect the central nervous system (CNS) are heterogeneous; they reflect the histopathologic spectrum and the various clinical presentations of these disorders.

Two broad categories can be identified:

(1) Disorders that mainly affect the nervous tissue in the CNS. These are often directed against the white matter, like multiple sclerosis (MS) or acute disseminated encephalomyelitis (ADEM), but may also be directed against white and gray matter (like Rasmussen's encephalitis), or may involve essentially the gray matter like some forms of cerebellitis, and may even selectively affect specific neuronal populations (e.g. neurons of the basal ganglia in Sydenham's chorea);

(2) Disorders that mainly affect the blood vessels. The damage to the vessel wall may cause vessel occlusion resulting in ischaemia; it may also cause disruption of the blood-brain barrier with possible damage to the tissue surrounding the blood vessels by an antigen-antibody reaction. Systemic and primary CNS vasculitides belong to this group of disorders.

Other disorders display intermediate or mixed neuroradiologic and pathologic features, and their mechanism remains rather obscure, as in Behçet's disease. Immune-mediated disorders may also affect the peripheral nervous system, like the Guillain-Barré syndrome.

From the neuroradiological standpoint, the immune-mediated disorders of the CNS are best studied using magnetic resonance imaging (MRI) which provides a detailed morphological demonstration of the involved areas and may demonstrate disruption of the blood-brain barrier. Computed tomography (CT) has a limited role in the diagnostic work-up of these disorders; it may be useful in the rare event of stroke-like presentation of a vasculitis. The role of angiography in the evaluation of vasculitis is still debated.

We shall now discuss the neuroradiological aspects of the most common immune-mediated disorders of the CNS that occur at paediatric age.

Multiple sclerosis

MS is rather rare in adolescents but may present even in childhood. MRI findings in paediatric MS cases do not differ from those observed in adults; there is perhaps a greater tendency to large, swollen plaques in the acute phase. Demyelinating plaques most often develop in the subependymal regions around the medullary veins of the deep white matter, resulting in the characteristic ovoid periventricular lesions, with the long axis perpendicular to the profile of the lateral ventricles; they may also affect the subcortical arcuate fibres. Involvement of the corpus callosum is common. In the posterior fossa, plaques at various levels of the brainstem and in the cerebellum are often seen.

Compared to the normal surrounding brain tissue, MS plaques are usually iso- or slightly hypointense on T1-weighted images and hyperintense on proton density and T2-weighted images. After contrast medium administration, both solid and ring-like patterns of enhancement may be seen in acute plaques; however, enhancement is highly variable and is typically transient, lasting a few days or a few weeks. At the first episode, there is no way of distinguishing with certainty demyelinating plaques of MS from demyelinating lesions of ADEM: large lesions, all enhancing, point to ADEM; smaller, disseminated lesions, some enhancing and some not, thus suggesting different ages and possible previous asymptomatic plaques, point to MS. Accurate clinical history is essential, but often only the follow-up will allow discrimination between MS and ADEM (Kesselring *et al.*, 1990).

Acute disseminated encephalomyelitis

ADEM is also characterized by perivenous demyelination in the brain and often in the spinal cord, associated with variable degrees of inflammatory cell infiltration. The process may be diffuse or very extensive and may even lead to petechial haemorrhages. On MRI, it may be indistinguishable from MS; clinical features are, therefore, very important in suggesting the correct diagnosis. The most typical presentation of ADEM follows an episode of viral infection or a vaccination; occurrence is more common in children and adolescents than in adults. ADEM usually runs a non-progressive monophasic course. The lesions may remarkably regress or even resolve without residual nervous tissue damage; rapid regression after a prompt course of steroid therapy is considered a good support to the diagnosis. However, when severe and extensive involvement of the nervous tissue has occurred, regression of the acute inflammatory changes may leave a severely damaged brain with permanent clinical sequelae (Andreula *et al.*, 1997).

In the acute phase of the disease, MRI usually demonstrates multiple, scattered lesions affecting

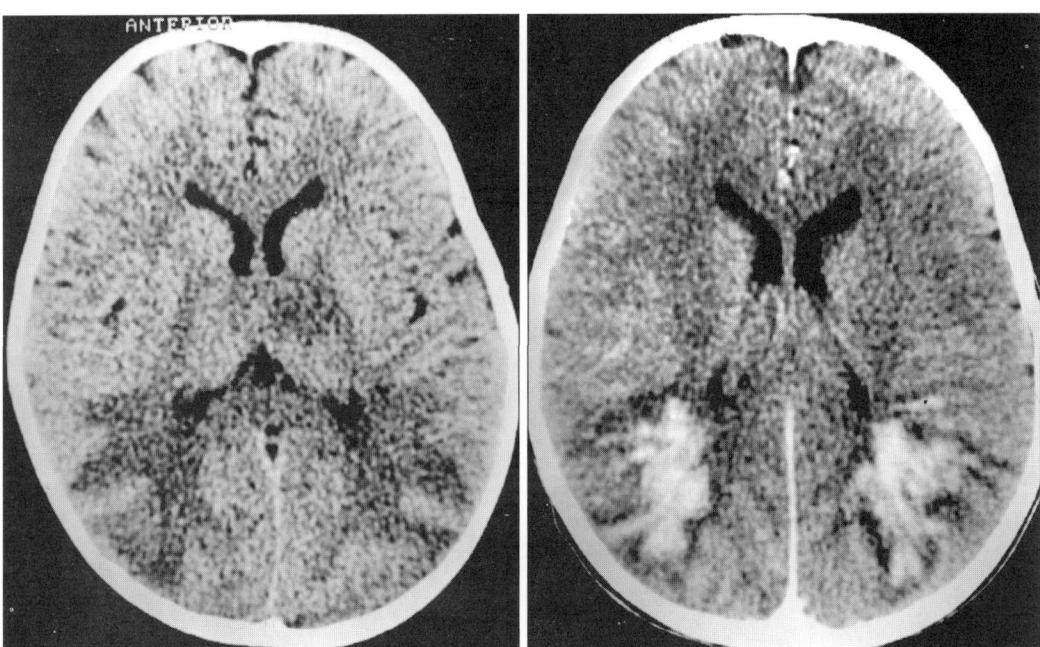

Fig. 1. ADEM in a 4-year-old girl after mycoplasma pneumoniae infection.

CT scan (A and B) demonstrates two large, hypodense areas involving the white matter of both parieto-occipital regions; a mild mass effect is present. Marked, central enhancement of both lesions is seen on post-contrast CT study (B). MRI obtained a few days later (C, axial T2-weighted image) confirms the white matter lesions, which are hyperintense. Follow-up MRI obtained 6 months later (D, axial T2-weighted image) shows marked reduction of the lesions with some decrease of the bulk of white matter; the lateral ventricles are slightly enlarged. The gray matter has been spared.

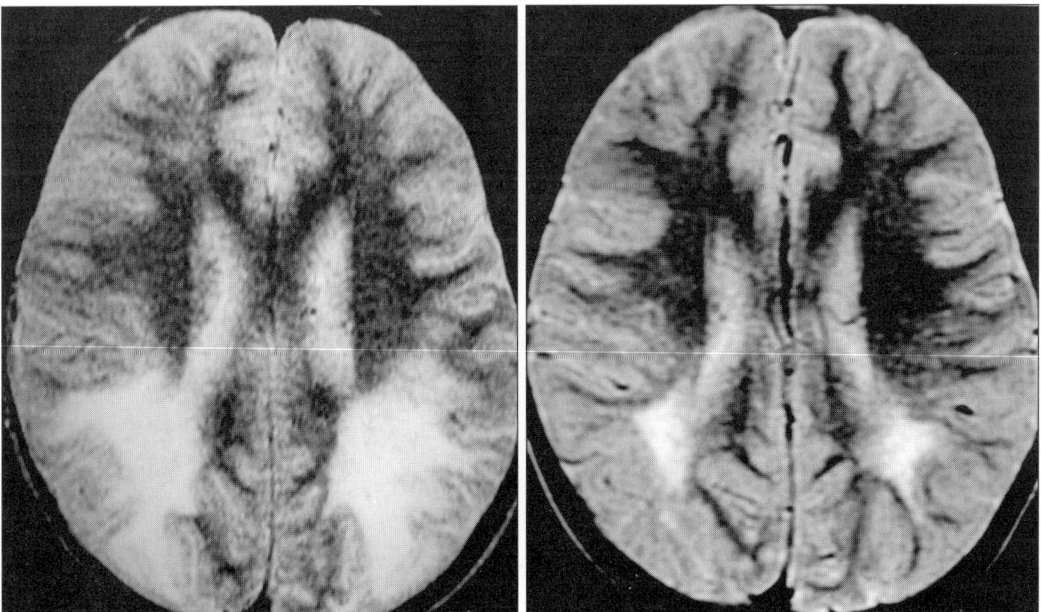

the subcortical white matter of one or both hemispheres; sometimes, gray matter of the cortex or deep cerebral nuclei, brainstem, cerebellar white matter and spinal cord are also involved. The lesions, often large, show only mild or no mass effect. As in MS, areas of demyelination are iso- or hypointense on T1-weighted images and hyperintense on proton density and T2-weighted images. The pattern of enhancement may be varied: patchy, ring-like or a combination of both, probably because of confluence of lesion of various size (Fig. 1). Enhancement may rapidly disappear and absence of enhancement does not rule out the diagnosis of ADEM (Mader et al., 1996; Caldemeyer & Azzarelli, 2000).

The clinician and the neuroradiologist are confronted with a difficult diagnostic challenge when a polyphasic presentation occurs. Shortly after the initial acute phase, in which a series of lesions with the same amount or pattern of enhancement are seen, new clinical findings and new enhancing lesions on MRI may appear, while the previously demonstrated lesions may show regression in size and enhancement. It is now accepted that the 'monophasic' characteristic of ADEM should not be intended in the very strict sense of a single episode; the 'monophasic' course of ADEM may comprise a cluster of episodes within a brief period of time which may last up to 4–6 months (Fig. 2).

We have observed, however, cases with post-viral acute onset of a disease which fulfilled the criteria of ADEM both clinically and neuroradiologically, in which the final diagnosis had to be changed. Regression of lesions was documented by repeat MRI studies and MRI residual findings remained stable for 2 or 3 years, after which new lesions appeared; the following relapsing-remitting course changed the diagnosis from ADEM to MS. It is impossible to say whether the first episode represented an ADEM, or was the onset of MS, or the following MS was triggered by ADEM; it is also impossible to state how long a patient with a diagnosis of ADEM should be examined with MRI to be sure that the acute episode is not followed by other lesions indicating MS. We advise MRI follow-up 1 year after the conclusion of the acute episode, with a need to repeat MRI only if new clinical findings appear.

An even more difficult and confusing problem is that of 'recurring' ADEM; differentiation from MS may be impossible or may require a very long follow-up (Andreula et al., 1997). On the other hand, demyelinating lesions seen on MRI, suspected of representing the onset of MS because of lack of preceding viral infection or vaccination, should be considered with caution; isolated episodes that can be considered as ADEM may not be heralded by evident viral infection; the label of MS should never be given on MRI findings alone but always requires careful clinical evaluation and follow-up.

In most cases of ADEM, the lesions affect the white matter; however, as has already been mentioned, cortex and deep gray matter may be involved (Caldemeyer & Azzarelli, 2000)

Fig. 2 (facing). ADEM, polyphasic, protracted course, vs. MS in an 11-year-old girl. MRI, axial T2-weighted sections, from three different examinations (A-D). On the first examination (A), large, multiple areas of hyperintensity involving the white matter of the frontal lobes, the periventricular regions, and the left parietal region, with different degrees of swelling, are present. On the examination obtained 3 months later (B), most of the lesions have regressed, but a new large lesion in the left fronto-parietal white matter has developed. On follow-up MRI obtained 8 months after onset of the disease (C, D), regression of all previously seen lesions with residual abnormalities of the white matter is seen (C); however, some new areas of signal abnormalities are found (arrowheads), without clinical symptoms (D). Subsequent examinations obtained at another institution and clinical follow-up 1 year later demonstrated stable conditions. Further follow-up will be necessary to differentiate ADEM from MS.

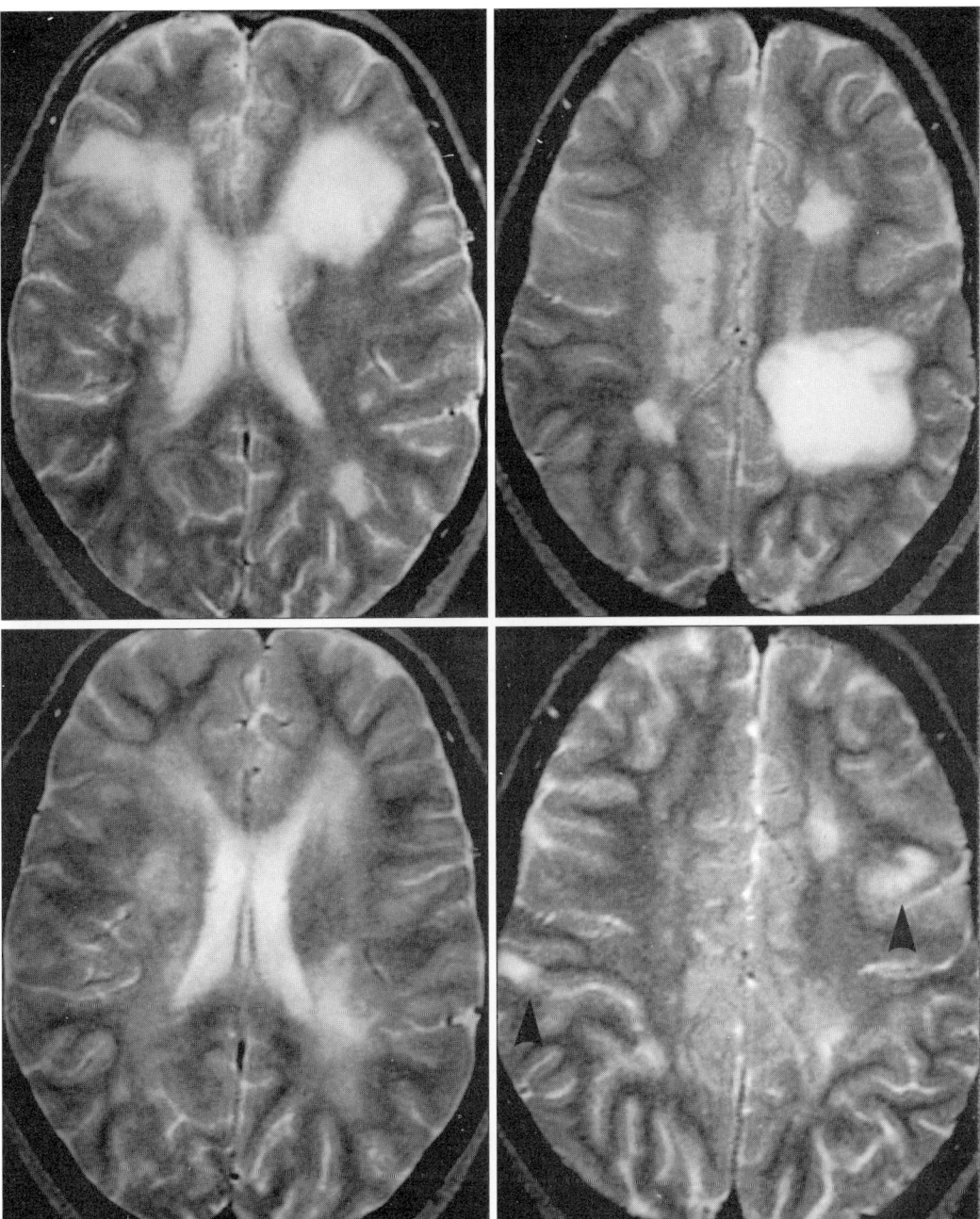

(Fig. 3). In our experience, ADEM occurred following chicken pox, measles, infection by mycoplasma pneumoniae, or simple upper respiratory infection, presumably viral, but of undetermined aetiology. It should also be clear that acute episodes of neurological deficits following viral infections – that can be labeled on clinical grounds as ADEM – may lack MRI manifestations. MRI, however, remains the best tool to demonstrate nervous tissue involvement in ADEM and its evolution.

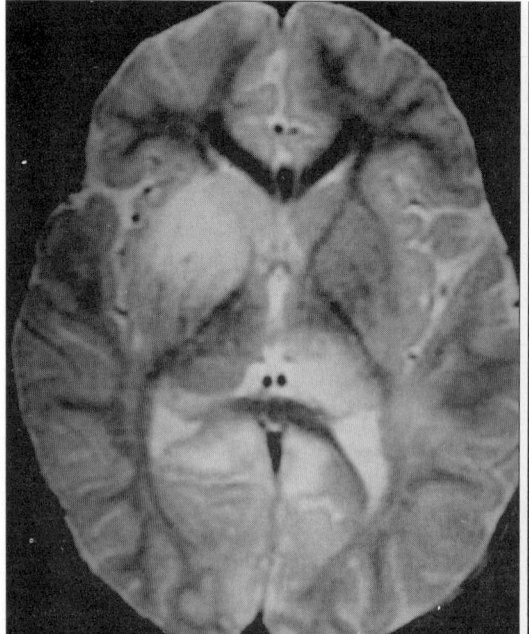
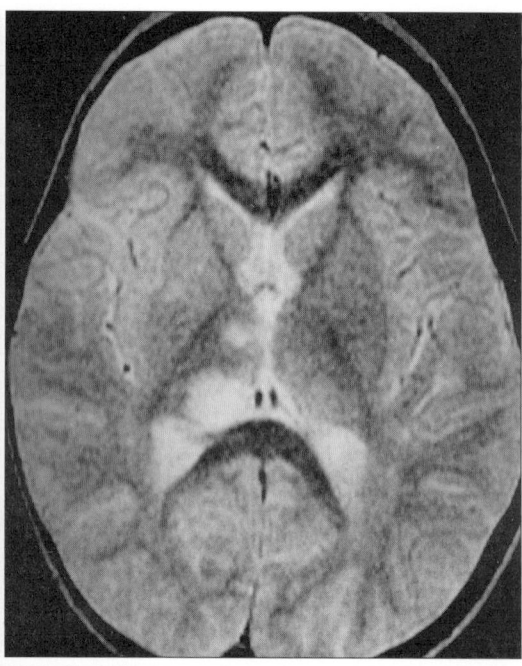
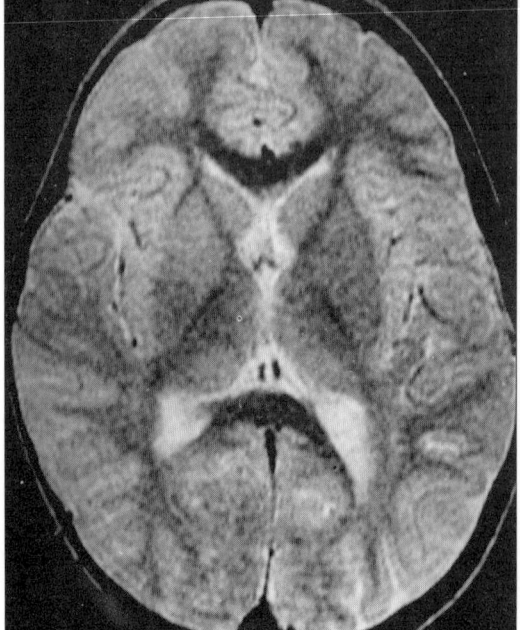

Fig. 3. ADEM after gastrointestinal infection, with involvement of the gray matter, and polyphasic course. MRI, axial T2-weighted sections at the same level, from 3 different examinations (A-C).

Initial MRI examination (A) shows lesions involving the right lenticular nucleus, the left thalamus, the left paratrigonal white matter, and the posterior interhemispheric regions, bilaterally. Follow-up MRI one month later (B) shows regression of the lesions with two new hyperintense areas in the right thalamus. Follow-up MRI obtained 3 years later (C) shows regression of all lesions with minimal residual white matter abnormalities in the left paratrigonal region and normal lateral ventricles.

Rasmussen's encephalitis

Rasmussen's encephalitis is a progressive inflammatory process of unknown aetiology, clinically characterized by intractable focal seizures, progressive hemiparesis, and intellectual deterioration; pathological studies show perivascular cuffs of lymphocytes, microglial nodules and

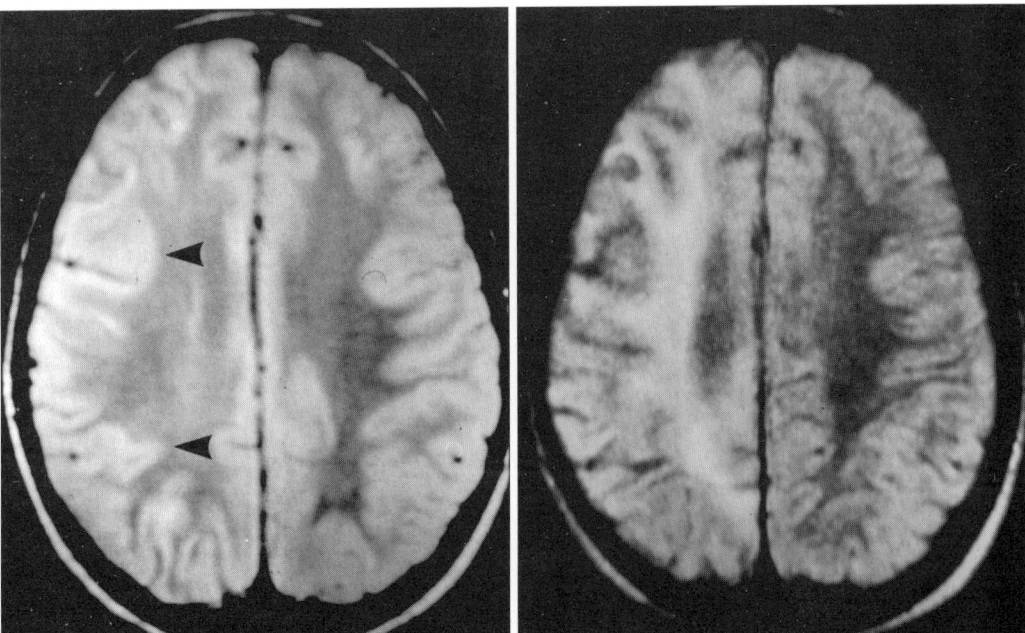

Fig. 4. Rasmussen's encephalitis in a 6-year-old girl. On the first MRI examination, axial proton density image (A) shows minimal cortical hyperintensity in the right frontal and parietal regions (arrowheads) and mild involvement of the subjacent white matter. Follow-up MRI obtained 12 months later (B, axial proton density image) shows right frontal cortical atrophy and extensive hyperintensity of the right frontal and parietal white matter.

mild meningitis, curiously confined to one cerebral hemisphere. Recently, autoantibodies to glutamate receptor GluR3 have been detected (Rogers *et al.*, 1994), suggesting a possible autoimmune process triggered by a virus. The end stage of the disease is characterized by cortico-subcortical atrophy affecting one cerebral hemisphere, even if minor involvement of the other hemisphere has been occasionally reported.

MRI findings differ according to disease stage. At the onset of the disease, MRI is often normal. During the follow-up, serial scans show progressive focal or hemispheric atrophy, and T2-weighted images may demonstrate the presence of progressively extending areas of increased signal intensity in the cortex and adjacent white matter and in the basal ganglia; the head of the caudate nucleus is often precociously affected (Tien *et al.*, 1992; Bhatjiwale *et al.*, 1998) (Figs. 4 and 5). No enhancement is seen after contrast medium administration.

No definite biologic or pathologic markers have been demonstrated; so far, continuous partial epilepsy and unilateral hemispheric involvement are considered the distinguishing features of Rasmussen's encephalitis. MRI, therefore, is an important tool in suggesting or confirming the clinical diagnosis and in monitoring the progression of the disease; it may obviate the necessity of brain biopsy.

Sydenham's chorea

In most patients with CNS involvement in the course of rheumatic fever manifested by choreic, sometimes unilateral, movements, no abnormalities can be detected by MRI. Given the clinical

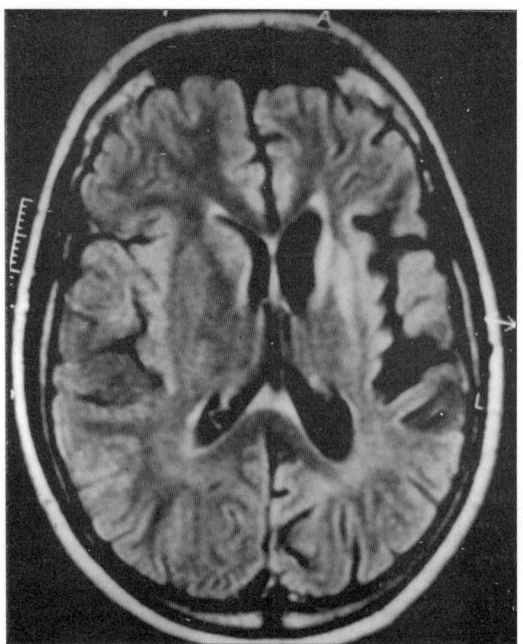

Fig. 5. Rasmussen's encephalitis in a different patient with involvement of the left hemisphere. Axial FLAIR image at the level of the basal ganglia shows atrophy and signal abnormalities of the head of caudate nucleus and putamen, in addition to involvement of the insular and fronto-parietal, opercular cortex.

manifestations, there is no question that the basal ganglia are affected even if MRI is normal. In only very few cases have MRI lesions been reported, usually confined to the head of the caudate nucleus and adjacent anterior part of the putamen, contra-lateral to the side affected by choreic movements. The lesions appear as areas of hyperintensity in proton density and T2-weighted images; post-contrast enhancement is observed and may last longer than is usually seen in vascular, ischaemic lesions; in addition, the evolution of lesions does not lead to a malacic area, such as is found in ischaemia (Kienzle et al., 1991; Klawans, 1991). Therefore, although vasculitis can be present, the abnormalities observed in the head of caudate nucleus and anterior part of the putamen are thought to result mainly from an autoimmune cross-reaction against antigens expressed by the neuronal population of this part of the neostriatum. In fact, it has been demonstrated that these striatal neurons share antigenic properties with the β-haemolytic streptococcal bacterial membrane (Husby et al., 1976).

Bilateral striatal necrosis

Infantile bilateral striatal necrosis is a heterogeneous condition sometimes associated with or attributed to mitochondrial dysfunction; it may follow an acute febrile illness and is, therefore, included among the parainfective encephalitides (Goutières & Aicardi, 1982; Roig et al., 1990). It is characterized by destructive lesions of the basal ganglia that affect the neostriatum; on MRI, the lesions appear as symmetrical areas of hypointensity in T1-weighted images, and hyperintensity in proton density and T2-weighted images. The nuclei which are always affected are the putamina; the caudate nuclei are less frequently involved. In our series of more than 10 cases, we observed involvement of both nuclei or of the putamen only, while the head of the caudate nucleus was never involved alone (Fig. 6). This sequence of involvement suggests a greater vulnerability of the putamen than of the caudate nucleus.

Because of the similarities of these lesions with those observed in mitochondrial disorders, particularly in Leigh's disease (Savoiardo et al., 1991), our patients affected by infantile bilateral striatal necrosis were tested for mitochondrial disease: none of the patients proved positive for mitochondrial disorders.

Another interesting point is that the lesions of the neostriatum in infantile striatal necrosis seem to have little or no progression after the first observation, even if clinical progression of dystonia may continue. The lesions seem to be complete early on in the course of the disease; by analogy with other conditions, clinical progression may be attributed to abnormal sprouting of the surviving neurons in the damaged nuclei (Nardocci *et al.*, 1996).

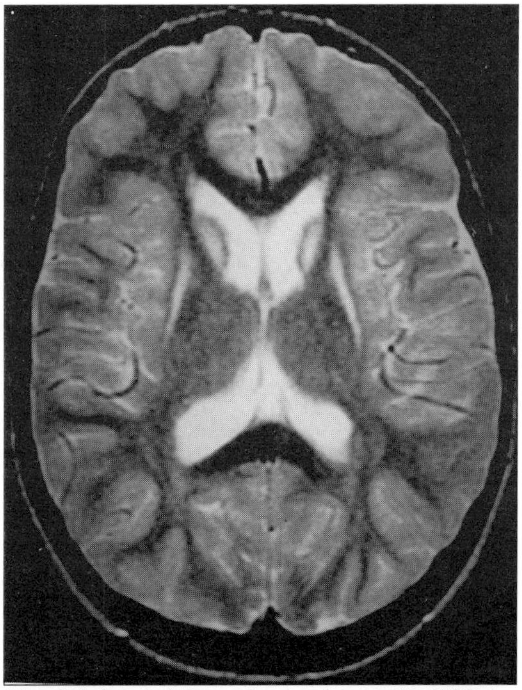

Vasculitis

Vasculitides may affect the CNS as a secondary manifestation of a diffuse, systemic disorder that affects the blood vessels; they may be caused by all infectious meningitides, by parasites and drugs. More rarely, isolated or primary angiitis of the CNS occurs.

Most of these diseases, such as connective tissue disorders, systemic lupus erythematosus, giant-cell arteritis, affect adults, but some of these diseases may also occur in adolescents and children.

In many cases the diagnosis is obvious, for instance in a patient with tuberculous meningitis who develops a stroke. In other cases the diagnosis is difficult and requires a series of laboratory tests and even brain biopsy (Chu *et al.*, 1998; Alrawi *et al.*, 1999).

On MRI, the diagnosis of vasculitis may be suspected when multiple areas of infarct are seen, accompanied by leptomeningeal post-contrast enhancement and enhancement extending deep into the brain along the penetrating medullary arteries. However, when small-size vessels are involved, deep, subcortical areas of abnormal signal intensity may be observed (Greenan *et al.*, 1992) that may be indistinguishable from areas of demyelination; coexistent involvement of gray matter, either in the basal ganglia, thalami, or cortex may suggest the diagnosis of possible vasculitis (Hurst & Grossman, 1994) (Fig. 7).

Fig. 6. Infantile bilateral striatal necrosis. MRI. Axial T2-weighted image shows symmetrical hyperintensity of the putamina and heads of the caudate nuclei, with marked putaminal atrophy.

A possible mechanism leading to vasculitis and cortical involvement is related to deposition of immune complexes in the vessel walls following an infection. This mechanism has been demonstrated by brain biopsy in a child following *Campylobacter jejuni* enteritis (Nasralla *et al.*, 1993); in addition to vasculitic changes in the cortex, electron-dense deposits in the basement membranes of the blood vessels, consistent with immune complex deposition, were demonstrated by electron microscopy. Wider use of brain biopsy could probably clarify many more cases in which the diagnosis remains unproven; prompt response to steroid therapy, however, may make the recourse to biopsy unwarranted (Fig. 8).

The role of angiography versus MRI in the diagnosis of vasculitis is debated (Harris *et al.*, 1994; Pomper *et al.*, 1999). The segmental narrowing and dilatation of the larger leptomeningeal arteries is rarely seen. When present, it establishes the diagnosis (Yuh *et al.*, 1999). We observed this finding in only one paediatric case, an adolescent who had, according to her, used unknown drugs for the first time for recreational use and developed a stroke with haemorrhage in the basal ganglia. However, since in CNS vasculitis small-size vessels that escape angiographic demon-

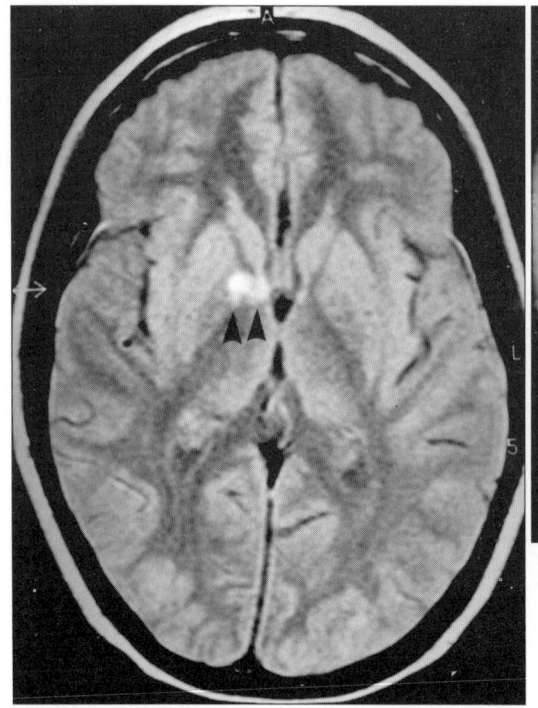 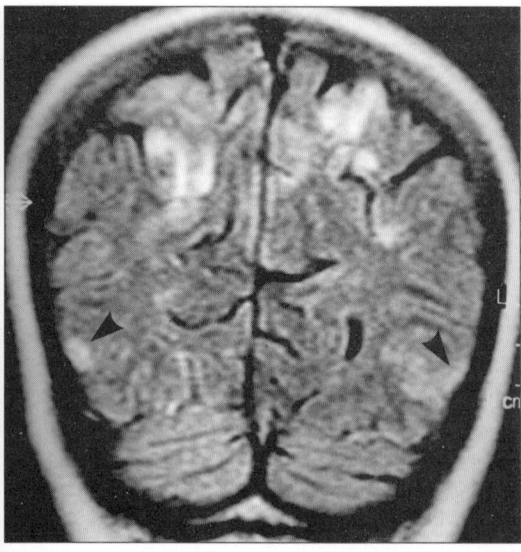

Fig. 7. Probable vasculitis in a patient with SLE. MRI: axial proton density section (A) shows a hyperintense lesion involving the genu of the right internal capsule and the adjacent medial part of the globus pallidus (arrowheads), consistent with the territories of the perforating branches from the posterior communicating artery and middle cerebral artery. Coronal FLAIR image (B) shows cortical and subcortical hyperintensities mainly centred on the watershed parietal areas; other small cortical areas are also involved (arrowheads).

stration are more commonly affected, a normal angiogram does not rule out the diagnosis of vasculitis.

The vascular narrowing characteristic of vasculitis may result in ischaemic but not infarcted areas, that may escape demonstration by conventional MRI. Therefore, the diagnosis of CNS vasculitis often relies on clinical parameters, on response to immunosuppressive therapy, and on new functional imaging techniques, such as perfusion and diffusion imaging, which can assess the disease process at the microcirculatory level with detection of hypoperfusion, early ischaemia or infarction (Yuh *et al.*, 1999).

In our experience, the 'vasculitic-like' condition that we encountered more frequently in paediatric age was the primary antiphospholipid syndrome (PAPS).

Antiphospholipid antibodies are circulating immunoglobulins associated with a hypercoagulable state (Del Papa *et al.*, 1997; Parisi *et al.*, 1998). Patients with these antibodies may develop stroke, even multiple strokes, with both arterial and venous occlusions. Many of them do not present clinical features of vasculitis, but some of them do; histologic demonstration of a lymphocytic infiltrate with typical features of vasculitis has been reported (Provenzale *et al.*, 1998), but, in the majority of the PAPS cases, a non-inflammatory vasculopathy rather than a vasculitis has been demonstrated.

In PAPS, MRI may demonstrate single or multiple areas of signal abnormalities mostly involving the basal ganglia or the cortex, suggesting medium-vessel occlusions (Fig. 9). Large vessels, however, can also be involved (Provenzale *et al.*, 1998).

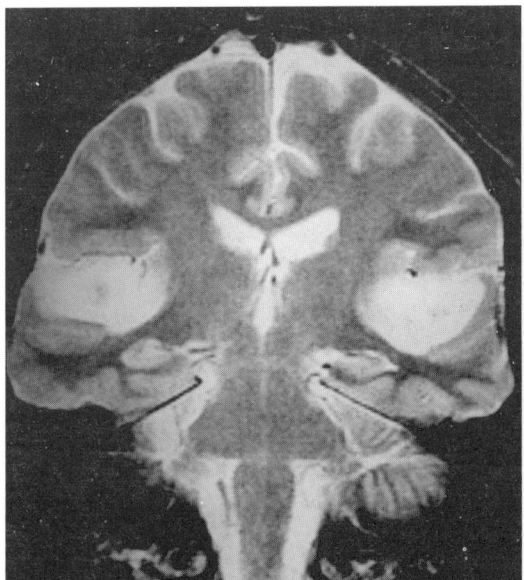
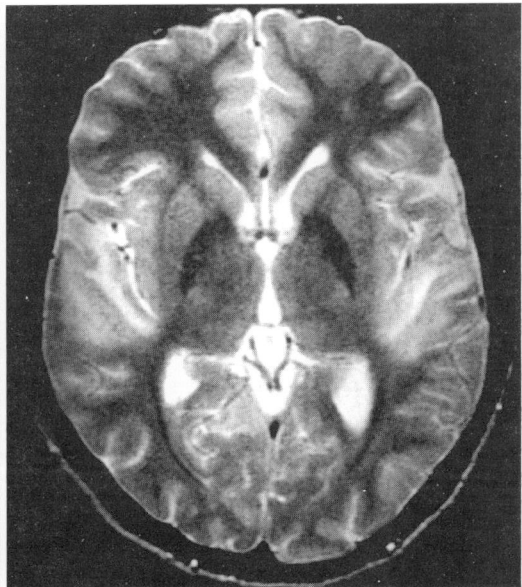

Fig. 8. MRI of possible vasculitis in a patient with acute cortical swelling involving both temporal opercula and inferior insular regions (A, coronal T2-weighted section). Rapid regression of the lesions after steroid therapy is seen in the follow-up examination (B, axial T2-weighted image), followed by complete resolution on the third examination (C). Diagnosis remains unproven.

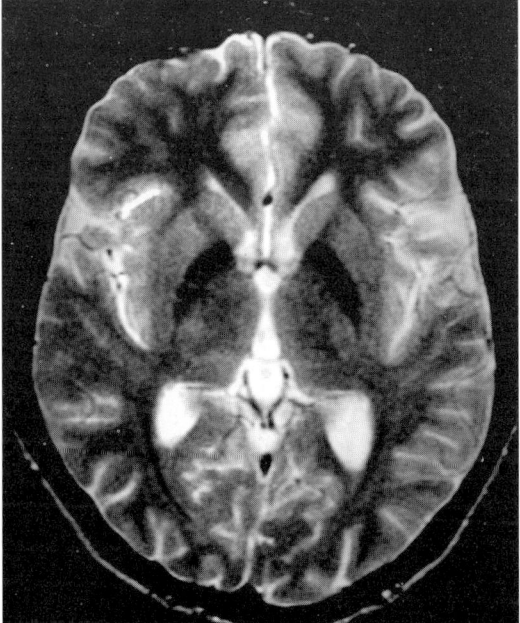

Another rather obscure systemic vasculitis, i.e. Behçet's disease, can affect the CNS in approximately 30 per cent of the cases. Both the arterial and venous systems are involved, with a venous predominance. This may explain some of the characteristic MRI findings, consisting in brainstem and diencephalic involvement, secondary to the peculiar venous drainage of this region (Koçer et al., 1999). No lesions are seen in arterial territory distribution. The involvement of the upper brainstem is usually central or bilateral and asymmetrical, with frequent post-contrast marginal or irregular enhancement. The lesions may evolve into necrotic areas. Supratentorial subcortical or periventricular white matter lesions and meningeal thickening may also occur

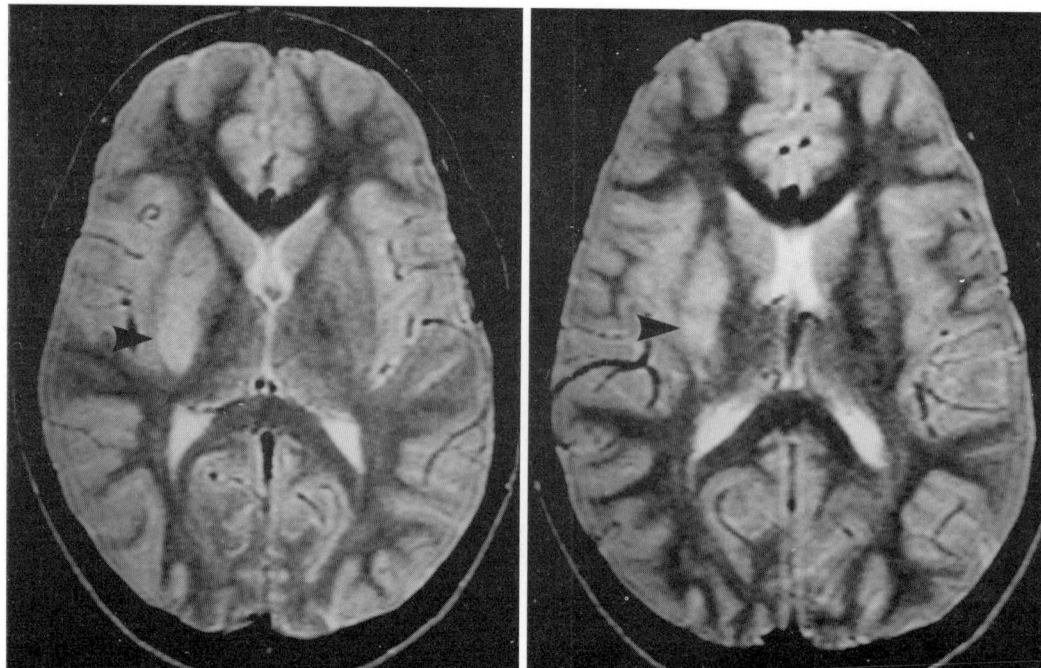

Fig. 9. PAPS. MRI in an 11-year-old boy, with acute onset of mild left hemiparesis. Axial T2-weighted sections (A and B) show involvement of the right putamen (arrowheads), suggesting a vascular distribution. Elevated antiphospholipid antibodies were the only abnormal finding.

(Gumà et al., 1998). Complete regression of large white matter lesions may be observed after prompt steroid treatment.

Conclusions

In many patients with a suspected immune-mediated disorder, MRI is the most informative neuroradiological examination: it may demonstrate peculiar patterns that confirm the clinical diagnosis, the evolution of the lesions and their response to therapy. It may also demonstrate the complications that immunosuppressive treatment may cause – for instance, in patients who develop infections or progressive multifocal encephalopathy (PML) as a consequence of the treatment itself (Fig. 10). Prompt recognition of the complication and avoidance of misinterpretation of the new findings – otherwise attributed to worsening of the primary disease – are essential in adopting the correct treatment. A close collaboration with the paediatric neurologist or the clinician in charge of the patient is absolutely necessary for a correct interpretation of neuroradiological findings.

Acknowledgements: We wish to thank Dr. N. Nardocci, paediatric neurologist, and Dr. A. Salmaggi, neuroimmunologist, for their frequent, helpful discussions.

References

Alrawi, A., Trobe, J.D., Blaivas, M. & Musch, D.C. (1999): Brain biopsy in primary angiitis of the central nervous system. *Neurology* **53,** 858–860.

Andreula, C.F., Recchia Luciani, A.N.M. & Milella, D. (1997): Magnetic resonance imaging in the diagnosis of acute disseminated encephalomyelitis (ADEM). *Int. J. Neuroradiol.* **3,** 21–34.

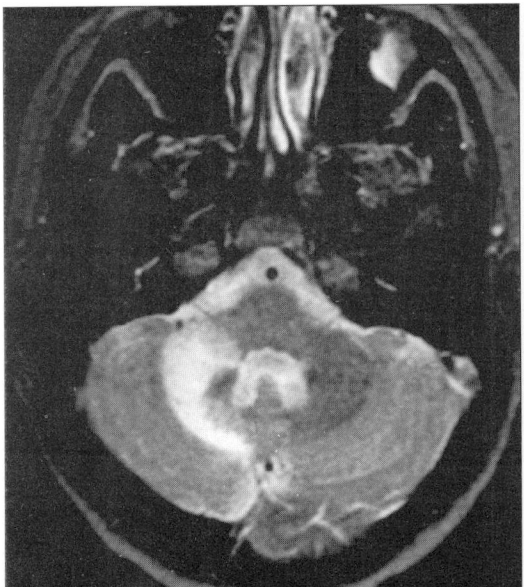
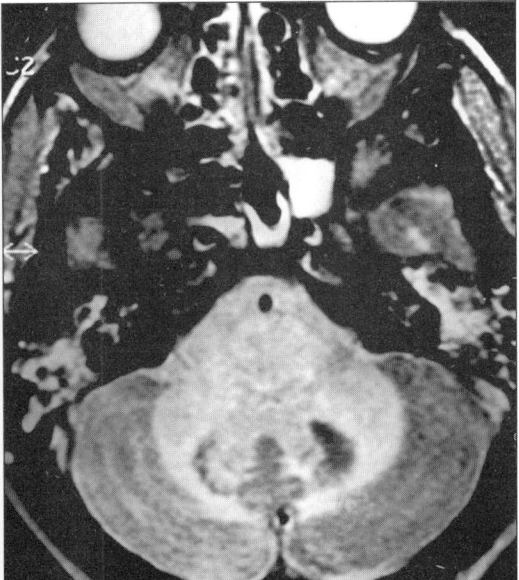
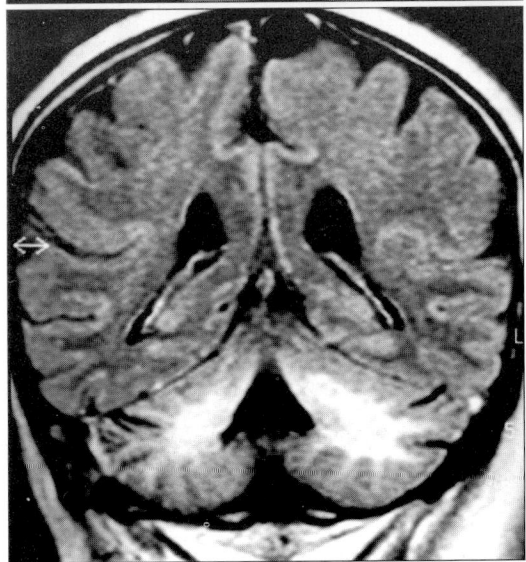

Fig. 10. MRI in a young woman affected by SLE since adolescence, submitted to repeated cycles of immunosuppressive treatment. Recent onset of cerebellar signs. Involvement of the right middle cerebellar peduncle and right cerebellar white matter seen in axial T2-weighted section of first MRI (A) was interpreted as a possible sign of arteritis. This misinterpretation led to more aggressive treatment. Progression of the lesion with involvement of brainstem and cerebellar white matter led to the correct diagnosis of PML, proven by detection by PCR of JC virus genomic material in the CSF (B: axial T2-weighted, and C: coronal FLAIR images of a late follow-up study).

Bhatjiwale, M.G., Polekey, C., Cox, T.C.S., Dean, A. & Deasy, N. (1998): Rasmussen's encephalitis: neuroimaging finding in 21 patients with a closer look at the basal ganglia. *Pediatr. Neurosurg.* **29**, 141–148.

Caldemeyer, K.S. & Azzarelli, B. (2000): Adult white matter disease. In: *Neuroimaging: clinical and physical principles*, eds. R.A. Zimmermann, W.A. Gibby, & R.F. Carmody, pp. 741–743. New York: Springer-Verlag.

Chu, C.T., Gray, L., Goldstein, L.B. & Hulette, C.M. (1998): Diagnosis of intracranial vasculitis: a multi-disciplinary approach. *J. Neuropathol. Exp. Neurol.* **57**, 30–38.

Del Papa, N., Guidali, L., Sala, A., Buccellati, C., Khamashta, M.A., Ichikawa, K., Koike, T., Balestrieri, G., Tincani, A., Hughes, G.R. & Meron, P.L. (1997): Endothelial cells as target for antiphospholipid antibodies. Human polyclonal and monoclonal anti-beta 2-glycoprotein antibodies react *in vitro* with endothelial cells through beta 2-glycoprotein I and induce endothelial activation. *Arthritis Rheum.* **40**, 551–561.

Goutières, F. & Aicardi, J. (1982): Acute neurological dysfunction associated with destructive lesions of the basal ganglia in children. *Ann. Neurol.* **12**, 328–332.

Greenan, T.J., Grossman, R.I. & Goldberg, H.I. (1992): Cerebral vasculitis: MR imaging and angiographic correlation. *Radiology* **182**, 65–72.

Gumà, A., Aguilera, C., Acebes, J., Arruga, J. & Pons, L. (1998): Meningeal involvement in Behçet disease: MRI. *Neuroradiology* **40**, 512–515.

Harris, K.G., Tran, D.D., Sickels, W.J., Cornell, S.H. & Yuh, W.T.C. (1994): Diagnosing intracranial vasculitis: the role of MR and angiography. *Am. J. Neuroradiol.* **15**, 317–330.

Hurst, R.W. & Grossman, R.I. (1994): Neuroradiology of central nervous system vasculitis. *Sem. Neurol.* **14**, 320–340.

Husby, G., van de Rijn, I., Zabriskie, J.B., Abdin, Z.H. & Williams, R.C. Jr. (1976): Antibodies reacting with cytoplasm of subthalamic and caudate nuclei neurons in chorea and acute rheumatic fever. *J. Exp. Med.* **144**, 1094–1110.

Kesselring, J., Miller, D.H., Robb, S.A., Kendall, B.E., Moseley, I.F., Kingsley, D., Du Boulay, E.P.G.H. & McDonald, I. (1990): Acute disseminated encephalomyelitis. MR findings and the distinction from multiple sclerosis. *Brain* **113**, 291–302.

Kienzle, G.D., Breger, R.K., Chun, R.W.M., Zupanc, M.L. & Sackett, J.F. (1991): Sydenham chorea: MR manifestations in two cases. *Am. J. Neuroradiol.* **12**, 73–76.

Klawans, H.K. (1991): Chorea: whither comest it? *Am. J. Neuroradiol.* **12**, 77.

Koçer, N., Islak, C., Siva, A., Saip, S., Akman, C., Kantarci, O. & Hamuryudan, V. (1999): CNS involvement in neuro-Behçet syndrome: an MR study. *Am. J. Neuroradiol.* **20**, 1015–1024.

Mader, I., Stick, W., Ettlin, T. & Probst, A. (1996): Acute disseminated encephalomyelitis: MR and CT features. *Am. J. Neuroradiol.* **17**, 104–109.

Nardocci, N., Zorzi, G., Grisoli, M., Rumi, V., Broggi, G. & Angelini, L. (1996): Acquired hemidystonia in childhood: a clinical and neuroradiological study of thirteen patients. *Pediatr. Neurol.* **15**, 108–113.

Nasralla, C.A.W., Pay, N., Goodpasture, H.C., Lin, J.J. & Svoboda, W.B. (1993): Postinfectious encephalopathy in a child following Campylobacter jejuni enteritis. *Am. J. Neuroradiol.* **14**, 444–448.

Parisi, L., Valente, G., Fantozzi, R., Serrao, M., Castagnoli, C., Valletta, L. & Tramutoli, R. (1998): Manifestazioni neurologiche nella sindrome da anticorpi antifosfolipidi. *Riv. Neurobiologia* **44**, 315–322.

Pomper, M.G., Miller, T.J., Stone, J.H., Tidmore, W.C. & Hellmann, D.B. (1999): CNS vasculitis in autoimmune disease: MR imaging findings and correlation with angiography. *Am. J. Neuroradiol.* **20**, 75–85.

Provenzale, J.M., Barboriak, D.P., Allen, N.B. & Ortel, T.L. (1998): Antiphospholipid antibodies: findings at arteriography. *Am. J. Neuroradiol.* **19**, 611–616.

Rogers, S.W., Andrews, P.I. & Gahring, L.C. (1994): Autoantibodies to glutamate receptor GluR3 in Rasmussen's encephalitis. *Science* **265**, 648–651.

Roig, M., Macaya, A., Munell, F. & Capdevilla, A. (1990): Acute neurological dysfunction associated with destructive lesions of the basal ganglia: a benign form of infantile bilateral striatal necrosis. *J. Pediatr.* **117**, 578–581.

Savoiardo, M., Uziel, G., Strada, L., Grisoli, M. & Wang, G. (1991): MRI findings in Leigh's disease with cytochrome-*c*-oxidase deficiency. *Neuroradiology* **33** (Suppl.), 507–508.

Tien, R.D., Ashdown, B.C., Lewis Jr, D.V., Atkins, M.R. & Burger, P.C. (1992): Rasmussen's encephalitis: neuroimaging findings in four patients. *Am. J. Roentgenol.* **158**, 1329–1332.

Yuh, W.T.C., Ueda, T. & Maley, J.E. (1999): Perfusion and diffusion imaging: a potential tool for improved diagnosis of CNS vasculitis. *Am. J. Neuroradiol.* **20**, 87–89.

Chapter 21

Use of magnetization transfer imaging to study multiple sclerosis and other immune-mediated disorders of the CNS

Marco Rovaris and Massimo Filippi

Neuroimaging Research Unit, Department of Neurosciences, Istituto Scientifico H San Raffaele, via Olgettina 60, 20132 Milan, Italy

Summary

Magnetization transfer imaging (MTI) is a magnetic resonance imaging (MRI) technique with a higher specificity than conventional T2-weighted scans to the heterogeneous pathological substrates of multiple sclerosis (MS) lesions. This review outlines the contribution of MTI in the study of lesion evolution and in the assessment of disease burden in MS and other immune-mediated diseases.

MTI studies of individual MS lesions confirm the pathological heterogeneity of T2-weighted MRI abnormalities and the potential role of unenhanced T1-weighted hypointensities as specific markers of localized severe white matter disruption. Correlative cross-sectional and longitudinal studies using MTI and gadolinium (Gd)-enhanced MRI reveal that MTI findings may vary in lesions with different patterns of enhancement, and that MTI abnormalities are closely related to the onset and recovery of blood-brain barrier disruption in new MS plaques. Measures obtained from MTI scans using whole-brain histogram analysis are highly correlated with the extent of MS abnormalities on conventional MRI scans and predict patients' clinical disability well, since they are sensitive to the amounts of both macro- and microscopic MS disease burden in the whole brain and in specific regions.

MTI studies suggest that: (a) MTI is sensitive to different stages of white matter lesion pathology and pathological evolution; and (b) in comparison with conventional MRI, MT histogram analysis can provide a more global assessment of disease burden in MS and other immune-mediated disorders of the central nervous system, since it encompasses both macro- and microscopic pathology.

Magnetization transfer imaging: basic principles

Magnetization transfer imaging (MTI) is a magnetic resonance imaging (MRI) technique that has recently been applied to the study of multiple sclerosis (MS) (McGowan et al., 1998). The physical basis of MTI is the exchange of magnetization from immobile protons, bound in a macromolecular matrix, to free water protons (McGowan *et al.,* 1998). Low-magnetization transfer ratio (MTR) indicates a reduced capacity of the molecules in the brain tissue matrix to exchange magnetization with the surrounding (MRI visible) water molecules. Although, in MS, this may be caused either by a reduction in the integrity of macromolecular matrix reflecting damage to the myelin or to the axonal membrane (McDonald *et al.,* 1992), or by a dilution of the macromolecules brought about by inflammatory oedema (McDonald *et al.,* 1992), studies with animal models (Dousset *et al.,* 1992, 1995) reported that MTR reduces only slightly with oedema but more strongly with severe demyelination and axonal loss in lesions of experimental allergic encephalomyelitis (Dousset *et al.,* 1992) or lysolecithin-induced demyelination (Dousset *et al.,* 1995).

MTI has three main advantages over conventional T2- and T1-weighted MRI in the study of MS. First, it provides both morphological and pathological information with a higher specificity than conventional MRI (McGowan *et al.,* 1998). Secondly, it enables us to assess the 'invisible' disease burden in the so-called normal-appearing white matter (NAWM), i.e. the brain tissue which does not show macroscopic abnormalities on conventional MRI (Filippi *et al.,* 1995a; Loevner *et al.,* 1995). Thirdly, with the application of magnetization transfer (MT) histogram methods (van Buchem *et al.,* 1996), it provides, from a single procedure, multiple parameters influenced by both the macro- and microscopic disease burden.

Several metrics can be obtained from MTI scans. The first step in the analysis is the creation of calculated MT images or MTR maps, which are derived from two sets of images, acquired with and without an off-resonance saturation pulse. MTR maps are derived pixel-by-pixel according to the equation MTR = $(M_0 - M_S) / M_0 \times 100$ (Dousset *et al.,* 1992), in which M_0 is the intensity of a given pixel without the saturation pulse, and M_S is the intensity of the same pixel when the saturation pulse is applied. MS lesions, which usually have lower MTR than NAWM (Dousset *et al.,* 1992), appear as areas of hypointensity on MTR maps. From these maps, the average MTR for specific regions of interest (ROIs) can be obtained. As a further step, the average lesion MTR for a given patient can be calculated. Moreover, using semi-automated thresholding techniques for lesion segmentation of digital images (Rovaris *et al.,* 1997; van Waesberghe *et al.,* 1998a), the load of these lesions (i.e. their total volume) can be assessed. From each MTI scan, histograms of MTR values can also be derived, using an image analysis method which was developed by van Buchem *et al.* (1996). Histograms of pixel intensity are created from the calculated MT images, after a preliminary manual or semi-automatic image segmentation aimed at excluding all the non-cerebral tissues (e.g. skull, orbital tissue, etc.). To reduce the effects of image noise and also cerebrospinal fluid (CSF) signal, all the pixels with very low MTR (i.e. from 0 to 5–10 per cent) are also excluded from the analysis. Then, the data set of MTR values is displayed as a histogram, which is usually normalized to the total number of brain voxels to allow comparisons of histograms from subjects with different brain volumes. For each histogram, several parameters can be calculated (van Buchem *et al.,* 1996): the height and position of the histogram peak (i.e. the most common MTR value in the brain), the average MTR, and the MTR corresponding to the 25th, 50th and 75th percentiles of the histogram (MTR25, MTR50 and MTR75), that indicate the MTR at which the integral of the histogram is 25 per cent, 50 per cent and 75 per cent of the total, respectively. MT histograms can be obtained both for the whole brain and for specific regions (e.g. frontal lobe, cerebellum, brainstem, etc.), which can be segmented according to standard neuroanatomical references.

MTI in the study of individual lesions

Conventional T2-weighted MRI scans have a high sensitivity in revealing MS lesions, but they lack specificity to further characterize the stages of the pathological process in individual lesions (Filippi & Miller, 1996). Oedema, demyelination, gliosis and axonal loss (McDonald *et al.*, 1992), all lead to a similar appearance of hyperintensity on T2-weighted images. On the other hand, chronic hypointense areas on unenhanced T1-weighted images show severe tissue disruption (van Walderveen *et al.*, 1998), but lesion hypointensity may also occur acutely and transiently in the case of inflammatory oedema and subsequently return to isointensity (van Waesberghe *et al.*, 1998b). Finally, gadolinium (Gd)-enhanced T1-weighted images allow active lesions to be separated from inactive lesions (Miller *et al.*, 1993), since enhancement occurs as a result of increased blood-brain barrier (BBB) permeability (Kermode *et al.*, 1990), but they do not enable us to distinguish purely oedematous-active from demyelinating lesions. Therefore, MTI findings have been correlated with conventional MRI abnormalities in several cross-sectional and longitudinal studies aimed at elucidating the variability of pathology in MS lesions and its evolution over time.

Several studies have demonstrated that MTR values for MS lesions visible on T2-weighted MRI are significantly lower than in NAWM, although their range is wide. Dousset *et al.* (1992) studied 209 T2-weighted hyperintense lesions in 15 MS patients and reported an average lesion MTR of 26.3 per cent, with a lower mean value in secondary progressive (SP) (23.3 per cent) than in relapsing-remitting (RR) (27.6 per cent) MS patients. Average MTR in NAWM was 37.1 per cent in MS patients and 41.8 per cent in healthy controls. Gass *et al.* (1994) found that MS lesions of 40 patients with different forms of MS had an average MTR lower than that of ischaemic lesions from patients with small-vessel disease, and that the average lesion MTR was significantly higher in benign MS compared to SP-MS. A recent, longitudinal study (Rocca *et al.*, 1999) showed that, over a three year follow-up period, new lesions in patients with SP-MS presented a more severe and significant MTR reduction than do those in patients with RR-MS. Campi *et al.* (1996b), studying 292 lesions from 21 MS patients, found an average MTR of 41.2 per cent, whereas the average for NAWM in healthy controls was 50.7 per cent. Interestingly, in the latter study (Campi *et al.*, 1996b), average MS lesion MTR was significantly lower than that measured for T2-weighted hyperintense lesions on MRI scans from patients with systemic lupus erythematosus (SLE) (43.4 per cent), which show a similar degree of T2-weighted hyperintensities. The latter data have been confirmed by a recent report from Rovaris *et al.* (2000), who found that average lesion MTR is significantly lower in patients with MS than in patients with SLE and Wegener's granulomatosis and in patients with neuropsychiatric SLE (NSLE) than in those with SLE. Decreased MTR has also been found for NAWM areas that are adjacent to focal T2-weighted MS lesions (Filippi *et al.*, 1995a; Loevner *et al.*, 1995); MTR progressively increased with distance from MS lesions to the cortical gray matter and MTR was lower for patients with more disabling MS courses. The latter findings suggest that the actual size of MS lesions is greater than that visible on T2-weighted images (Filippi *et al.*, 1995a) and that the demyelinating 'penumbra' detected by MTI techniques might be relevant in determining patients' disability. From all these studies, it is evident that decreased MTR corresponds well with T2-weighted hyperintensity and that a wide range of pathological substrates underlie the non-specific conventional MRI signal changes. On the basis of the MTI results obtained with animal models of demyelination (Dousset *et al.*, 1995), where MTR decrease was found to be minimal in acute, non-demyelinating inflammatory lesions, it may be argued that T2-weighted MS lesions with lower MTR are expressions of more severe demyelination. This is confirmed by the lower MTR found in MS lesions of patients with a more disabling disease course (Gass et al., 1994; Rocca et al., 1999) and by the robust, inverse correlation between average lesion MTR and severity of neurological impairment (Gass et al., 1994).

Pathological studies have confirmed that hypointense lesions on T1-weighted MRI correspond to areas of tissue disorganization due to demyelination and/or axonal loss (van Walderveen et al., 1998). The potential of T1-weighted MRI abnormalities as pathologically specific MRI markers of MS severity has been emphasized by cross-sectional (van Walderveen et al., 1995) and longitudinal (Truyen et al., 1997) studies, and confirmed by studies using MTI. Lower MTR has been reported in hypointense lesions than in lesions that are isointense to NAWM on T1-weighted scans (van Waesberghe et al., 1998b; Hiehle et al., 1995), and MTR has been found to be inversely correlated with the degree of hypointensity, i.e. MTR is more reduced for very hypointense lesions (Hiehle et al., 1995). Van Waesberghe et al. (1997) demonstrated that MTR in MS lesions was significantly correlated with their longitudinal relaxation rates and signal intensities normalized to both NAWM and CSF on T1-weighted MRI, thus concluding that these MRI measures may all be considered markers of severe tissue destruction. More recently, the same authors (van Waesberghe et al., 1999) performed a correlative study between MTI findings and post-mortem brain specimens from 17 MS patients and confirmed that both MTR and T1 contrast ratio correlate strongly with axonal density in MS lesions and NAWM. In addition, they found that both MTR and T1 contrast ratio correlate well with the degree of demyelination within MS lesions. Van Waesberghe et al. (1998b) also compared the natural course of active MS lesions on serial unenhanced T1-weighted and MTI scans. They found that the patterns described for active lesions on both baseline and follow-up unenhanced T1-weighted and MTI scans were highly correlated. For MS lesions that changed from hypointense to isointense when Gd enhancement ceased, MTR increased significantly during a 6-month follow-up, whereas a strongly decreased MTR at the time of initial enhancement was predictive of a persistent T1-weighted hypointensity and lower MTR after six months.

Gd enhancement of MS lesions, which indicates local BBB disruption, may show two typical patterns: homogeneous and ring-like (Kermode et al., 1990; Bruck et al., 1997). The latter is thought to reflect peripheral inflammation and complete central demyelination, and can be caused by reactivation at the periphery of chronic lesions (Bruck et al., 1997). The relationship between the enhancement patterns of MS lesions and their MTR has been extensively investigated. Petrella et al. (1996) studied 42 MS lesions and found that the MTR for homogeneously enhancing lesions was significantly higher than in the central portion of ring-like enhancing lesions. These results were confirmed by Campi et al. (1996a), who measured MTR in 65 enhancing and 292 non-enhancing MS lesions: they found no differences between the MTR of enhancing and non-enhancing lesions, but found that MTR was significantly lower for ring-like than for homogeneously enhancing lesions. A recent longitudinal study (van Waesberghe et al., 1998b) also confirmed that ring-like enhancing lesions had the lowest MTR, both at baseline and at follow-up, after enhancement ceased. Moreover, ring-enhancing lesions had significantly greater enhancement areas than homogeneously enhancing lesions, and all were hypointense on both baseline and follow-up unenhanced T1-weighted scans. Longitudinal studies correlating MTI and enhanced T1-weighted MRI using monthly (van Waesberghe et al., 1998b; Filippi et al., 1998b; Dousset et al., 1998; Lai et al., 1997) or weekly (Silver et al., 1998) scanning schedules found that new enhancing lesions all show a reduction of MTR, which may subsequently show a partial or complete recovery. MTR recovery mainly occurs during the first few weeks after new lesion formation, which is consistent with pathological reports of remyelination in nascent MS lesions (Prineas *et al.*, 1993). A recent investigation (Filippi *et al.*, 1998b) of the correlation between MTR and enhanced MRI used a triple dose (TD) of Gd, a technique which reveals a substantial number of active MS lesions not seen with standard dose (SD) Gd (Filippi *et al.*, 1996; Filippi *et al.*, 1998c), and showed that new lesions enhancing only after TD had significantly higher MTR than those enhancing with SD (Filippi *et al.*, 1998b). Mean MTR in enhancing lesions recovered significantly during a 3-month follow-up period and, at each time point during this follow-up, MTR in TD lesions was significantly higher than in SD lesions (Filippi *et al.*, 1998b). These results highlight the pathological heterogeneity of enhancing MS lesions, and indicate a less severe tissue damage in those lesions with less severe BBB disruption.

MTI in the assessment of disease burden

Conventional T2-weighted MRI plays a major role in the assessment of MS disease burden (Filippi & Miller, 1996; Filippi *et al.*, 1995b). Although in cross-sectional studies of MS patients the correlation between clinical disability and brain T2-weighted lesion load (LL) is only moderate (van Walderveen *et al.*, 1995; Filippi *et al.*, 1995b; Gawne-Cain *et al.*, 1998), some longitudinal studies (Paty *et al.*, 1993; Zhao *et al.*, 1997) have shown a relationship between the percentage change in T2-weighted MRI LL and clinical evolution. Hypointense LL measured on unenhanced T1-weighted images, which has the potential for higher pathological specificity (van Walderveen *et al.*, 1998), has also shown a stronger correlation with MS clinical impairment (van Walderveen *et al.*, 1995) and its progression over time (Truyen *et al.*, 1997).

Measures of MS disease burden that can be derived from MTI scans include MTI LL (Rovaris *et al.*, 1997; van Waesberghe *et al.*, 1998a) and MTR histogram-derived parameters (van Buchem *et al.*, 1996). Several studies (Rovaris *et al.*, 1997; van Waesberghe *et al.*, 1998a; Rovaris *et al.*, 1998; Filippi *et al.*, 1998a) have shown that MTI, T2- and T1-weighted LL differ considerably, and the measurement reproducibilities also differ. One possible explanation for these conflicting findings is that the identification of MS lesions on MTI scans is rather subjective, albeit supported by the presence of corresponding abnormalities on T2-weighted images. On MTR maps, MS lesions, due to their low MTR, may show varying degrees of hypointensity, whereas several areas of white matter, which are isointense on T2-weighted images, also have reduced MTR (Filippi *et al.*, 1995a) and look relatively hypointense on MTI scans. The proportion of T2-weighted lesions that can be identified as MTI abnormalities may, therefore, vary widely according to the criteria used for lesion identification and delineation. A 'conservative' approach leads to an MTI LL lower than the corresponding T2-weighted LL, with a similar measurement repeatability (Rovaris *et al.*, 1997). On the other hand, the inclusion of diffuse white matter abnormalities extending beyond the borders of focal lesions weakens the pathological specificity of MTI findings, leading to MTI LL higher than T2-weighted LL (van Waesberghe *et al.*, 1998a), and also to poorer measurement reproducibility. On the basis of these studies, the volume of hypointense lesions on MTI scans would seem not to be a reliable MRI measure of disease burden in MS. The limitations of MTI LL as an MRI outcome measure in MS are reinforced by its modest correlations with clinical disability (Rovaris *et al.*, 1997; Rovaris *et al.*, 1998), that are similar or even lower than for T2-weighted LL (van Waesberghe *et al.*, 1998a; Filippi *et al.*, 1998a).

A more convenient way to assess global MS disease burden on MTI scans is to use MT histogram analysis (van Buchem *et al.*, 1996). As already noted, this is a highly automated technique able to provide several metrics reflecting both macro- and microscopic MS pathology in the whole brain or in selected regions. The data from two recent studies (Philips *et al.*, 1998; Rovaris *et al.*, 1999) showed that a reduction of MT histogram peak height is strongly correlated with both an increasing volume of MS lesions seen on T2-weighted MRI and a greater degree of brain atrophy. As expected, T2- and T1-weighted lesion volumes also influence the average brain MTR. The robust correlations between MS disease burden on conventional MRI and MT histogram metrics confirm that the latter technique can be used as a reliable method to assess disease severity in MS. Moreover, the major influence that brain atrophy has on the MT histogram supports the hypothesis that MT histogram analysis may also provide information about the more severe MS pathological processes (either macro- and microscopic) which lead to loss of brain parenchyma.

Several studies demonstrated that brain MT histogram measures can distinguish MS patients from healthy controls (van Buchem *et al.*, 1996; Filippi *et al.*, 1999a; Rocca *et al.*, 1999). MS patients typically have lower average MTR, histogram peak height and position than normal subjects. However, MT histogram parameters may be different in the various clinical forms of MS, as demonstrated by Filippi *et al.* (1999a) in a cross-sectional study of 93 MS patients with different clinical phenotypes. Patients with clinically isolated syndromes suggestive of MS have MT histogram-derived metrics similar to those from healthy controls, whereas primary progressive MS patients have signficantly lower histogram peak height with normal peak position and only slightly reduced average MTR. RR-MS patients have lower average MTR and peak height than benign MS, whose histograms are similar to those of healthy subjects. Patients with SP-MS had the lowest MT measures. On the basis of these results (Filippi *et al.*, 1999a), it can be concluded that MT histogram-derived measures can provide insights into the pathogenesis of the different MS phenotypes. For instance, the reported findings suggest that, in primary progressive MS, a subtle but widespread damage of the NAWM seems to be the major contributor to the neurological impairment. Other studies have found that MT histogram metrics are also well correlated with the presence of neuropsychological impairment in MS patients (Comi *et al.*, 1999; Rovaris *et al.*, 1998; van Buchem *et al.*, 1998) and that MT histogram parameters from the cerebellum and brainstem of MS patients are significant predictors of disability in these functional systems (Iannucci *et al.*, 1999). The potential use of MT histogram analysis to provide paraclinical outcome measures for monitoring MS clinical trials has been investigated in a preliminary, baseline versus treatment study by Richert *et al.* (1998). These authors found that, in eight RR-MS patients, a 6-month treatment with interferon (IFN) beta-1b immediately reduces enhancing lesion frequency, causes a more gradual reduction in T2-weighted LL but has no effect on MT histogram peak position. This suggests that longer follow-up periods could be required to detect a significant effect of IFN treatment on MT histogram measures or that IFN does not prevent the more destructive aspects of the MS pathology.

Since, in all the aforementioned studies, slabs of whole brain tissue were used to create MT histograms, the relative contributions of macroscopic lesions and of subtle NAWM abnormalities to the overall MS disease burden were not clearly disentangled. However, the macroscopic lesions segmented on T2-weighted images can be superimposed onto the co-registered MTR maps and the areas corresponding to the segmented lesions can be nulled out, thus obtaining MTR maps of normal-appearing brain tissue (NABT) (Tortorella *et al.*, 2000). Recent studies using such an approach demonstrated that NABT MT histogram measures are different in the different MS clinical phenotypes (Tortorella *et al.*, 2000). Using a multivariate analysis of several MRI and MTI variables, Filippi *et al.* (2000b) found that average MTR of the NABT was the only factor that significantly predicted cognitive impairment in a group of 20 MS patients. In another study, comparing NABT MT histogram findings from patients with MS or systemic autoimmune diseases (SAD), Rovaris et al. (2000) found that MS patients had significantly lower average MTR than all patients with SAD but those with NSLE had significantly lower peak height and location than SLE patients. These results indicate that microscopic brain tissue damage is relevant in MS patients, but, apart from patients with NSLE, it seems to be absent in patients with other SAD, even in the presence of macroscopic MRI lesions or clinical evidence of CNS involvement.

Recent advances in MTI acquisition techniques lead to an improved quality for MT-calculated images of the cervical spinal cord. Using cervical cord MT histogram analysis, it has been reported that, in MS patients, MT histogram measures correlate well with locomotor disability (Filippi et al., 1999b) and do not differ from those obtained in patients with Devic's neuromyelitis optica (Filippi et al., 2000a).

References

Bruck, W., Bitsch, A., Kolenda, H., Bruck, Y., Stiefel, M. & Lassmann, H. (1997): Inflammatory central nervous system demyelination: correlation of magnetic resonance imaging findings with lesion pathology. *Ann. Neurol.* **42,** 783–793.

Campi, A., Filippi, M., Comi, G., Scotti, G., Gerevini, S. & Dousset, V. (1996a): Magnetization transfer ratios of contrast-enhancing and nonenhancing lesions in multiple sclerosis. *Neuroradiology* **38,** 115–119.

Campi, A., Filippi, M., Gerevini, S., Ciboddo, G., Comi, G., Scotti, G. & Dousset, V. (1996b): Multiple white matter lesions of the brain. Magnetization transfer ratios in systemic lupus erythematosus and multiple sclerosis. *Int. J. Neuroradiol.* **2,** 134–140.

Comi, G., Rovaris, M., Falautano, M., Santuccio, G., Martinelli, V., Rocca, M.A., Possa, F., Leocani, L., Paulesu, E. & Filippi, M. (1999): A multiparametric study of frontal lobe dementia in multiple sclerosis. *J. Neurol. Sci.* **171,** 135–144.

Dousset, V., Grossman, R.I., Ramer, K.N., Schnall, M.D., Young, L.H., Gonzalez-Scarano, F., Lavi, E. & Cohen, J.A. (1992): Experimental allergic encephalomyelitis and multiple sclerosis: lesion characterization with magnetization transfer imaging. *Radiology* **182,** 483–491.

Dousset, V., Brochet, B., Vital, A., Gross, C., Benazzouz, A., Boullerne, A., Bidabe, A.M., Gin, A.M. & Caille, J.M. (1995): Lysolecithin-induced demyelination in primates: preliminary *in vivo* study with MR and magnetization transfer. *AJNR Am. J. Neuroradiol.* **16,** 225–231.

Dousset, V., Gayou, A., Brochet, B. & Caille, J.M. (1998): Early structural changes in acute MS lesions assessed by serial magnetization transfer studies. *Neurology* **51,** 1150–1155.

Filippi, M. & Miller, D.H. (1996): MRI in the differential diagnosis and monitoring the treatment of multiple sclerosis. *Curr. Opin. Neurol.* **9,** 178–186.

Filippi, M., Campi, A., Dousset, V., Baratti, C., Martinelli, V., Canal, N., Scotti, G. & Comi, G. (1995a): A magnetization transfer imaging study of normal-appearing white matter in multiple sclerosis. *Neurology* **45,** 478–482.

Filippi, M., Horsfield, M.A., Tofts, P.S., Barkhof, F., Thompson, A.J. & Miller, D.H. (1995b): Quantitative assessment of MRI lesion load in monitoring the evolution of multiple sclerosis. *Brain* **118,** 1601–1612.

Filippi, M., Yousry, T., Campi, A., Kandziora, C., Colombo, B., Voltz, R., Martinelli, V., Spuler, S., Bressi, S., Scotti, G. & Comi, G. (1996): Comparison of triple dose versus standard dose gadolinium-DTPA for detection of MRI enhancing lesions in patients with MS. *Neurology* **46,** 379–384.

Filippi, M., Rocca, M.A., Horsfield, M.A. & Comi, G. (1998a): A one year study of new lesions in multiple sclerosis using monthly gadolinium-enhanced MRI: correlations with changes of T2 and magnetization transfer lesion loads. *J. Neurol. Sci.* **158,** 203–208.

Filippi, M., Rocca, M.A., Rizzo, G., Horsfield, M.A., Rovaris, M., Minicucci, L., Colombo, B. & Comi, G. (1998b): Magnetization transfer ratios in MS lesions enhancing after different doses of gadolinium. *Neurology* **50**, 1289–1293.

Filippi, M., Rovaris, M., Capra, R., Gasperini, C., Yousry, T.A., Sormani, M.P., Prandini, F., Horsfield, M.A., Martinelli, V., Bastianello, S., Kuhne, I., Pozzilli, C. & Comi, G. (1998c): A multi-center longitudinal study comparing the sensitivity of monthly MRI after standard and triple dose gadolinium-DTPA for monitoring disease activity in multiple sclerosis: implications for phase II clinical trials. *Brain* **121**, 2011–2020.

Filippi, M., Iannucci, G., Tortorella, C., Minicucci, L., Horsfield, M.A., Colombo, B., Sormani, M.P. & Comi, G. (1999a): Comparison of MS clinical phenotypes using conventional and magnetization transfer MRI. *Neurology* **52**, 588–594.

Filippi, M., Rocca, M.A., Moiola, L., Martinelli, V., Ghezzi, A., Capra, R., Salvi, F., & Comi, G. (1999b): MRI and MTI changes in the brain and cervical cord from patients with Devic's neuromyelitis optica. *Neurology* **53**, 1705–1710.

Filippi, M., Bozzali, M., Horsfield, M.A., Rocca, M.A., Sormani, M.P., Iannucci, G., Colombo, B. & Comi, G. (2000a): A conventional and magnetization transfer MRI study of the cervical cord in patients with multiple sclerosis. *Neurology* **54**, 207–213.

Filippi, M., Tortorella, C., Rovaris, M., Bozzali, M., Possa, F., Sormani, M.P., Iannucci, G. & Comi, G. (2000b): Changes in the normal-appearing brain tissue and cognitive impairment in multiple sclerosis. *J. Neurol. Neurosurg. Psychiatry* **68**, 157–161.

Gass, A., Barker, G.J., Kidd, D., Thorpe, J.W., MacManus, D.G., Brennan, A., Tofts, P.S., Thompson, A.J., McDonald, W.I. & Miller, D.H. (1994): Correlation of magnetization transfer ratio with disability in multiple sclerosis. *Ann. Neurol.* **36**, 62–67.

Gawne-Cain, M.L., O'Riordan, J.I., Coles, A., Newell, B., Thompson, A.J. & Miller, D.H. (1998): MRI lesion volume measurement in multiple sclerosis and its correlation with disability: a comparison of fast fluid-attenuated inversion recovery (fFLAIR) and spin echo sequences. *J. Neurol. Neurosurg. Psychiatry* **64**, 197–203.

Hiehle, J.F., Grossman, R.I., Ramer, K.N., Gonzalez-Scarano, F. & Cohen, J.A. (1995): Magnetization transfer effects in MR-detected multiple sclerosis lesions: comparison with gadolinium-enhanced spin-echo images and non-enhanced T1-weighted images. *AJNR Am. J. Neuroradiol.* **16**, 69–77.

Iannucci, G., Minicucci, L., Rodegher, M., Sormani, M.P., Comi, G. & Filippi, M. (1999): Correlations between clinical and MRI involvement in multiple sclerosis: assessment using T1, T2 and MT histograms. *J. Neurol. Sci.* **171**, 121–129.

Kermode, A.G., Tofts, P., Thompson, A.J., MacManus, D.G., Kendall, B.E., Kingsley, D.P.E., Moseley, I.F., Rudge, P. & McDonald, W.I. (1990): Heterogeneity of blood-brain barrier changes in multiple sclerosis: an MRI study with gadolinium-DTPA enhancement. *Neurology* **40**, 229–235.

Lai, H.M., Davie, C.A., Gass, A., Barker, G.J., Webb, S., Tofts, P.S., Thompson, A.J., McDonald, W.I. & Miller, D.H. (1997): Serial magnetization transfer ratios in gadolinium-enhancing lesions in multiple sclerosis. *J. Neurol.* **244**, 308–311.

Loevner, L.A., Grossman, R.I., Cohen, J.A., Lexa, F.J., Kessler, D. & Kolson, D.L. (1995): Microscopic disease in normal-appearing white matter on conventional MR imaging in patients with multiple sclerosis: assessment with magnetization-transfer measurements. *Radiology* **96**, 511–515.

McDonald, W.I., Miller, D.H. & Barnes, D. (1992): The pathological evolution of multiple sclerosis. *Neuropathol. Appl. Neurobiol.* **18**, 319–334.

McGowan, J.C., Filippi, M., Campi, A. & Grossman, R.I. (1998): Magnetisation transfer imaging: theory and application to multiple sclerosis. *J. Neurol. Neurosurg. Psychiatry* **64** (Suppl. 1), S66–S69.

Miller, D.H., Barkhof, F. & Nauta, J.J.P. (1993): Gadolinium enhancement increased the sensitivity of MRI in detecting disease activity in MS. *Brain* **116**, 1077–1094.

Paty, D.W., Li, D.K.B., MS/MRI Study Group & IFN-beta MS Study Group (1993): Interferon beta 1b is effective in relapsing-remitting multiple sclerosis 2: MRI analysis results of a multicenter, randomized, double-blind, placebo-controlled trial. *Neurology* **43**, 662–667.

Petrella, J.R., Grossman, R.I., McGowan, J.C., Campbell, G. & Cohen, J.A. (1996): Multiple sclerosis lesions: relationship between MR enhancement pattern and magnetization transfer effect. *Am. J. Neuroradiol.* **17**, 1041–1049.

Phillips, M.D., Grossman, R.I., Miki, Y., Wei, L., Kolson, D.L., van Buchem, M.A., Polansky, M., McGowan, J.C. & Udupa, J.K. (1998): Comparison of T2 lesion volume and magnetization transfer ratio histogram analysis and of atrophy and measures of lesion burden in patients with multiple sclerosis. *AJNR Am. J. Neuroradiol.* **19**, 1055–1060.

Prineas, J.W., Barnard, R.O., Kwon, E.E., Shorer, L.L. & Cho, E.S. (1993): Multiple sclerosis: remyelination of nascent lesions. *Ann. Neurol.* **33**, 137–151.

Richert, N.D., Ostuni, J.L., Bash, C.G., Duyn, J.H., McFarland, H.F. & Frank, J.A. (1998): Serial whole-brain magnetization transfer imaging in patients with relapsing-remitting multiple sclerosis at baseline and during treatment with interferon beta 1b. *AJNR Am. J. Neuroradiol.* **19**, 1705–1713.

Rocca, M.A., Mastronardo, G., Rodegher, M., Comi, G. & Filippi, M. (1999): Long-term changes of magnetization transfer-derived measures from patients with relapsing-remitting and secondary-progressive multiple sclerosis. *AJNR Am. J. Neuroradiol.* **20**, 821–827.

Rovaris, M., Bozzali, M., Rodegher, M., Tortorella, C., Comi, G. & Filippi, M. (1999): Brain MRI correlates of magnetization transfer imaging metrics in patients with multiple sclerosis. *J. Neurol. Sci.* **166**, 59–63.

Rovaris, M., Filippi, M., Calori, G., Rodegher, M., Campi, A., Colombo, B. & Comi, G. (1997): Intra-observer reproducibility in measuring new putative MR markers of demyelination and axonal loss in multiple sclerosis: a comparison with T2-weighted images. *J. Neurol.* **244**, 266–270.

Rovaris, M., Filippi, M., Falautano, M., Minicucci, L., Rocca, M.A., Martinelli, V. & Comi, G. (1998): Relation between MR abnormalities and patterns of cognitive impairment in multiple sclerosis. *Neurology* **50**, 1601–1608.

Rovaris, M., Viti, B., Ciboddo, G., Gerevini, S., Capra, R., Iannucci, G., Comi, G. & Filippi, M. (2000): Brain involvement in systemic immune-mediated diseases: a magnetic resonance and magnetization transfer imaging study. *J. Neurol. Neurosurg. Psychiatry* **68**, 170–177.

Silver, N.C., Lai, M., Symms, M.R., Barker, G.J., McDonald, W.I. & Miller, D.H. (1998): Serial magnetization transfer imaging to characterize the early evolution of new MS lesions. *Neurology* **51**, 758–764.

Tortorella, C., Viti, B., Bozzali, M., Sormani, M.P., Rizzo, G., Gilardi, M.F., Comi, G. & Filippi, M. (2000): A magnetization transfer histogram study of normal appearing brain tissue in multiple sclerosis. *Neurology* **54**, 186–193.

Truyen, L., van Waesberghe, J.H.T.M., van Walderveen, M.A.A., van Oosten, B.W., Polman, C.H., Hommes, O.R., Adèr, H.J.A. & Barkhof, F. (1997): Accumulation of hypointense lesions ('black holes') on T1 spin-echo MRI correlates with disease progression in multiple sclerosis. *Neurology* **47**, 1469–1476.

van Buchem, M.A., McGowan, J.C., Kolson, D.L., Polansky, M. & Grossman, R.I. (1996): Quantitative volumetric magnetization transfer analysis in multiple sclerosis: estimation of macroscopic and microscopic disease burden. *Magn. Reson. Med.* **36**, 632–636.

van Buchem, M.A., Grossman, R.I., Armstrong, C., Polansky, M., Miki, Y., Heyning, F.H., Boncoeur-Martel, M.P., Wei, L., Udupa, J.K., Grossman, M., Kolson, D.L. & McGowan, J.C. (1998): Correlation of volumetric magnetization transfer imaging with clinical data in MS. *Neurology* **50**, 1609–1617.

van Waesberghe, J.H.T.M., Castelijns, J.A., Scheltens, P., Truyen, L., Lycklama à Nijeholt, G.J., Hoogenraad, F.G., Polman, C.H., Valk, J. & Barkhof, F. (1997): Comparison of four potential MR parameters for severe tissue destruction in multiple sclerosis lesions. *Magn. Reson. Imaging* **15**, 155–162.

van Waesberghe, J.H.T.M., van Buchem, M.A., Filippi, M., Castelijns, J.A., Rocca, M.A., van der Boom, R., Polman, C.H. & Barkhof, F. (1998a): MR outcome parameters in multiple sclerosis: comparison of surface-based thresholding segmentation and magnetization transfer ratio histographic analysis in relation to disability (a preliminary note). *AJNR Am. J. Neuroradiol.* **19,** 1857–1862.

van Waesberghe, J.H.T.M., van Walderveen, M.A.A., Castelijns, J.A., Scheltens, P., Lycklama à Nijeholt, G.J., Polman, C.H. & Barkhof, F. (1998b): Patterns of lesion development in multiple sclerosis: longitudinal observations with T1-weighted spin-echo and magnetization MR. *AJNR Am. J. Neuroradiol.* **19,** 675–683.

van Waesberghe, J.H.T.M., Kamphorst, W., De Groot, C.J.A., van Walderveen, M.A.A., Castelijns, J.A., Ravid, R., Lycklama à Nijeholt, G.J., van der Valk, P., Polman, C.H., Thompson, A.J. & Barkhof, F. (1999): Axonal loss in multiple sclerosis lesions: magnetic resonance imaging insights into substrates of disability. *Ann. Neurol.* **46,** 747–754.

van Walderveen, M.A.A., Barkhof, F., Hommes, O.R., Polman, C.H., Tobi, H., Frequin, S.T.F.M. & Valk, J. (1995): Correlating MRI and clinical disease activity in multiple sclerosis: relevance of hypointense lesions on short TR/short TE (T1-weighted) spin-echo images. *Neurology* **45,** 1684–1690.

van Walderveen, M.A.A., Kamphorst, W., Scheltens, P., van Waesberghe, J.H.T.M., Ravid, R., Valk, J., Polman, C.H. & Barkhof, F. (1998): Histopathologic correlates of hypointense lesions on T1-weighted spin-echo MRI in multiple sclerosis. *Neurology* **50,** 1282–1288.

Zhao, G.J., Li, D.K.B., Wolinsky, J.S., Koopmans, R.A., Mietlowski, W., Redekop, W.K., Riddehough, A., Cover, K. & Paty, D.W. (1997): Clinical and magnetic resonance imaging changes correlate in a clinical trial monitoring cyclosporine therapy for multiple sclerosis. The MS study group. *J. Neuroimaging* **7,** 1–7.

Chapter 22

Corticosteroids

Maria Bardare

Paediatric Rheumatology Centre, First Paediatric Clinic, University of Milan, via Commenda 9, 20122 Milan, Italy

Summary

Even in neurologic immune-mediated disorders, as in other inflammatory diseases, there is a place for corticosteroids. Indeed, in some encephalopathies these drugs can be life-saving. There is no definite indication to use a specific steroid, but the medium half-life preparations are preferred. Steroids can be grouped into mineralcorticoids and glucocorticoids, the latter being the ones employed in inflammatory disorders, due to their minor sodium-retaining effect.

Glucocorticoids (GC) can be administered either per os or i.v.: this latter route, especially if doses as high as 30 mg/kg/day of methylprednisolone are used ('pulse' therapy), allows a more rapid response and a sparing of steroids later, but may be associated to more important side effects. The doses of GC range from low (0.1–0.4 mg/kg/day of prednisone) to medium (0.5–1.0 mg/kg/day) to high (1.5–2.0 mg/kg/day), according to the severity of the disease.

Treatment duration depends on the course of the neurologic disorders, but long-term therapy is likely to provoke more frequently adverse effects, such as growth impairment and osteoporosis. To minimize these side effects one must follow a few simple rules: to use steroids only in well-established conditions; to employ medium half-life preparations; to prescribe the minimum effective dose in one morning administration; to reduce treatment duration to the minimum.

Mechanisms of action

Glucocorticoids (GC) are the strongest anti-inflammatory substances presently known, and they prevent or suppress inflammation at pharmacological doses through different mechanisms, playing an immunomodulatory role in the complex immunoneuroendocrine network (Wilckens, 1995; Chrousos, 1995; Wilder, 1995). In fact, GC inhibit the production of adhesion molecules and of cytokines such as IL1, IL2, IL4, IL5, IL6, TNFalpha and IFN, all of which are involved in the inflammatory process; the release of platelet-activating factor (PAF), prostaglandins and leukotrienes is also inhibited through the block of phospholipase (reviewed by Spahn & Kamada, 1995). Moreover, GC downregulate the expression of HLA I and II class on immunocompetent cells, decrease the antibody production (only for long-term administration) and alter the ratio in the CD4/CD8 lymphocyte subpopulations. In addition, GC display vasoconstrictive properties and, decreasing capillary permeability, inhibit plasma exudation, so reducing the concentration of chemotactic and inflammatory factors (Szefler, 1991; Spahn & Kamada, 1995).

GC exert their therapeutic effect via genomic action, which involves binding to a cytosolic receptor (GR) after passing through the cell membrane. The binding generally results in an increase of the transcription rate of certain genes, which leads to increased production of the target proteins, such as lipocortin 1 (which inhibits phospholipase A2) (Goulding & Guyre, 1993).

Recently Buttgereit et al. (1998) have hypothesized two further non-genomic mechanisms which could explain the rapid action of some steroids without requiring new protein synthesis: (1) GC could act directly on membrane-bound steroid receptors; (2) they could dissolve in membranes and affect the physicochemical membrane properties and the activities of the membrane-associated proteins. This latter mechanism could provide an explanation for the good therapeutic effect of high-dose glucocorticoid treatment ('pulse' therapy) of severe immune-mediated diseases.

Choice of steroid

The most important characteristics of the different GC are listed in Table 1. The choice between the GC is optional, but the medium half-life compounds are preferred; prednisone and prednisolone are considered the standard preparations and are the most cost-effective substances. Among the others, triamcinolone has a low sodium-retaining effect, but causes myopathy more frequently, as do the fluorinated substances (Michels, 1997); deflazacort is a relatively recent preparation which appears to produce a bone-sparing effect but has a lower potency (Loftus et al., 1993). Steroids with longer half-life (e.g. dexamethasone) have a prolonged effect on hypothalamic-pituitary-adrenal (HPA) axis and should be avoided for long-term treatments (Michels, 1997).

Table 1. Some more commonly used corticosteroids

Compound	Anti-inflammatory effect	Approximate potency mg	Sodium-retaining potency	Biological half-life h[1]	Regular daily dose above which HPA axis[2] suppression is likely	
					Male	Female
Hydrocortisone	1	20	1	8–12	20–30	15–25
Prednisolone	4	5	0.25	18–36	7.5–10	7.5
Methylprednisolone	5	4	±	18–36	7.5–10	7.5
Triamcinolone	5	4	±	18–36	7.5–10	7.5
Betamethasone	25–30	0.6	±	36–54	1–1.5	1–1.5
Dexamethasone	25	0.8	±	36–54	1–1.5	1–1.5

[1]Biological half-lives are based on the duration of pituitary adrenal suppression;
[2]These values are given only as a guideline and are dependent on total body surface area.

Routes of administration and dosage

The route of administration and the dosage are very important: GC can be administered either per os or i.v. as pulse therapy. This latter route gives more rapid results and allows to spare

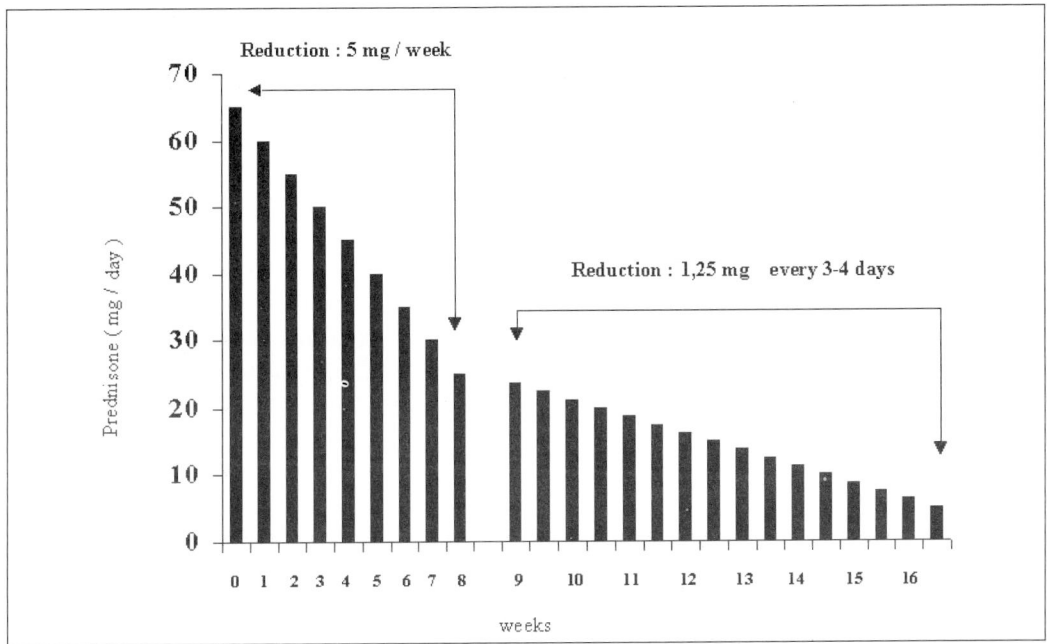

Fig. 1. Schedule for withdrawal of steroids after long-term treatment.

steroids later (giving smaller quantities of GC per os), but is associated to heavier short-term side effects (Table 2).

The medium dosage of prednisone ranges from 0.5–1 mg/kg/day, while the high dosage ranges from 1.5–2 mg/kg/day, with a maximum of 60–70 mg/day. Low dosage is considered to range from 0.1–0.4 mg/kg/day.

The alternate-day regimen has the least side effects and inhibition of HPA axis, but is not sufficiently effective in controlling the disease in its active phase. For long-term maintenance therapy, alternate-day regimen or low doses of prednisone, such as 0.1mg/kg/day, can work.

Whenever possible, the daily dose of GC should be administered in the morning, between 7 and 8 a.m., in order to keep the disturbances in the HPA axis as controlled as possible, but in some particularly severe cases the daily doses can be distributed into two or three individual doses, at least for a brief length of time. The overall duration of GC therapy depends on the type and on the course of the disease, but should be as short as possible.

Tapering GC after long-term treatment is very difficult because of the possible and frequent disease rebounds, and dose reduction must be carried out very slowly and carefully: a possible schedule of reduction, according to the experience of our Rheumatology Centre, is proposed in Fig. 1.

Side effects

The side effects of steroids are well known and frequent and can be associated both to high-dose short-term and long-term treatment (Tables 2 and 3) (Cochrane, 1983).

The adverse effects in adults and children (reviewed by Melo-Gomes, 1993) are similar, but the suppression of growth is the only serious GC side effect specific to childhood. Growth impairment occurs almost universally when divided doses of GC are used, and even with low doses such as 5 mg/day or 0.4 mg/kg/day of prednisone, especially in long-term treatments.

Another frequent and dangerous side effect is osteoporosis, which can provoke multiple collapse of vertebral bodies and bone necrosis. Osteoporosis can be prevented using an alternate-day regimen or a GC with bone-sparing effect, such as deflazacort (Loftus *et al.*, 1993); calcium, vitamin D and biphosphonates may be usefully employed to prevent or to treat osteoporosis.

Table 2. Side effects of corticosteroids, which may be of sudden onset, associated with short-term, high-dose therapy (≥ 40 mg prednisolone, 200 mg hydrocortisone)

Hypokalaemic alkalosis (exacerbated by hyperventilation)
Clinical diabetes mellitus (excacerbated by parenteral feeding)
Hyperosmolar non-kinetic coma
Hypertension
Sodium and water retention (oedema) – exacerbated by the use of intermittent positive pressure ventilation
Mental disturbances including severe psychoses
Cerebral oedema (especially in young children)
Proximal myopathy
Glaucoma
Pancreatitis
Peptic ulceration and gastrointestinal haemorrhage (unproven side effects)

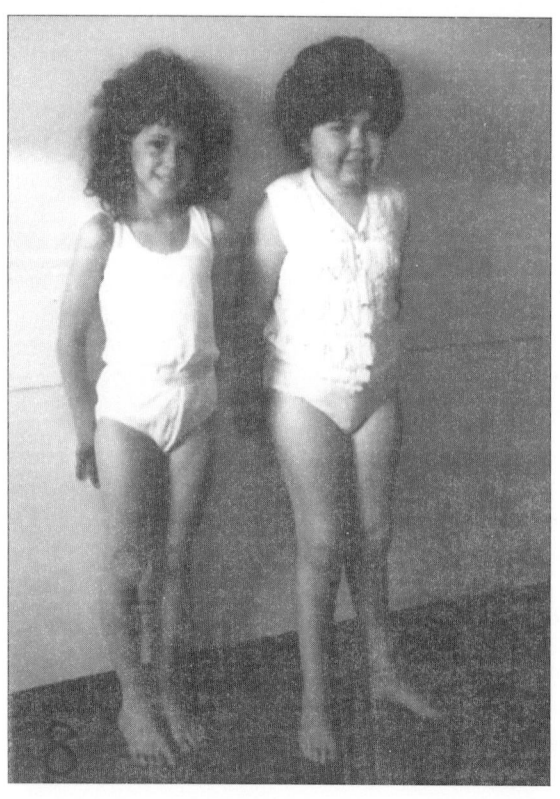

Fig. 2. The girl on the right is 13 years old and has been treated long-term with steroids: the other is 8 years, and was never administered steroids.

Table 3. Side effects of corticosteroids more likely to be associated with long-term administration (10–20 mg prednisolone or equivalent). Sudden onset side effects may also occur.

Osteoporosis with vertebral compression and multiple bone fractures
Aseptic necrosis of bone
Cerebral atrophy
Development of latent epilepsy
Variations in mood – depression, anxiety and lability of mood
Posterior sub-capsular cataracts
Hyperlipidaemia with perhaps increased incidence of gallstones
Centripetal obesity (lemon on a tooth pick appearance)
Growth failure in children and adolescents
Secondary amenorrhoea
Suppression of hypothalamic-pituitary-adrenal axis
Impaired wound healing with subcutaneous tissue atrophy
Diminished immune response leading to increased vulnerability to bacterial and opportunistic organisms

The typical cushingoid appearance, with centripetal obesity, hirsutism, cutaneous striae and acne, occurs also with doses as low as 10 mg/day of prednisone.

Another complication of long-term steroid treatment is posterior subcapsular cataract: periodic ophthalmologic controls are advisable.

In conclusion, GC are potent anti-inflammatory agents which can be useful, and sometimes life-saving, also in neurologic immune-mediated diseases. As GC have many side effects of varying severity, the goal to be achieved is to exploit the treatment potential of GC while avoiding as much as possible their adverse effects. To attain this goal, GC must be used only in well-established indications, at the minimum effective dose, with a daily morning administration and, if possible, with alternate-day regimen and whenever possible for the shortest time.

References

Buttgereit, F., Wehling, M. & Burmester, G.-R. (1998): A new hypothesis of modular glucocorticoid actions. *Arthritis Rheum.* **41,** 761–767.

Cochrane, G.M. (1983): Systemic steroids in asthma. In: *Steroids in asthma*, ed. T.J.H. Clark, pp. 103–120. Auckland: ADIS Press.

Chrousos, G.B. (1995): The hypothalamic- pituitary-adrenal axis and immune- mediated inflammation. *N. Eng. J. Med.* **332,** 1351–1362.

Goulding, N.J. & Guyre, P.M. (1993): Glucocorticoids, lipocortins and the immune response. *Curr. Opin. Immunol.* **5,** 108–113.

Loftus, J.K., Reeve, J., Hesp, R., David, J., Ansell, B.M. & Woo, P.M.M. (1993): Deflazacort in JCA. *J. Rheumatol.* **20** (Suppl. 37), 40–42.

Melo-Gomes, J.A. (1993): Problems related to systemic glucocorticoid therapy in children. *J. Rheumatol.* **20** (Suppl. 37), 35–39.

Michels, H. (1997): Is there a renaissance of corticosteroid therapy? *Rev. Rhumatisme* (English edition) **64** (Suppl. 10), 183S–185S.

Spahn, J. & Kamada, A.K. (1995): Special considerations in the use of glucocorticoids in children. *Pediatrics Rev.* **16,** 266–272.

Szefler, S.J. (1991): Glucocorticoid therapy: clinical pharmacology. *J. Allergy Clin. Immunol.* **88,** 147–165.

Wilckens, T. (1995): Glucocorticoids and immune function: physiological relevance and pathogenic potential of hormonal dysfunction. *Trends Pharmacol. Sci.* **16,** 193–197.

Wilder, R.L. (1995): Neuroendocrine-immune system interactions and autoimmunity. *Annu. Rev. Immunol.* **13,** 307–338.

Chapter 23

Intravenous immunoglobulins

Rosa Maria Dellepiane and Cristina Panisi

First Paediatric Clinic, University of Milan, via Commenda 9, 20122 Milan, Italy

Summary

Intact unmodified intravenous immunoglobulins (IVIG) have been available since the 1980s. They are chemically intact and have the same immunologic properties as the pooled immunoglobulin concentrates from which they were produced. IVIG derive from a large healthy donor pool and contain more than 95 per cent monomeric intact IgG and negligible IgM and IgA quantities. Since the first successful experience by Imbach who treated idiopathic thrombocytopenic purpura in children, a wide range of indications for IVIG was described for diseases with known or presumed autoimmune origin. The opportunity to infuse very high doses of IVIG revealed their immunomodulating pharmacological effects. IVIG have been widely used in neurological diseases during the last decade. In controlled clinical trials IVIG have been effective in treating Guillain-Barré syndrome, chronic inflammatory demyelinating polyneuropathy, and multifocal motor neuropathy. In other controlled or open-label trials and case reports, IVIG produced improvement in patients with relapsing-remitting multiple sclerosis, acute myasthenic crisis, inclusion-body myositis, steroid-resistant dermatomyositis, intractable childhood epilepsy. Evidence is also anedoctal or not fully substantiated. Apart from the immunomodulatory effect, evidence exists that IVIG may promote remyelination. IVIG is an extremely expensive therapy and its use should be limited to diseases for which a positive effect has been proven in controlled trials.

Introduction

Intravenous immunoglobulins (IVIG) represent a real therapeutic success of the last fifty years. In the 1940's Cohn and Oncley first set up the cold-ethanol fractionation system of human plasma (Cohn *et al.*, 1946; Oncley *et al.*, 1949). This technique allows the isolation of the gammaglobulinic component, pure at 95 per cent, from other plasmatic components (Fig. 1). This fraction still serves today as starting material for most industrial preparations of IVIG. Subsequently, in the 1950s, immunoglobulins were available only for intramuscular use ('standard' immunoglobulins). Their employment in replacement therapy of immune deficiency diseases revealed serious disadvantages. In fact immunoglobulins are slowly absorbed into the circulation from the tissue and are subject to degradation by local proteolysis. In addition, even when small amounts of immunoglobulins are injected into tissue, they may produce painful local irritation and in immunodeficient patients, who need regular immunoglobulin substitution, adverse reactions may occur even with intramuscular injection (Barandun *et al.*, 1975)

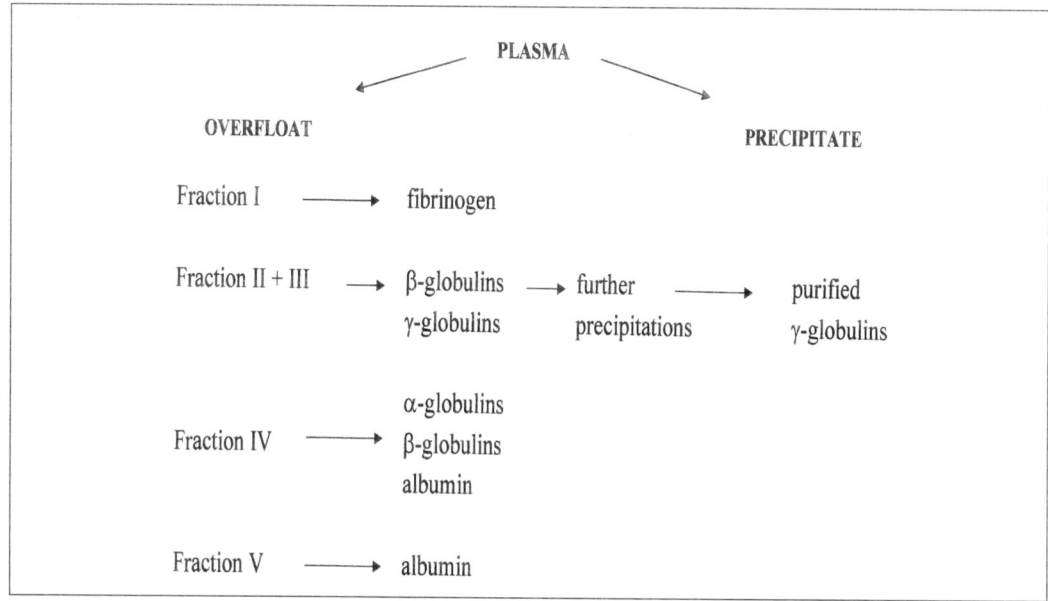

Fig. 1. Cold plasma fractionation method with ethanol.

However, over the past 30 years, various methods to modify immunoglobulin solution have been devised to produce products suitable for intravenous use. The methods (summarized in Table 1) include enzymatic treatment, addition of chemical groups to prevent aggregation, reduction, sulphonation, reduction and alkylation, addition of stabilizers, column filtration, and precipitation of aggregates by polyethylene glycol (Deutsch *et al.*, 1970; Morell, 1986; Romer *et al.*, 1982; Gronski *et al.*, 1983; van Furth *et al.*, 1984).

Table 1. Generations of commercial Ig for i.v. use

First generation	Papaine-pepsine mediated enzymatic fragmentation. *Immunochemical characteristics:* Intact Fab fragment Fc fragment destroyed
Second generation	Chemical treatment: betapropiolactone, sulphonation, alkylation. *Immunochemical characteristics:* Intact Fab fragment Fc functioning compromised
Third generation	Aggregrate selective removal through pH 4 and traces of pepsine, pH 4 only, polyethylene-glycol, ion-exchange resin. *Immunochemical characteristics:* Intact Fab fragment Fc functioning compromised

From the 1980s intact unmodified preparations (third-generation immunoglobulins) have been available for intravenous use (Stiehm, 1979; Eibl & Wedgwood, 1989). They are chemically intact and have the same immunologic properties as the pooled immunoglobulin concentrates from which they were produced. The production methods have almost entirely removed aggregates, liable for serious adverse reactions.

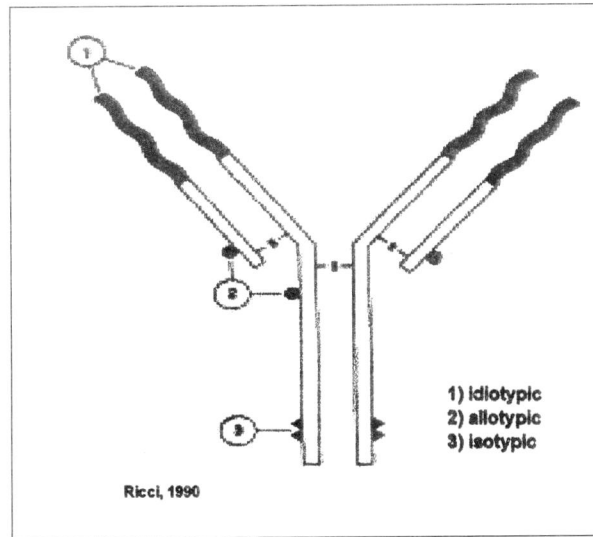

Fig. 2. Heterogeneity of immunoglobins.

Fc-fragment integrity is important for the biological Fc-mediated properties of human immunoglobulins. They are binding to C1q, cytotropic activity, transport through membranes (placenta, enteric and bronchial mucosa), control on catabolism rate, binding to membrane receptors (of macrophages, mast-cells, etc.), helping action to B-cells, binding to staphylococcal protein A.

Commercially available IVIG preparations derive from a large healthy donor pool (5–10,000 plasma units); they contain more than 95 per cent monomeric intact IgG and negligible IgM and IgA quantities (in concentrations below to 2.5 per cent).

Immunoglobulins have an isotypic heterogeneity (for the different heavy and light chains classes and subclasses), an allotypic heterogeneity (presence or lack of a genetic marker as variants of heavy chain constant regions), and an idiotypic heterogeneity (for the variation in the variable domain, particularly in the hypervariable regions) (Fig. 2). Idiotypes are usually specific for the individual antibody clone (Roitt, 1989).

The large donor pool ensures the diversity of IgG molecules in the preparation that by far exceeds the repertoire of a single human being. In one gram of IgG there are about 4×10^{18} molecules with 10×10^6 different antibody specificity. This diversity may be of importance for the therapeutic effect. In fact all the other drugs have, at most, one or two active substances (Ricci, 1990).

Today intravenous immunoglobulins are employed as follows: (1) replacement therapy of primary or secondary immunodeficiencies; (2) prophylaxis/therapy of some infectious diseases; (3) therapy of some immune-mediated diseases. This last use originates from an occasional observation of Imbach et al. (1981). In fact they first noticed that in agammaglobulinaemic children with idiopathic thrombocytopenic purpura, the application of high-dose replacement therapy with IVIG was followed by a rapid increase of platelet count. The opportunity to infuse very high doses of IVIG has revealed their immunomodulating pharmacological effects.

The potential mechanisms involved in immunomodulating effects of IVIG are summarized in Table 2.

In immune-mediated diseases the commonly used dose schedule is 400 mg/kg for five consecutive days or 2 g/kg in two daily doses of 1 g/kg each, provided that the patient does not have such underlying conditions as congestive heart failure, renal insufficiency, or high serum viscosity.

In 1990 the National Institutes of Health organized the Consensus Development Conference that indicated two conditions in which the employment of IVIG was unanimously accepted: acute PTI and Kawasaki disease (NIH Consensus Conference, 1990).

Table 2. Possible mechanisms of IVIG action (from Stangel, 1998 – modified)

Anti-idiotype Ab (Jayne et al., 1993; Jefferis, 1993; Ronda et al., 1994)	Anti-idiotype Ab against auto-Ab can bind these and neutralize them
Inhibition of Ab production of B-cells (Bijsterbosch and Klaus, 1985)	Anti-idiotype Ab can bind on membrane-bound Ab on the surface of B-cells and shut down the immunoglobulin production
Inhibition of CD5-positive cells (Vassilev et al., 1993)	CD5 is expressed on a subset of B-cells that synthesize low-affinity polyreactive auto-Ab
Blockage of Fc receptors (Heyman, 1990)	Intact IgG can bind to receptors of cells of the reticuloendothelial system
Modulation of T-cell activation via soluble molecules (Gross-Wilde et al., 1992; Blasczyck et al., 1993; Perosa et al., 1995)	Soluble CD4, CD8 and MHC molecules contained in IVIG preparations can act as antagonists of the T-cell receptor and thus block activation
Anti-idiotypic effect on TCR (Marchalonis et al., 1992)	Ab against the TCR β-chain can block T-cell activation and inhibit activation and clonal expansion of cytotoxic T-cells stimulated by superantigens
Enhancement of CD8 positive suppressor T-cell function (Delfraissy et al., 1985; Leung et al., 1987; Ballow et al., 1989)	Such increase was noted after IV administration of Ig
Neutralization of superantigens (Takei et al., 1993)	Neutralizing Ab to bacterial and viral superantigens have been shown to be present in IVIG
Neutralization of toxins and pathogens (Masson, 1993)	Direct binding of antigens that initiate or perpetuate autoimmune reaction
Modulation of cytokines production by immune cells (Andersson et al., 1993; Klaesson et al., 1993; Ruiz de Souza et al., 1995)	Modulation of expression of various cytokines was shown *in vitro* after addition of IVIG to lymphocyte cultures (reduction of IL-1 in Kawasaki syndrome, reduction of TNF-α in experimental allergic encephalomyelitis in animal models, dose-depending decrease of IL-6, IL-2, IL-3, IL-10, TNF-β)
Induction of production of IL-1 receptor antagonists (Rouiz de Souza et al., 1995)	IL-1 plays a key role in the inflammatory cascade
Direct binding of cytokines (Svenson et al., 1993; Ross et al., 1995)	Binding Ab against IL-1, IL-6, IFN-γ and IFN-β were shown to be present in IVIG preparations
Inhibition of complement-mediated effects (Basta et al., 1989; Frank et al., 1992)	IgG can bind complement and thus inhibit the damage following complement activation
Increase of Ig catabolism (Masson, 1993)	The catabolic rate of immunoglobulins increases with higher serum concentrations and thus the half-life of auto-Ab is decreased

Since Imbach's successful experience IVIG have been used in a large number of other diseases with known or presumed autoimmune origin as cytopenias, coagulation disorders, vasculitis, organ-specific autoimmune diseases (Table 3) (Dwyer, 1992; Ronda et al., 1993; Ratko et al., 1995).

Table 3. IVIG in autoimmune diseases

Cytopenias
- Chronic idiopathic thrombocytopenic purpura (IPT)
- Autoimmune haemolytic anaemia
- Autoimmune neutropenia
- Aplastic anaemia

Coagulation disorders
- Anti-haemophylic Factor VIIIc inhibitors
- Antiphospholipid antibodies syndrome
- Recurrent spontaneous abortion

Vasculitides
- SLE
- Rheumatoid arthritis
- Polymiositis
- Wegener's granulomatosis
- Sjögren syndrome
- Haemolytic-uraemic syndrome (HUS)

Intestinal diseases
- Chron's disease
- Ulcerative colitis

Organ-specific autoimmune diseases
- Insulin-dependent diabetes
- Uveitis
- Steroid-dependent asthma

During the last decade, the clinical use of IVIG has also dramatically increased in neurological autoimmune diseases, although in many cases neither the pathomechanisms of the disease nor the mode of IVIG action are yet known (Stangel et al., 1998). This is probably due to the limited therapeutic effect of other immunosuppressive treatments in these diseases and the easy handling of IVIG with only few side effects. In contrast to the widespread use of IVIG, only a few well designed controlled trials have been reported (Table 4). In some neurological diseases, such as Guillain-Barré syndrome, chronic inflammatory demyelinating polyneuropathy (CIDP) and multifocal motor neuropathy (MMN), encouraging clinical evidence for the effectiveness is available. In other neurologic diseases (Table 5), evidence for the efficacy of IVIG therapy is either anedoctal or not fully substantiated (Marinos & Dalakas, 1997).

In Guillain-Barré syndrome, controlled clinical trials claimed that IVIG are at least as effective as plasma exchange (van der Meché et al., 1992; Bril et al., 1996; Stangel et al., 1998).

A large multicentre study comparing IVIG with plasma exchange and the combined use of both treatments has just been completed, demonstrating no difference between plasma exchange, IVIG and plasma exchange followed by IVIG (Plasma Exchange Trial Group, 1997). Therapy with IVIG may be preferred for patients in hospitals in which plasmapheresis is not immediately available and not routinely used with expertise, and in small children or patients who have poor venous access, sepsis, severe autonomic dysfunction, or unstable haemodynamics (Marinos & Dalakas, 1997).

Table 4. Neurologic diseases treated with IVIG (Marinos & Dalakas, 1997)

Controlled clinical trials:
- Guillain-Barré syndrome
- Chronic inflammatory demyelinating polyneuropathy (CIDP)
- Motorial multifocal neuropathy (MMN)
- Dermatomyositis

Proven clinical efficacy:
- Guillain-Barré syndrome
- CIDP
- Motorial multifocal neuropathy

Table 5. Preliminary results from controlled trials, open studies and case reports (Marinos & Dalakas, 1997)

- Amyotrophic lateral sclerosis
- Inclusion-body myositis
- Lambert-Eaton myasthenic syndrome
- Myasthenia gravis
- Rasmussen syndrome
- Intractable childhood epilepsy
- West syndrome
- Lennox-Gastaut syndrome
- Polymyositis
- Multiple sclerosis
- Optic neuritis
- Stiff-man syndrome
- Systemic vasculitis
- Paraneoplastic cerebellar degeneration
- Paraneoplastic encephalomyelitis and sensory neuropathy
- Autoimmune diabetic neuropathy
- Acute idiopathic dysautonomic neuropathy
- Adrenoleukodystrophy

Steroids are still the first choice for treating CIDP. The response to these agents is sometimes slow, and protracted therapy increases the risk for severe side effects. In a controlled, randomized, crossover study of IVIG or plasmapheresis in 20 patients with CIDP, the two therapies were equally effective in improving muscle strength and neuropathic symptoms and in increasing the amplitude of evoked muscle-action potentials (Dyck et al., 1994).

Plasma exchange and IVIG should be reserved for those who fail to respond to, or worsen on steroids or present unacceptable side effects. IVIG therapy is preferable because it is easier to administer than plasmapheresis. Plasmapheresis is best reserved for cases in which IVIG therapy is ineffective. In successful cases, studies are necessary to titrate the minimally effective intravenous immunoglobulin dose/time interval (Wills & Unsworth, 1998).

As shown in a controlled trial (Azulay *et al.*, 1994) and several open-label studies (Dalakas *et al.*, 1994; Chaudhry *et al.*, 1993; Nobile-Orazio *et al.*, 1993) MMN responds remarkably well to IVIG therapy. This is currently the treatment of choice. The GM1 antibody titres, present in 70 per cent of the patients, may remain unchanged.

At present it appears that the therapeutic schedule has to be set up for each patient individually. Some authors (Nobile-Orazio, 1996) suggest the combination of IVIG with cyclophosphamide.

In other neurological conditions, clinical results are discordant and further confirmations are necessary.

Although IVIG are a theoretically promising therapy in multiple sclerosis, the available evidence is not sufficient to recommend this treatment presently. However, some trials in patients with relapsing-remitting disease should be noted. Fazekas *et al.* (1997) observed a high efficacy with regard to reduction of relapse rate and even clinical improvement during the early phase of IVIG medication (controlled trial). Achiron *et al.* (1996) in an open trial observed reduction of relapse rate and severity and, in particular, reduction of number and diameter of demyelinating lesions shown by magnetic resonance imaging. Combined immunoglobulin and azathioprine reduce relapse rate and improve functional neurologic condition (Hossein & Seid, 1998) (open trial). In another small trial, five patients with persistent deficit after optic neuritis were treated with IVIG and vision improvement was observed in four of them (Van Engelen *et al.*, 1992).

An interesting aspect of IVIG in demyelinating inflammatory neuropathies is that not only an immune modulating mechanism has been proposed, but also a possible promotion of remyelination in the central nervous system (Noseworthy *et al.*, 1994).

IVIG promote remyelination not only by abrogation of the autoimmune attack but also by an effect on glial cells. Van Shaik *et al.* (1997) showed that IVIG induce growth arrest of normal human fibroblasts and Schwann cells *in vitro*. Myelin synthesis by Schwann cells is initiated concomitant with arrest of proliferation. In fibroblasts this growth arrest is accompanied by upregulation of GAS-3 expression (Schneider *et al.*, 1988). Initially GAS-3 was thought to be a regulatory gene for growth arrest. Subsequently, the gene was found to encode also for the myelin glycoprotein PMP-22. The correlation of IVIG-induced growth arrest and increased GAS-3/PMP-22 expression supports the suggestion that IVIG play a role in remyelination. This hypothesis is currently being investigated in human Schwann cells.

Most cases of myastenia gravis can be controlled by a combination of anticholinesterases (symptomatic treatment), steroids, azathioprine (immunosuppression) and thymectomy (in young or thymoma patients) (Wills & Unsworth, 1998). The routine use of IVIG as initial treatment of myasthenia gravis is currently not recommended, but it seems to have a similar therapeutic effect to that of plasma exchange during an acute myastenic crisis. In patients where plasma exchange is contraindicated or other therapies have failed, IVIG may be the treatment of choice (Stangel *et al.*, 1998; Drachman, 1994; Ratko *et al.*, 1995).

Several reports suggest that IVIG therapy may have a moderate-to-dramatic benefit within a short period of time in as many as 70 per cent of patients and an efficacy similar to that of plasmapheresis (Marinos & Dalakas, 1997; Così *et al.*, 1991; Gajdos, 1994). IVIG are better tolerated by patients with the acute exacerbations of myasthenia gravis. When compared to plasma exchange, IVIG have the advantages of not requiring special equipment or trained teams. Further studies are required to optimize the efficacy and clinical applications of IVIG therapy in specific stages of the illness.

There are basically three forms of inflammatory myopathies, namely polymyositis, dermatomyositis and inclusion-body myositis (Dalakas, 1991; Stangel et al., 1998). While the first two respond well to steroids and immunosuppression, the latter is often refractory to immunosuppressive therapy (Lotz et al., 1989). For dermatomyositis and polymyositis, IVIG should not be the first-line treatment. IVIG therapy is reserved for steroid-resistant patients or patients in whom steroid are contraindicated (Marinos & Dalakas, 1997; Dalakas et al., 1993). In a few patients with inclusion-body myositis IVIG have been claimed to be effective after established therapies have failed (Soueidan & Dalakas, 1993; Stangel et al., 1998). In a controlled, double-blind study of 19 patients (Dalakas et al., 1997), IVIG therapy produced an increase in muscle strength compared with placebo, but these gains were minor and not statistically significant. However, a modest, transitory, but functionally important improvement was noted in six of 19 patients (31.5 per cent).

Several controlled and uncontrolled studies regard intractable childhood epilepsy (ICE), an heterogeneous group of epileptic encephalopathies, nonresponders to treatment with conventional anticonvulsant therapy. In this group are very serious cases of West syndrome and Lennox-Gastaut syndrome. It is estimated that 10–20 per cent of childhood epilepsies are intractable (Duse et al., 1996; Livingston, 1991). The rate of responders to IVIG treatment in ICE is similar in most studies, about 50 per cent, but no reliable predictive marker of responsiveness has been found so far. Recurrent seizures may be caused by autoimmunity, immunodeficiency – most frequently selective IgA deficiency and IgG2 deficiency – or viral infections (Ugazio et al., 1990). Thus, IVIG may act in different ways: as a biological response modifier, as replacement therapy or as a source of antiviral antibodies, and these hypotheses are not mutually exclusive.

Recently, Rogers et al. (1994) found human and animal antibodies directed against the glutamate receptor of neurons. Twyman et al. (1995) subsequently demonstrated that GluR3 antibodies raised in the symptomatic rabbits after immunization with GluR3 or in sera from two patients with Rasmussen's encephalitis, a rare form of childhood epilepsy. During IVIG treatment in a patient with Rasmussen syndrome (one infusion every four months for 46 months) there was no progression in motor and cognitive signs, or in the incidence of seizures, and although the mechanism of their action is obscure it may well be related to the modification of an immunological disorder (Gordon, 1996). This confirms that immune mechanisms may be involved in the pathogenesis of some of childhood epileptic fits. Autoantibodies such as those present in the serum with Rasmussen's encephalitis or other immune markers may prove useful also to identify the subset of children with ICE most likely to benefit from treatment with IVIG (Duse et al., 1996).

In the last 20 years (1978–1998) we have treated with IVIG 145 patients affected by primitive immunodeficiency syndromes (60 patients), secondary immunodeficiency syndromes (35 patients, 27 HIV-infected), autoimmune diseases (39 patients), intractable childhood epilepsy (11 patients). As to intractable childhood epilepsy, from February 1985 to February 1987 we treated 11 patients, seven males and four females, with age range 20 months to 15 years and 10 months. The age at beginning was 6 days to 6 years; the duration of seizures ranged from 9 months to 14 years. Patients' characteristics are summarized in Table 6. All patients presented daily seizures of variable number and features. All patients were treated with one or more drug.

Table 6. Patients with intractable epilepsy admitted to First Paediatric Clinic I, Milan, Italy

Patients	Sex	Age	Onset	Diagnosis	Frequency of seizures
1 C.D.	M	5 y	7 m	Partial simple epilepsy and generalized clonic seizures	over 20/day
2. V.F.	M	15 y 2 m	4.5 m	Epileptic encephalopathy with partial simple seizures	over 20/day
3. L.R.	M	2 y	13 d	Continuous partial epilepsy	10–20/day
4. B.I.	F	6 y 6 m	2.5 m	Lennox–Gastaut syndrome	4–7/day
5. B.M.	M	20 m	7 m	Lennox–Gastaut syndrome	> 10 series/day
6. C.M.	M	2 y	6 d	Previous meningoencephalitis – West syndrome	over 20/day
7. I.F.	M	1 y 11 m	2 m	Lennox–Gastaut syndrome	> 10/day
8. B.F.	M	3 y	13 m	Lennox–Gastaut syndrome	over 20/day
9. C.L.	F	11 y	6 y	Generalized seizures of myoclonic-astasic type	over 20/day
10. C.C.	F	7 y	unknown	Generalized tonic seizures, partial simple seizures	> 8–10/day
11. C.P.	F	15 y 10 m	4 m	Previous encephalitis – Lennox–Gastaut syndrome	> 2–3/day

The dose and schedule of IVIG used was 200 mg/kg every 7 days for 1 month, followed by 200 mg/kg every 14 days for 1 month and subsequently every 21 days for 4 months (12 infusions in 6 months). Before treatment, neurological examination and EEG were performed. Furthermore, blood was taken for immunoglobulins, and IgG subclasses, C_3, C_4, IgE, autoantibodies, lymphocytic subsets were tested. EEG was repeated 48 h after the first, the third and fifth IVIG infusion. A daily diary for number, kind and duration of the attacks had to be maintained.

From blood sample serum, IgA deficiency associated with IgG3 deficiency was found in one patient (case no. 8 in Table 6); this patient was never treated with diphenylhydantoin as anticonvulsant. IgG3 deficiency was found in two patients (case nos. 5 and 7 in Table 6) while no alterations were found in the other eight patients.

EEG was abnormal in all patients; however, no patients showed significant changes in recordings after therapy.

Clinical results were evaluated according to the number of daily seizures and the improvement of neurological condition. Nine patients stopped IVIG treatment between the fourth and the sixth infusion because in five cases, including patient no. 7 (with IgG3 deficiency), there was no benefit:

- In three cases there was only temporary reduction of seizure number after the second infusion.

- In one case (patient no. 5 with IgG3 deficiency) increase of daily seizures was observed.

One patient stopped therapy after eight infusions. He presented persistent incomplete reduction of pretreatment sizures, but also increase of absences and appearance of a new kind of seizures. Only one patient, no. 8 with IgA and IgG3 deficiency, was administered all twelve IVIG infusions. He had significative reduction of seizures number after the first infusion. During the six months of the study there were alternate worsening (with more daily seizures) and improvement with one seizure every week. Furthermore psychological performance and behaviour improved. All clinical improvements disappeared one month after discontinuing IVIG infusions. In our experience IVIG treatment of intractable childhood epilepsy has an unfavourable cost/benefit ratio.

In conclusion, IVIG is a promising immunomodular therapy in a large number of neurological autoimmune disorders often unresponsive to other immunotherapies. However, because this therapy is extremely expensive, IVIG should be limited to diseases for which a positive effect has been proven in controlled trials. The dose (mg/kg), frequency and duration of treatment should be the minimum proven to be effective.

References

Achiron, A., Barak, Y., Goren, M., Gabbay, U., Miron, S., Rotstein, Z., Noy, S. & Sarova-Pinhas, I. (1996): Intravenous immune globulin in multiple sclerosis: clinical and neuroradiological results and implications for possible mechanisms of action. *Clin. Exp. Immunol.* **104** (Suppl. 1), 67–70.

Andersson, U.G., Bjork, L., Skansen-Saphir, U. & Andersson, J.P. (1993): Down-regulation of cytokine production and interleukin-2 receptor expression by pooled human IgG. *Immunology* **79**, 211–216.

Azulay, J.P., Blin, O., Pouget, J., Boucrout, J., Bille-Turc, F., Carles, G. *et al.* (1994): Intravenous immunoglobulin treatment in patients with motor neuron syndromes associated with anti-GM1 antibodies: a double-blind, placebo-controlled study. *Neurology* **44**, 429–432.

Ballow, M., White, W. & Desbonnet, B.A. (1989): Modulation of *in vitro* synthesis of immunoglobulin and the induction of suppressor activity by therapy with intravenous immune globulin. *J. Allergy Clin. Immunol.* **84**, 595–602.

Barandun, S., Castel, V., Makula, M.F., Morell A., Plan, R. & Skvaril, F. (1975): Clinical tolerance and catabolism of plasmin-treated gamma-globulin for intravenous application. *Vox Sang.* **28**, 157–175.

Basta, M., Langlois, P.F., Marques, M., Frank, M.M. & Fries, L.F. (1989): High-dose intravenous immunoglobulin modifies complement-mediated *in vitro* clearance. *Blood* **74**, 326–333.

Bijsterbosch, M.K. & Klaus, G.G.B. (1985): Crosslinking of surface immunoglobulin and Fc receptors on B lymphocytes inhibits stimulation of inositol phospholipid breakdown via the antigen receptors. *J. Exp. Med.* **162**, 1825–1836.

Blaszcyk, R., Westhoff, U. & Grosse-Wilde, H. (1993): Soluble CD4, CD8, and HLA molecules in commercial immunoglobulin preparations. *Lancet* **341**, 789–790.

Bril, V., Ilse, W.K., Pearce, R., Dhanami, A., Sutton, D. & Kong, K. (1996): Pilot trial of immunoglobulin versus plasma exchange in patients with Guillain-Barré syndrome. *Neurology* **46**, 100–103.

Cohn, E.J., Strong, L.E., Hughes,W.L., Mulford,D.J., Ashworth, J.N., Melin, M. & Taylor, H.L. (1946): Preparation and properties of serum and plasma proteins. IV. A system for the separation into fractions of the protein and lipoprotein components of biological tissues and fluids. *J. Am. Chem. Soc.* **68**, 459–475.

Chaudhry, V., Corse, A.M., Cornblath, D.R., Kunci, R.W., Drachman, D.B., Freimer, M.I. *et al.* (1993): Multifocal motor neuropathy: response to human immune globulin. *Ann. Neurol.* **33**, 237–242.

Così, V., Lombardi, M., Piccolo, G. & Erbetta, A. (1991): Treatment of myastenia gravis with high-dose intravenous immunoglobulin. *Acta Neurol. Scand.* **84**, 81–84.

Dalakas, M.C. (1991): Polymyositis, dermatomyositis and inclusion-body myositis. *New Engl. J. Med.* **325**, 1487–1498.

Dalakas, M.C., Illa, I., Dambrosia, J.M., Soueidan, S.A., Stein, D.P., Otero, C., Dinsmore, S.T. & McCrosky, S.A. (1993): A controlled trial of high-dose intravenous immune globulin infusions as treatment for dermatomyositis. *New Engl. J. Med.* **329**, 1993–2000.

Dalakas, M.C., Stein, D.P., Otero, C., Sekul, E., Cupler, E.J. & Sivakumar, K. (1994): Effect of high-dose intravenous immunoglobulin on amyotrophic lateral sclerosis and multifocal motor neuropathy. *Arch. Neurol.* **51**, 861–864.

Dalakas, M.C., Sonies, B., Dambrosia, J., Sekul, E.A., Cupier, E.J. & Sivakumar, K. (1997): Treatment of inclusion-body myositis with IVIg: a double-blind, placebo-controlled study. *Neurology* **48**, 712–716.

Delfraissy, J.F., Tchernia, G., Laurian, Y., Wallon, C., Galanaud, P. & Dormont, J. (1985): Suppressor cell function after intravenous gammaglobulin treatment in adult chronic idiopathic thrombocytopenic purpura. *Br. J. Haematol.* **60**, 315–322.

Deutsch, H.F. (1970): Problems and perspectives in the preparation of human immunoglobulin fractions. In: *Immunoglobulins: Biological aspects and clinical uses*, ed. E. Merler, pp. 317–331. Washington, DC: National Academy of Sciences.

Drachman, D.B. (1994): Myasthenia gravis. *New Engl. J. Med.* **330**, 1797–1810.

Duse, M., Notarangelo, D., Tiberti, S., Menegati, E., Plebani, A. & Ugazio, A.G. (1996): Intravenous immune globulin in the treatment of intractable childhood epilepsy. *Clin. Exp. Immunol.* **104** (Suppl. 1), 71–76.

Dyck, P.J., Litchy, W.J., Kratz, K.M., Suarez G.A., Low, P.A. & Pineda, A.A. (1994): A plasma exchange versus immune globulin infusion trial in chronic inflammatory demyelinating polyradiculoneuropathy. *Ann. Neurol.* **36**, 838–845.

Dwyer, J.M. (1992): Manipulating the immune system with immune globulin. *New Engl. J. Med.* **326**, 107–116.

Eibl, M.M. & Wedgwood, R.J. (1989): Intravenous immunoglobulins: a review. *Immunodeficiency Rev.* **1** (Suppl.), 1–42.

Frank, M.M., Basta, M. & Fries, L.F. (1992): The effects of intravenous immune globulin on complement-dependent immune damage of cells and tissues. *Clin. Immunol. Immunopathol.* **62**, S82–S86.

Fazekas, F., Deisenhammer, F., Strasser-Fuchs, S., Nahaler, G. & Mamoli, B., for the Austrian Immunoglobulin in Multiple Sclerosis Study Group (1997): Randomised placebo-controlled trial of monthly intravenous immunoglobulin therapy in relapsing-remitting multiple sclerosis. *Lancet* **349**, 589–593.

Gajdos, P. (1994): Intravenous immune globulin in myastenia gravis. *Clin. Exp. Immunol.* **97** (Suppl. 1), 49–51.

Gordon, N. (1996): Rasmussen's encephalitis. *Development. Med. Child Neurol.* **38**, 133–136.

Gronski, P., Hofstaetter, T., Kanzy, E.J., Luben, G. & Seiler, F.R. (1983): S-sulfonation: a reversible chemical modification of human immunoglobulins permitting intravenous application. I. Physicochemical and binding properties of S-sulfonated and reconstituted IgG. *Vox Sang.* **45**, 144–154.

Grosse-Wilde, H., Blasczyk, R. & Westhoff, U. (1992): Soluble HLA class I and class II concentrations in commercial immunoglobulin preparations. *Tissue Antigens* **39**, 74–77.

Heyman, B. (1990): The immune complex: possible ways of regulating the antibody response. *Immunol. Today* **11**, 310–313.

Hossein, K. & Seid, S.T. (1998): Combined immunoglobulin and azathioprine in multiple sclerosis. *Eur. Neurol.* **39**, 178–181.

Imbach, P., Barandun, S., d'Apuzzo, V., Baumgartner, C., Hirt, A., Morell, A., Rossi, E., Schoni, M., Vest, M. & Wagner, H.P. (1981): High-dose intravenous gammaglobulin for idiopathic thrombocytopenic purpura in childhood. *Lancet* **ii**, 1228–1231

Jayne, D.R.W., Esnault, V.L.M. & Lockwood, C.M. (1993): ANCA anti-idiotype antibodies and the treatment of systemic vasculitis with intravenous immunoglobulin. *J. Autoimmun.* **6**, 207–219.

Jefferis, R. (1993): Idiotypy and idiotypic networks: a time to redefine concepts. *Clin. Exp. Immunol.* **91**, 193–195.

Klaesson, S., Ringden, O., Markling, L., Remberger, M. & Lundkvist, I. (1993): Immune modulatory effects of immunoglobulins on cell-mediated immune responses *in vitro*. *Scand. J. Immunol.* **38**, 477–484.

Leung, D.Y.M., Burns, J.C., Newburger, J.W., Cotran, R.S. & Geha, R.S. (1987): Reversal of lymphocyte activation *in vivo* in the Kawasaki syndrome by intravenous gammaglobulin. *J. Clin. Invest.* **79**, 468–472.

Livingston, J.H. (1991): Management of intractable epilepsy. *Arch. Dis. Child.* **66**, 1454–1456.

Lotz, B.P., Engel, A.G., Nishino, H., Stevens, J. C. & Litchy, W.J. (1989): Inclusion body myositis. Observations in 40 patients. *Brain* **112**, 727–747.

Marchalonis, J.J., Kaymaz, H., Dedeoglu, F., Schluter, S.F., Yocum, D.E. & Edmundson, A.B. (1992): Human autoantibodies reactive with synthetic autoantigens from T-cell receptor β-chain. *Proc. Natl. Acad. Sci. USA* **89**, 3325- 3329.

Marinos, C. & Dalakas, M.D. (1997): Intravenous immune globulin therapy for neurologic diseases. *Ann. Intern. Med.* **126**, 721–730.

Masson, P.L. (1993): Elimination of infectious agents and increase of IgG catabolism as possible mode of action of IVIG. *J. Autoimmun.* **6**, 683–689.

Morell, A. (1986): Various immunoglobulin preparations for intravenous use. *Vox Sang.* **51** (Suppl. 2), 44–49.

NIH Consensus Conference (1990): Intravenous immunoglobulin. Prevention and treatment of disease. *J. Am. Med. Assoc.* **264**, 3189–3193.

Nobile-Orazio, E. (1996): Multifocal motor neuropathy. *J. Neurol. Neurosurg. Psychiatry* **60**, 599–604.

Nobile-Orazio, E., Meucci, N., Barbieri, S., Carpo, M. & Scarlato, G. (1993): High-dose intravenous immunoglobulin therapy in multifocal motor neuropathy. *Neurology* **43**, 537–543.

Noseworthy, J.H., O'Brien, P., Van Engelen, B.G.M. & Rodriguez, M. (1994): Intravenous immunoglobulin therapy in multiple sclerosis: progress from remyelination in the Theiler's virus model to a randomized, double-blind, placebo-controlled clinical trial. *J. Neurol. Neurosurg. Psychiatry* **57** (Suppl.), 11–14.

Oncley, J.L., Melin, M., Richert, D.A., Cameron, J.W. & Gross, P.M. (1949): The separation of antibodies, isoagglutinins, prothrombin, plasminogen, and β-lipoproteins into sub-fractions of human plasma. *J. Am. Chemi. Soc.* **71**, 541–550.

Perosa, F., Rizzi, R., Pulpito V. & Dammacco, F. (1995): Soluble CD4 antigen reactivity in intravenous immunoglobulin preparations: is it specific? *Clin. Exp. Immunol.* **99**, 16–20.

Plasma exchange Sandoglobulin Guillain-Barré syndrome trial group (1997): Randomized trial of plasma exchange, intravenous immunoglobulin, and combined treatments in Guillain-Barré syndrome. *Lancet* **349**, 225–230.

Ratko, T.A., Burnett, D.A., Foulke, G.E., Matuszewski, K.A., Sacher, R.A. & University Consortium Expert Panel. (1995): Recommendations for off-label use of intravenously administered immunoglobulin preparations. *J. Am. Med. Assoc.* **273**, 1865–1870.

Ricci, C. (1990): La terapia con Ig ev nelle malattie autoimmunitarie. In: *Le immunoglobuline endovena nella pratica clinica*, pp. 63–76. Turin: Minerva Medica.

Rogers, S.W., Andrews, P.I., Gahring, L.C., Whisenand, T., Cauley, K., Crain, B., Hughes, T.E., Heinemann, S.F. & McNamara, J.O. (1994): Autoantibodies to glutamate receptor GluR3 in Rasmussen's encephalitis. *Science* **265**, 648–651.

Roitt, I, Brostoff, J. & Male, D. (1989): Molecules which recognize antigen. In: *Immunology*, Chapter 5, pp. 1–11. London-New York: Gower Medical Publishing.

Romer, J., Morgenthaler, J.-J., Scherz, R. & Skvaril, F. (1982): Characterization of various immunoglobulin preparations for intravenous application. *Vox Sang.* **45**, 62–73.

Ronda, N., Hurez, V. & Kazatchkine, M.D. (1993): Intravenous immunoglobulin therapy of autoimmune and systemic inflammatory diseases. *Vox Sang.* **64**, 65–72.

Ronda, N., Haury, M., Nobrega, A., Coutinho, A. & Kazatchkine, M.D. (1994): Selectivity of recognition of variable (V) regions of autoantibodies by intravenous immunoglobulin (IVIg). *Clin. Immunol. Immunopathol.* **70**, 124–128.

Ross, C., Svenson, M., Hansen, M.B., Vejlsgaard, G.L. & Bendtzen, K. (1995): High avidity IFN-neutralizing antibodies in pharmaceutically prepared human IgG. *J. Clin. Invest.* **95**, 1974–1978.

Ruiz de Souza, V., Carreno, M.P. & Kaveri, S.V. (1995): Selective induction of interleukin-1 receptor antagonist and interleukin-8 in human monocytes by normal polyspecific IgG (intravenous immunoglobulin). *Eur. J. Immunol.* **25**, 1267–1273.

Schneider, C., King, R.M. & Philipson, L. (1998): Genes specifically expressed at growth arrest of mammalian cells. *Cell* **54**, 787–793.

Soueidan, S.A. & Dalakas, M.C. (1993): Treatment of inclusion-body myositis with high-dose intravenous immunoglobulin. *Neurology* **43**, 876–879.

Stangel, M., Hartung, H.P., Marx P. & Gold, R. (1998): Intravenous immunoglobulin treatment of neurological autoimmune diseases. *J. Neurol. Sci.* **153**, 203–214.

Stiehm, E.R. (1979): Standard and special human immune serum globulins as therapeutic agents. *Pediatrics* **63**, 301–319.

Svenson, M., Hansen, M.B. & Bendtzen, K. (1993): Binding of cytokines to pharmaceutically prepared human immunoglobulin. *J. Clin. Invest.* **92**, 2533–2539.

Takei, S., Arora, Y.K. & Walker, S.M. (1993): Intravenous immunoglobulin contains specific antibodies inhibitory to activation of T-cells by staphylococcal toxin superantigens. *J. Clin. Invest.* **91**, 602–607.

Twyman, R.E., Gahring, L.C., Spiess, J. & Rogers, S.W. (1995): Glutamate receptor antibodies activate a subset of receptors and reveal an agonistic binding site. *Neuron* **14**, 755–762.

Ugazio, A.G., Duse, M., Plebani, A., Notarangelo, L.D. & Tiberti, S. (1990): *Intravenous immunoglobulin: prevention and treatment of disease*, pp. 147–150. NIH Consensus Development Conference.

Van der Meché, F.G.A., Schmitz, P.I.M. & Dutch Guillain-Barré Study Group (1992): A randomized trial comparing intravenous immune globulin and plasma exchange in Guillain-Barré syndrome. *New Engl. J. Med.* **326**, 1123–1129.

Van Engelen, B.G.M., Hommes, C.R., Pinkers, A., Cruysberg, J.R.M., Barkhof, F. & Rodriguez, M. (1992): Improved vision after intravenous immunoglobulin in stable demyelinating optic neuritis. *Ann. Neurol.* **32**, 835–836.

Van Furth, R., Leijh, P.C.J. & Klein, F. (1984): Correlation between opsonic activity for various microorganisms and composition of gammaglobulin preparations for intravenous use. *J. Infect. Dis.* **149**, 511–517.

Van Schaik, I.N., Vermeulen, M. & Brand, A. (1997): Immunomodulation and remyelination: two aspects of human polyclonal immunoglobulin treatment in immune-mediated neuropathies? *Multiple Sclerosis* **3**, 98–104.

Vassilev, T., Gelin, C., Kaveri, S.V., Zilber, M.-T., Boumsell, L. & Kazatchkine, M.D. (1993): Antibodies to the CD5 molecule in normal human immunoglobulins for therapeutic use (intravenous immunoglobulins IVIg). *Clin. Exp. Immunol.* **92**, 369–372.

Wills, A.J. & Unsworth, D.J. (1998): A practical approach to the use of intravenous immunoglobulin in neurological disease. *Eur. Neurol.* **39**, 3–8.

Chapter 24

Cytotoxic and noncytotoxic immunosuppressive agents

Maria Grazia Sabbadini and Matteo Bellone

Department of Medicine, Istituto Scientifico H San Raffaele and University of Milan, via Olgettina 60, 20132 Milan, Italy

Summary

Cytotoxic immunosuppressive agents are drugs initially used for the treatment of neoplastic diseases, where the immunosuppressive activity resulted as a side effect of the drug. Cytotoxic and noncytotoxic immunosuppressive drugs are now widely used for prevention of allograft rejection, and for the treatment of immunomediated diseases (e.g. connective tissue diseases, vasculitis, demyelinating diseases). Their mechanisms of action are not fully understood, and they probably affect several processes involved in inflammation. The main characteristics and therapeutic indications of the most widely used cytotoxic and noncytotoxic immunosuppressive agents will be discussed here.

Introduction

Immunosuppressive cytotoxic agents, with the exclusion of azathioprine (AZA), have been initially used for the treatment of neoplastic diseases of haematopoietic origin, in which the immunosuppressive activity resulted as a side effect of the drug.

The goal of the immunosuppressive therapy in immunomediated diseases should be the selective deletion of pathogenic clones, leaving the immune response against exogenous antigens unaltered, as well as the function of the bone marrow. The widely used immunosuppressive agents are usually not able to select for the specificity of the clones, although they exert a much stronger cytotoxic activity against activated clones, like the ones involved in an autoimmune reaction. A more selective activity is exerted by noncytotoxic agents like cyclosporine A (CsA) or tacrolimus, which specifically inhibit the antigen-specific T-lymphocyte activation (Schreiber & Crabtree, 1992). This group of drugs has been initially used to sustain allograft transplantation. However, clinical trials now indicate that noncytotoxic immunosuppressive agents can be used effectively for the treatment of a variety of immunomediated disorders.

Both cytotoxic and noncytotoxic immunosuppressive agents are used in immunopathology at doses much lower than the ones used in cancer or transplantation, and this fact significantly reduces the frequency and intensity of the relevant side effects.

The mechanisms of immunosuppression mediated by cytototoxic and noncytotoxic agents are not fully understood. It is very likely that their effect is only partially mediated by the antiproliferative activity, and they probably affect several mechanisms involved in the inflammatory process (e.g. cell adhesion, cytokines and other mediator production).

Unfortunately, these drugs rarely cause disease resolution, and relapses are frequent after the drug is withheld.

Cytotoxic immunosuppressive agents

The cytotoxic drugs most commonly used in immunopathology belong to the family of alkylating agents [i.e. cyclophosphamide (CTX), and chlorambucil (CHB)], folic acid antagonists [i.e. methotrexate (MTX)], and purine analogues (i.e. AZA). More recently, leflunomide (LFM, an inhibitor of pirimidine synthesis) and mycophenolate mofetil (MMF, inhibitor of purine synthesis) have been introduced as immunosuppressive agents (Table 1).

Table 1. Cytotoxic agents used in immunomediated diseases

Class	Agent	Acronym
Alkylating agents	Cyclophosphamide	CTX
	Chlorambucil	CHB
Purine analogues	Azathioprine	AZA
	6-mercaptopurine	6-MP
Antimetabolites	Methotrexate	MTX
Purine inhibitor	Leflunomide	LFM
Pyrimidine inhibitor	Mycophenolate mofetil	MMF

Alkylating agents

Alkylating agents are a wide group of drugs among which the nitrogen mustards, the ethylenamines, the alkylsulphonates, and the nitrosureas. However, the nitrogen mustards, CTX and CHB in particular, are the only drugs of this family currently used for the treatment of autoimmune diseases. Alkylating agents substitute alkyl radicals into other molecules, forming covalent bounds with purine and pyrimidine residues, and therefore altering the structure and function of proteins and nucleic acids. They may exert a toxic effect during the entire cell cycle, although their activity is stronger during the late G1 or S phases (Chabner et al., 1996).

Unfortunately, these drugs have potent toxic side effects, and their use is associated with increased frequency of neoplasm.

Cyclophosphamide

CTX is a pro-drug, and it requires activation in the liver by the oxidase system P-450. The principal active metabolites of CTX are the nitrogen mustard phosphoramide and acrolein, which act by cross-linking DNA and blocking cell replication. CTX can alkylate molecules also in non-replicating cells, but its cytotoxic effect is active only during cell replication. CTX acts both on T- and B-lymphocytes, therefore impairing the cellular and the humoral immune response.

CTX is a potent immunosuppressive agent usually indicated in the most difficult clinical situations as in systemic vasculitis (Wegener's granulomatosis, classic polyarteritis nodosa, microscopic polyangiitis, and Churg-Strauss's allergic granulomatosis; Cupps, 1992), and in central nervous system (CNS) (Neuwelt *et al.*, 1995) or renal involvement in systemic lupus erythematosus (SLE) (Steinberg & Steinberg, 1991). CTX is also used for other vasculitides like Takayasu's arteritis (Kerr *et al.*, 1994) and CNS primitive angiitis (Calabrese *et al.*, 1997) when steroid resistance is manifested, or to control particularly aggressive leukocytoclastic vasculitis.

CTX has been used in severe rheumatoid arthritis (RA) especially when associated with vasculitis. Owing to its toxic and oncogenic effects (Radis *et al.*, 1995), CTX is currently substituted by MTX and CsA. CTX is also used in early progressive pulmonary fibrosis associated with systemic sclerosis (Silver *et al.*, 1993), dermatomyositis/polymyositis (al-Janadi *et al.*, 1989) and multiple sclerosis.

CTX is generally administered either orally (2–2.5 mg/kg per day) or as intermittent intravenous boluses (0.5–1 g/m^2). Oral administration is usually indicated for vasculitis (Hoffman & Fauci, 1994), and clinical effects are seen within 2 to 3 weeks after starting the therapy.

The first demonstration of the efficacy of CTX in the treatment of vasculitis has been reported in 1983 by Fauci *et al.* (1983) on 85 patients affected by Wegener's granulomatosis, a vasculitis with upper respiratory tract, lung, and renal involvement, and poor prognosis. The association of CTX and glucocorticoids produced remission in 80 per cent of the patients. In the following years CTX has been successfully tested in other severe vasculitides like classic polyarteritis nodosa, microscopic polyangiitis, Churg-Strauss's allergic granulomatosis, Goodpasture's syndrome and ANCA-positive glomerulonephritis (Hoffman & Fauci, 1994). The treatment of severe vasculitis should be prolonged for at least 12–18 months after the remission has been reached, to avoid flares of disease.

Intermittent pulse boluses are used when a prolonged treatment is indicated. This regimen has been used successfully for the treatment of SLE nephritis. A clinical trial involving more than 100 SLE patients with diffuse proliferative (WHO class IV) and extensive or necrotizing focal proliferative (WHO class III) lupus nephritis, and followed for up to ten years, showed that CTX treatment reduces the probability of progression to renal failure (Steinberg & Steinberg, 1991). Intermittent pulse boluses are also used for the CNS involvement in SLE, where it can be associated with plasmapheresis to obtain a faster therapeutic effect.

Intermittent pulse doses of CTX allow reduction of toxic side effects (Table 2), probably because a reduced cumulated amount of drug is reached, compared with oral administration.

Table 2. Toxic side effects of cyclophosphamide therapy

Most frequent	Less frequent
Gonadal suppression	Pulmonary interstitial fibrosis
Bone marrow suppression	Cutis pigmentation
Haemorrhagic cystitis	Hepatic toxicity
Infectious diseases	Oncogenesis
Gastrointestinal intolerance	
Hypogammaglobulinaemia	
Alopecia	
Teratogenicity	

This type of administration also allows a more efficient prevention of haemorragic cystitis, that occurs in 25–50 per cent of the patients chronically treated with CTX *per os* (Cupps, 1990) and is caused by a direct toxic effect of acrolein on the uroepithelium. Chronic treatment with CTX is associated also with the development of bladder carcinoma, which is predicted to occur in 15 per cent of the long-term treated patients (Talar-Williams *et al.*, 1996). Prevention of bladder toxicity is obtained by the combination of a high urinary flux (> 3000 ml/day) and agents acting on SH groups like mesna (usually associated with i.v. administration) or acetyl-cysteine for the entire period required for the clearance of the drug (the plasma half life of CTX is 6–7 h; Fraiser *et al.*, 1991).

Other relevant side effects of CTX are dose-related marrow suppression (predominantly neutropenia), alopecia, and gastrointestinal intolerance (nausea and emesis). Less frequently, pulmonary interstitial fibrosis, liver toxicity and cutis pigmentation may occur.

However, one of the most relevant side effects of CTX is the gonadal suppression. Indeed, CTX interferes with spermatogenesis and follicle maturation, and induces oligospermia or azoospermia and oligomenorrhea or amenorrhea, respectively (Boumpas *et al.*, 1993).

Finally, CTX is considered a mutagenic and teratogenic agent, and even low-dose chronic administration is associated with increased incidence of haematopoietic, cutaneous and bladder neoplasm. It also increases the incidence of *Herpes zoster* and opportunistic infections (e.g. *Pneumocystis carinii*). *Pneumocystis carinii* prevention is recommended in long-term therapies (i.e. 6 months), especially in association with high daily doses of glucocorticoids, and is obtained by trimetoprim (800 mg, three times per week).

Chlorambucil

CHB has been used for more than twenty years for the treatment of immunomediated diseases (Steinberg, 1993). CHB is another alkylating agents in which the methyl group of the mustard is replaced by phenylbutyric acid. The mechanism of action of this agent is similar to CTX, and at high doses it suppresses all myeloid components. It has been reported, however, that CHB at lower doses is able to inhibit lymphopoiesis more selectively than granulopoiesis.

In the past it has been actively used in severe RA (Patanian *et al.*, 1988), in several forms of transition to lymphoproliferative diseases, like mixed cryoglobulinaemia and cryoagglutinine disease (O'Duffy *et al.*, 1984). CHB has been considered the drug of choice for, and successfully used to control, in association with glucocotricoids, the ocular and meningo-encephalic involvement in Behçet's disease. CsA is now considered the immunosuppressive agent of first choice for uveitis in Behçet's disease.

CHB is still used, in association with glucocorticoids, to control relapsing and/or resistant membranous glomerulonephritis. In this case, CHB is administered for three months, followed by alternating with three months of high-dose glucocorticoids (Ponticelli *et al.*, 1995).

On the other hand, a controlled study in patients affected by systemic sclerosis (scleroderma) showed that CHB is ineffective on the cutaneous evolution of the disease (Furst *et al.*, 1989). It can only be administered *per os* at a recommended dose of 0.06–0.2 mg/kg per day. Before the advent of safer cytotoxic drugs, CHB has been used for indications similar to CTX.

Unfortunately, CHB has higher bone marrow suppressive and oncogenetic effects than CTX.

CHB is a mutagenic and teratogenic agent, and induces sterility. On the other hand, it does not induce bladder toxicity, and alopecia and gastrointestinal intolerance are less associated with

CHB therapy. Owing to these factors, and to the short half life (i.e. 90 min), its use has been limited.

Purine analogues

Purine analogues are considered less potent immunosuppressive drugs than alkylating agents, but also less toxic and easier to handle. This is probably the reason for their extensive use in immunomediated diseases.

Of the two most frequently used purine analogues (i.e. 6-ME and AZA), AZA is the currently and almost exclusively used.

Azathioprine

AZA is probably the only cytostatic agent initially used as immunosuppressive drug, at the beginning in the prevention of allograft rejection, and subsequently for the treatment of immunomediated diseases.

AZA differentiates from 6-ME (an analogue of hypoxanthine) because it has an imidazole group attached to the S, which makes it more resistant to tissue oxidative inactivation.

AZA is rapidly metabolized in the liver to 6-ME, which is the active agent. Due to its analogy with hypoxanthine, 6-ME works as substrate for the hypoxantine-guanine phosphoribosyltransperase, determining the production of false metabolites, which eventually inhibit DNA synthesis (Chabner et al., 1996).

The toxic effect is more pronounced against leukocytes than marrow cells, and in particular against monocytes, of which both replication and accumulation at the inflammatory site are blocked. Indeed, AZA appears to have a noticeable anti-inflammatory effect, independent from the action of the specific immune response.

Despite its low immunosuppressive activity, AZA is widely used due to its limited toxicity. Indeed, there is probably no immunomediated disease where AZA has not been used and is currently indicated (e.g. RA, SLE, connective tissue diseases, systemic vasculitis, inflammatory bowel disease). In most of these clinical settings, AZA allows tapering of glucocorticoids needed to maintain the patient in remission.

AZA has been used for decades in RA, because it is able to delay the bone damage associated with the disease (Cash & Kippel, 1994), but it is currently substituted by MTX.

AZA is the most widely used immunosuppressive agent in SLE patients, although only a few controlled studies have evaluated AZA efficacy in this disease. AZA is usually used in all non-severe clinical manifestations (e.g. arthritis, sierositis, haematologic and muco-cutaneous manifestations), which are not controlled by glucocorticoids or antimalarial drugs (Fox & McCune, 1994). Because the clinical effects are usually appreciated within 4 to 8 weeks after commencement of the therapy, AZA is not indicated in acute or severe manifestations of SLE. Indeed, AZA efficacy in lupus nephritis is still under debate. Based on the NIH study (Steinberg & Steinberg, 1991), AZA appears to be less efficient than CTX, and modestly more efficient than glucocorticoids in preventing long-term impairment of renal function.

In systemic vasculitis, AZA is used in patients for which CTX is not indicated (e.g. elderly, pervious toxicity by CTX, pregnancy). In Behçet's disease, AZA has been used to prevent disease flares. A retrospective study reported a long term reduced impairment of the visual function in Behçet's disease patients treated with AZA when compared to glucocorticoids alone

(Hamuryudan et al., 1997). It has also been successfully used in Horton's arteritis, when relapses occur at the tapering or withdrawal of glucocorticoids.

AZA or 6-ME are also considered the immunosuppressive agents of choice, to induce remission and control flares in inflammatory bowel diseases (Pearson et al., 1995). In polymyositis/dermatomyositis AZA is currently used for long-term treatments in substitution for MTX (Villalba & Adams, 1996).

AZA is well absorbed when administered orally, and is used at the dose of 2–2.5 mg/kg per day. Myelosuppression (leukopenia rather than thrombocytopenia and anaemia) is the most relevant toxic side effect, and it is usually monitored to adjust the dose of the drug (Table 3). However, at the recommended dose, leukopenia and megaloblastic anaemia are quite infrequent. At higher doses also mucositis and hepatotoxicity may appear. The most common toxic side effects are rash, urticarial reactions and gastrointestinal intolerance. In some cases, probably due to an allelic variant of the thyopurine methyltransferase gene, an idiosyncratic reaction can occur with severe bone marrow suppression and/or hepatotoxicity (Black et al., 1998). In this case a rapid fall in white blood cells and/or increase of AST/ALT may follow within a week of initiation of therapy. The simultaneous administration of xanthine oxidase inhibitors (e.g. allopurinol) decreases the metabolism of the drug, and increases its toxicity.

Table 3. Toxic side effects of azathioprine therapy

Bone marrow suppression
Hepatotoxicity
Gastrointestinal intolerance
Infectious disease complications
Urticarial reactions
Rashes
Oncogenesis (reduced in autoimmune diseases)

AZA is teratogenic in experimental animals. However, the clinical experience in women carrying renal allografts has not documented a higher incidence of foetal abnormalities. AZA has been used sometimes in SLE patients during the last semester of pregnancy, but it cannot be considered safe for the foetus.

AZA does not appear to act on gonadal function, although this effect has not been fully evaluated.

AZA can be used in patients with impaired renal function, although dosage must be regulated according to the reduced clearance of the drug.

Although in patients receiving an allograft and treated with AZA an increased relative risk of neoplasm (especially non-Hodgkin lymphomas) has been documented, in patients with immunomediated diseases this risk does not appear relevant (Connel et al., 1994).

Anti-metabolites

The family of anti-metabolites is constituted by immunosuppressive agents with selected inhibitory actions on several key enzymatic functions.

Methotrexate

MTX is the most frequently used anti-metabolite in immunomediated diseases. MTX is a folic acid antagonist, whose action is exerted on the dihydrofolate reductase enzyme. Binding and inhibition of dihydrofolate reductase cause the block in the synthesis of dihydrofolate and tetraydrofolate, and eventually of the thymidylate and inosinic acid synthesis. Moreover, MTX blocks the conversion of glycine to serine, and homocysteine to methionine. The cytostatic effect is exerted only at high doses, usually indicated in cancer therapy, and is evident in the S phase of the cell cycle (Chabner et al., 1996). Its immunosuppressive and anti-inflammatory effects are due primarily to the inhibition of the protein synthesis (in particular the synthesis of IL-1, IL-8, and TNFa), which is evident already at the dose used to treat autoimmune diseases (Chang, 1994).

MTX has been initially approved for the treatment of severe psoriasis, psoriatic arthritis, and RA (Willkens & Watson, 1982). It is currently considered the 'gold standard' for the treatment of RA (O'Dell, 1997). The positive results obtained in this disease have suggested its use also in other chronic polyarthritis (e.g. juvenile RA, Reiter's syndrome, spondyloarthropathies, etc).

MTX is also used in several connective tissue diseases and cell-mediated chronic inflammatory diseases (Weinblatt, 1995), e.g. polymyositis, dermatomyositis, primary biliary cirrhosis, and sarcoidosis. In polymyositis/dermatomyositis and other pathological conditions, MTX is usually used instead of AZA when a more profound and rapid immunosuppression is required, without the need of alkylating agents (Oddis & Medsger, 1989). MTX is indicated for both pulmonary and cutaneous involvement in sarcoidosis and, when used in association with glucocorticoids, it can allow faster tapering of the latter. A prospective study on sarcoidosis patients has demonstrated the efficacy of MTX in contrasting the impairment of lung function induced by the disease (Lower & Baughman, 1995).

In SLE patients, MTX has only rarely been used, especially in association with low doses of CsA. Finally, MTX is indicated in the treatment of systemic vasculitis (e.g. Wegener's granulomatosis and Takayasu's arteritis), when the disease is resistant to, or reactivates after withdrawal of CTX treatment (Hoffman et al., 1992, 1994).

For rheumatic diseases, MTX is used at the dose of 5–25 mg once a week, either by oral or parenteral route. It can be taken either in one, two or three portions at 12-h intervals. The three-portion administration is used in psoriatic patients to better control the replication cycle of keratinocytes, but it has no real indication in other immunomediated diseases. The two-portion administration appears to reduce the gastrointestinal symptoms frequently associated with oral administration. When doses higher then 20 mg are indicated, the parenteral administration is preferred, owing to decreased oral bioavailability of the drug at higher doses. A positive response is expected within 2–8 weeks, at which the initial dose can be increased if no clinical response has been achieved and no toxicity has occurred. As for many immunosuppressant drugs, the dose of MTX is slowly reduced when a satisfactory clinical response is obtained.

The drug is excreted mostly in the urine, and its dosage must be reduced in patients with impaired renal function.

The long-term administration of MTX may be associated with relevant toxic side effects, but serious toxicity has been rare (Table 4). Although the occurrence of hepatic fibrosis and cirrhosis in psoriatic patients treated with MTX is high, Kremer et al. (1994) reported a much lower frequency of hepatotoxicity in RA patients. Hepatotoxicity appears to be dose-related, and increases with the ingestion of ethanol and in the presence of other cytopathic factors (e.g. hepatitis C virus).

Table 4. Toxic side effects of methotrexate therapy

Bone marrow suppression
Hepatic fibrosis and cirrhosis
Pulmonary toxicity
Gastrointestinal intolerance
Stomatitis
Teratogenicity

Table 5. Toxic side effects of cyclosporine A therapy

Reversible and irreversible nephrotoxicity
Hypertension
Gastrointestinal intolerance
Gum hypertrophy
Hirsutism
Hepatotoxicity

Table 6. Indications for cytotoxic agents in immunomediated diseases

Agent	Indication
Cyclophosphamide	Sistemic vasculitis (Wegener's granulomatosis, polyarteritis nodosa, Churg-Strauss's allergic granulomatosis and Takayasu's arteritis resistant to steroids); CNS and renal involvement in SLE; ANCA-positive glomerulonephritis; early progressive pulmonary involvement in systemic sclerosis and dermatomyositis/polymyositis.
Chlorambucil	Behçet's disease; vasculitis associated with lymphoproliferative diseases; idiopathic membranous glomerulonephritis.
Azathioprine	Systemic lupus erythematosus; rheumatoid arthritis; Behçet's disease; sistemic vasculitis when CTX is not indicated; dermatomyositis/polymyositis; Crohn's disease.
Methotrexate	Rheumatoid arthritis; severe psoriasis and psoriatic arthritis; dermatomyositis/polymyositis; sistemic vasculitis (Wegener's granulomatosis and Takayasu's arteritis) when CTX is not indicated; sarcoidosis; systemic lupus erythematosus; inflammatory bowel diseases.
Cyclosporine A	Behçet's disease; rheumatoid arthritis; membranous glomerulonephritis.

Bone marrow toxicity may cause leukopenia, thrombocytopenia and megaloblastic anaemia, and it occurs in less than 5 per cent of patients treated with MTX. Renal insufficiency, folic acid deficiency, acute infections, and the concomitant use of trimethoprim/sulphamethoxazole or probenecid may increase the occurrence of haematopoietic toxic effects.

At the dosage used for the treatment of immunomediated diseases, MTX does not exert gonadal toxic effects, although it is teratogenic.

On the other hand, acute and chronic pulmonary toxicity has been reported in patients treated with low doses of MTX, with clinical manifestations ranging from bilateral interstitial infiltrates to fibrosis.

The most frequent toxic side effects of MTX, however, are anorexia, nausea, vomiting, diarrhoea and weight loss. Symptoms in most patients are mild, usually occur at the beginning of the therapy, and may diminish with long-term exposure. MTX may also cause stomatitis, with erythema, painful ulcers, or erosions.

Most of the toxic side effects of the drug are generally reversible if the drug is promptly withdrawn. Folic acid therapy (at a dose < 50 per cent of the MTX dose) administered in the following 24 h may improve hepatic and gastrointestinal tolerability, as well as stomatitis (Morgan et al., 1994). MTX does not appear to have oncogenic activity.

Mofetil micophenolate

MMF is an ester of the agent micophenolate, recently approved by the FDA for the prevention of acute renal allograft rejection. It is rapidly metabolized to micophenolic acid, which is its active metabolite. Micophenolic acid is a potent reversible and non-competitive inhibitor of the inosine monophosphate dehydrogenase enzyme (Wu, 1994). *In vitro*, the micophenolic acid selectively inhibits the *de novo* synthesis of purine nuclotides, and the cell proliferation. Because nucleotide shortage may influence the glycosilation of membrane glycoproteins, the micophenolic acid may also cause relevant changes in the structure and function of adhesion molecules. This mechanism may explain the reduced adhesion of activated T-lymphocytes to activated endothelial cells after their incubation with micophenolic acid. A reduced adhesion potential of T-lymphocytes and monocytes may in part explain the immunosuppressive effect of the drug (Ransom, 1995).

MMF does not cause renal toxicity and does not increase CsA or tacrolimus renal toxicity. Therefore, MMF can be used in association with those agents to prevent acute allograft rejection. The use of MMF in renal transplant from cadavers (at a dose of 2–3 g/day) has allowed a consistent reduction of acute allograft rejection (Mathew, 1998). The association of MMF with tacrolimus has reduced the occurrence of acute liver rejection by 40 per cent (Eckhoff et al., 1998).

MMF, especially at high doses, can exert some gastrointestinal toxicity, and causes leukopenia, anaemia, and thrombocytopenia in a dose-dependent manner. It may also increase the incidence of opportunistic infections.

Controlled clinical trials are still not available in immunomediated diseases, although sporadic reports have documented positive results in the treatment of blistering autoimmune diseases, RA, Takayasu's arteritis and lupus nephritis resistant to the common immunosuppressive agents (Dooley et al., 1999). Leukopoenia is far less frequent in these patients than in transplanted recipients.

MMF is usually used in autoimmunity at 1–2 g/day orally in two doses.

Leflunomide

LFM is an inhibitor of the pyrimidine synthesis. Its active metabolite A77 1726, the only known immunosuppressive metabolite, selectively inhibits B- and T-lymphocyte proliferation (Cao et al., 1995). Its mechanism of action is not fully understood. A77 1726 exerts a noncytotoxic and reversible immunosuppressive effect, probably through the inhibition of the synthesis of growth factors, or the production of immunomodulatory cytokines (e.g. the transforming growth factor-β1) (Cherwinki et al., 1995; Seimasko et al., 1996). Recently is has been also reported that A77 1726 can act on the *de novo* pyrimidine nucleotide synthesis, probably through the inhibition of the enzyme dihydroorotate dehydrogenase, that is required for the synthesis of the uridine 5'-monophosphate (Williamson et al., 1995). Indeed, this inhibitory effect can drastically impair several vital cellular functions (e.g. RNA, DNA, glycoproteins and phospholipids synthesis).

LFM is actually experimented in phase III clinical trials in RA patients. Preliminary reports have documented a therapeutic effect comparable to or even better than sulphasalazine (Mladenovic et al., 1995; Smolen et al., 1999).

Usually a starting dose of 100 mg per day for three days, given parenterally, is followed by an oral dose of 20 mg per day.

Noncytotoxic immunosuppressive agents

The advent of immunosuppressive agents able to selectively act on T-lymphocytes, such as CsA and tacrolimus (FK506), without haematopoietic toxicity represented a major breakthrough in the prevention of allograft rejection, and has induced immunopathologists to test these agents also on immunomediated diseases. Although tacrolimus and sirolimus (rapamycin) have been used so far in experimental trials only, well-defined indications exist for the use of CsA in rheumatologic and dermatologic diseases.

Cyclosporine A

CsA is a cyclic endecapeptide. Because of its chemical structure in which some aminoacids are unconventional or modified, it has a fairly good (20–50 per cent) gastrointestinal absorption, and it does not need to be activated *in vivo*. The agent is lipophilic, easily penetrates the cellular membrane, and binds a family of proteins called cyclophillins. Because cyclophillins are abundant in lymphoid tissues, the drug is particularly effective on lymphocytes. The complex CsA/cyclophillin blocks calcineurin, a Ca^{++}-dependent phosphatase required for the nuclear traslocation and assembly of the cytoplasmic component NF-AT. The direct consequence is the inhibition of the transcription of early T-cell activation genes, like IL-2, IL-3, IL-4, IFN-γ and GM-CSF genes. The effect of the drug is reduced in already activated lymphocytes, where NF-AT traslocation is functioning already. CsA may also exert an anti-inflammatory activity, blocking the release of histamine and the *de novo* synthesis of leukotriens.

CsA has been successfully used for the treatment of immunomediated uveitis resistant to glucocorticoids (Behçet's disease and sympathic ophthalmitis), especially owing to its rapid effects (Nussenblatt et al., 1985). The agent has been also used in several dermatologic diseases (e.g. psoriasis, atopic dermatitis, chronic urticaria) with very good results.

Recently, an Italian study has compared CsA with other 'disease modifier' agents (MTX was not included) in the treatment of RA (Pasero et al., 1996). The study showed that CsA is comparably effective in eliminating joint inflammation, and is superior in slowing the progression of bone erosions. At the dosage used (2.5–4 mg/kg) no severe toxic side effects were evident. Other studies propose associating CsA with MTX when patients are resistant to the latter.

Only small controlled studies are available on the use of CsA in SLE patients, although the results are quite encouraging, especially in reducing disease activity and the dose of glucocorticoids (Takuda et al., 1994).

CsA has been tested in other autoimmune diseases, among which primary biliary cirrhosis, chronic active hepatitis, dermatomyositis/polymyositis, inflammatory bowel diseases, and type I diabetes mellitus, often when drugs of first choice had failed.

Although positive results have been described on the cutaneous score in systemic sclerosis patients treated with CsA (Gisslinger et al., 1991), this drug has to be used with caution in systemic sclerosis patients, owing to CsA nephrotoxicity, and recent reports describing the precipitation of renal involvement in association with CsA treatment.

The absence of bone marrow toxicity has allowed the use of this agent in association with other immunosuppressive agents. Another advantage in the use of this agent is its rapid efficacy. A clinical response indeed is expected within a few weeks.

The drug is usually administered orally at a dose of 2.5–5 mg/kg per day in two portions, but it can also be administered parenterally.

The most relevant toxic side effects are hypertension (seen in more than 30 per cent of the patients) and nephrotoxicity (in 25–75 per cent of the patients). Hypertension is easily controlled by pharmacologic treatment, but it may require tapering or discontinuation of the therapy. Renal injury (i.e. tubular atrophy, interstitial fibrosis or arteriolar alterations) may be irreversible. Because the renal toxicity is dose-related, an accurate control of the renal function is required to taper the dosage to need. Indeed, nephrotoxicity is less frequent in autoimmune patients treated with lower CsA doses than in organ transplant recipients (Feutren & Mihatsch, 1992). Care should be taken during CsA treatment to avoid the association with other nephrotoxic agents, or drugs able to interfere with CsA bioavailability.

CsA is prothrombotic, owing to an increased aggregability of the platelets and reduced prostacycline synthesis by endothelial cells. The drug may also cause hirsutism, gum hyperplasia, and gastrointestinal toxicity. Gum hyperplasia does not seem to be a direct effect of the drug, but the consequence of a 'hyper-reactivity' to the gingival bacterial flora, and it can be prevented with accurate oral hygiene.

Among other less frequent toxic side effects of the drug are tremors, seizures, increase of hepatic transaminase activities, concentration of bilirubin in plasma, headache, paraesthesias, flushing, sinusitis, gynecomastia, conjunctivitis and tinnitus.

Although a relatively low incidence of malignancies is associated with CsA therapy, the association of CsA with other immunosuppressive agents may cause malignant lymphoma, or EBV-related lymphomas, that resolve after withdrawal of the drug.

CsA does not appear to be teratogenic, but owing to its embryotoxicity in animals, it should be avoided in pregnant women.

Tacrolimus (FK 506)

Tacrolimus is an antibiotic produced by the fungus *Streptomyces tsukubaensis*, with immunosuppressive effects similar to those of CsA but at doses 10 to 100 times lower.

The drug acts similarly to CsA, inhibiting the calmodulin/calcineurin system through a different cytoplasmic receptor, the FK-binding protein. Tacrolimus drastically reduces IL-2 production by T-lymphocytes.

As CsA, tacrolimus is incompletely adsorbed when given orally, and it is metabolized in the liver by the cytochrome P-450.

Since 1994, tacrolimus has been used as immunosuppressive agent of first choice to prevent rejection in liver transplants (Abbasoglu et al., 1997). Several multicentric studies have now evaluated the efficacy of tacrolimus, in alternative to CsA, in the prevention of renal and cardiac allograft rejection, or as rescue agents for acute allograft rejections resistant to CsA treatment.

Compared to CsA, tacrolimus does not have well-defined indications in immunomediated diseases. Recently, its use has been suggested for the treatment of cutaneous immunomediated diseases like psoriasis. In this disease, tacrolimus appears to inhibit IL-8 receptor expression on keratinocytes.

Toxic side effects are in part comparable to the ones found in CsA-treated patients. Nephrotoxicity, hyperglycaemia, headache, insomnia and gastrointestinal intolerance have been described so far.

General considerations in the use of cytotoxic and noncytotoxic agents in immunomediated diseases

Why use them

All the immunosuppressive agents may cause toxic side effects, of which several are severe (e.g. oncogenesis), difficult to prevent, and dose-related. Indeed, owing to the intrinsic characteristic of the autoimmune diseases, immunosuppressive therapy must be continued for months and years, to prevent flares. Therefore the line between risk and benefit of the immunosuppressive therapy is extremely fine, and the therapeutic choice for the clinician may be difficult.

When to start

Three levels of indication can be considered: (i) when a rapid and strong immunosuppressive effect is wanted to treat severe and steroid-resistant manifestations of the disease; (ii) to control a chronic disease when tapering of the glucocorticoids is required; and (iii) to prevent relapses.

What to use

A specific immunosuppressive drug for each immunomediated disease does not exist. The mechanism of action of a drug in a specific disease is often understood only after its initial use. Therefore, many of the current indications are based solely on clinical experience. However, the following generalization may be made.

- CTX appears to be particularly effective in diseases in which polymorphonucleates are involved (e.g. several systemic necrotizing vasculitides, leukocytoclastic vasculitis, and immunocomplex-mediated diseases).

- CsA has a specific activity on T-lymphocytes, and it is particularly indicated in cell-mediated diseases.

- It is conceivable that the immunosuppressive activity of purine and pyrimidine synthesis inhibitors is exerted through the interference with cytokine and chemokine synthesis, or with the cell membrane expression of adhesion molecules relevant for the adhesion and migration of leukocytes. These agents are therefore indicated for the treatment of cell- and cytokine-mediated immune diseases.

The rapidity and severity of onset are also relevant criteria in the choice of the agent, and the most potent and rapidly effective immunosuppressive drugs are used for the most severe and life threatening (e.g. CTX for the treatment of organ ischaemia due to vasculitis).

A rough estimate of rapidity may allow the following succession: glucocorticoids in bolus > CsA > CTX > MTX > AZA.

How to use them

Owing to their toxic side effects, immunosuppressive agents should be used for the shortest possible period of time. The dose is usually tapered as soon as clinical remission is reached. Unfortunately, many diseases require a prolonged treatment time at full regimen (e.g. 1 year or more for vasculitis and 2–3 years for lupus nephritis). In the meanwhile the patient should be carefully monitored by physical examination and laboratory tests. For most of the immunosuppressive drugs, cell blood count + differential, hepatic transaminases, urinalysis, plasma creatinine should be checked every 3–4 weeks at the beginning of the therapy, and every 2–3 months subsequently. For CsA, an increase of plasma creatinine < 30 per cent from the baseline value is tolerated, but also plasma urea should be monitored. When CTX is used at intermittent pulse boluses, the nadir of white cells should be carefully followed with cell blood counts between days 10 and 14. AZA treatment requires a control of cell blood count + differential and hepatic transaminases within the first two weeks of treatment to identify ipersensitivity and idiosyncratic reactions. Once a year an X-ray examination of the chest should be performed for patients undergoing MTX therapy.

References

Abbasoglu, O., Levy, M.F., Brkic, B.B., Testa, G., Jeyarajah, D.R., Goldstein, R.M. et al. (1997): Ten years of liver transplantation. *Transplantation* **64,** 1801–1807.

al-Janadi, M., Smith, C.D. & Karsh, J. (1989): Cyclophosphamide treatment of interstitial pulmonary fibrosis in polymyositis/dermatomyositis. *J. Rheumatol.* **16,** 1592–1596.

Black, A.J., McLeod, H.L., Capell, H.A., Powerie, R.H., Matowe, L.K., Pitchard, S.C., Collie-Duguid, E.S.R. & Reid, D.M. (1998): Thiopurine methyltransferase genotype predicts therapy-limiting severe toxicity from azathioprine. *Ann. Intern. Med.* **129,** 716–718.

Boumpas, D.T., Austin, H.A. 3rd, Vaughan, E.M., Yarboro, C.H., Klippel J.H. & Balow, J.E. (1993): Risk for sustained amenorrhea in patients with systemic lupus erythematosus receiving intermittent pulse cyclophosphamide therapy. *Ann. Intern. Med.* **119,** 366–369.

Calabrese, L.H., Duna. G.F. & Lie, J.T. (1997): Vasculitis in central nervous system. *Arthritis Rheum.* **40,** 1189–1201.

Cao, W.W., Kao, P.N., Chao, A.C., Gardner, P.N.J. & Morris, R.E. (1995): Mechanism of the antiproliferative action of leflunomide. *Heart Lung Transplant.* **14,** 1016–1030.

Cash, J.M. & Kippel, J.H. (1994): Second-line drug therapy for rheumatoid arthritis. *N. Engl. J. Med.* **330,** 1368–1375.

Chabner, B.A., Allegra, C.J., Curt, G.A. & Calabresi, P. (1996): Antineoplastic agents. In: *Goodman & Gilman's. The pharmacological basis of therapeutics* (9th edn.), eds. J.G.Hardman & L.E. Limbird, pp. 1233-1263. New York: McGraw-Hill.

Chang, D.-M. (1994): Mechanisms of methotrexate action in rheumatoid arthritis. *Rheumatol. Rev.* **3,** 43–48.

Cherwinki, H.M., McCarley, D., Schatzman, R., Devens, B. & Ransom, J.T. (1995): The immunosoppressant leflunomide inhibits lymphocyte progression through cell cycle by a novel mechanism. *J. Pharmacol. Exp. Ther.* **272,** 460–468.

Connel, W.R., Kamm, M.A., Dickson, M., Balkwill, A.M., Ritchie, J.K. & Lennard-Jones, J.E. (1994): Long-term neoplasia risk after azathioprine treatment in inflammatory bowel disease. *Lancet* **343**, 1249–1252.

Cupps, T.R. (1990): Cyclophosphamide: to pulse or not to pulse? *Am. J. Med.* **89**, 399–401.

Cupps, T.R. (1992): Systemic vasculitis. In: *Current therapy in allergy, immunology & rheumatology*, pp. 211–230, eds. L.S. Goodman, L.E. Limbird, P. Milinoff, A.G. Gilman, J.G. Hardman, Lichtenstein & A.S. Fauci. Mosby Year Book. New York: McGraw Hill.

Dooley, M.A., Cosio, F.G., Nachman, P.H., Falkenhain, M.E., Hogan, S.L., Falk, R.J. & Herbert, L.A. (1999): Mycophenolate mofetil therapy in lupus nephritis: clinical observations. *J. Am. Soc. Nephrol.* **10**, 833–839.

Eckhoff, D.E., McGuire, B.M., Frenette, L.R., Contreras, J.L., Hudson, S.L. & Bynon, J.S. (1998): Tacrolimus (FK506) and mycophenolate mofetil combination therapy versus tacrolimus in adult liver transplantation. *Tranplantation* **65**, 180–187.

Fauci, A.S., Haynes, B.F., Katz, P. & Wolf, S.M. (1983): Wegener granulomatosis: prospective clinical and therapeutic experience with 85 patients for 21 years. *Ann. Intern. Med.* **98**, 76–85.

Feutren, G. & Mihatsch, M.J. (1992): Risk factors for cyclosporine-induced nephropathy in patients with autoimmune diseases. International Kidney Biopsy Registry of Cyclosporine in Autoimmune Diseases. *N. Engl. J. Med.* **326**, 967–969.

Fox, D.A. & McCune, W.J. (1994): Immunosuppressive drug therapy of systemic lupus erythematosus. In: *Systemic lupus erythematosus*, ed. W.J. McCune, vol. 20:1, pp. 265–299. Rheumatic Disease Clinics of North America. Philadephia, WB Saunders.

Fraiser, L.H., Kanekal, S. & Kehrer, J.P. (1991): Cyclophosphamide toxicity. Characterising and avoiding the problem. *Drugs* **42**, 781–795.

Furst, D.E., Clements, P.J., Hillis, S., Lachenbruch, P.A., Miller, B.L., Sterz, M.G. *et al.* (1989): Immunosuppression with chlorambucil, versus placebo, for scleroderma. Results of a three-year, parallel, randomised, double-blind study. *Arthritis Rheum.* **32**, 584–593.

Gisslinger, H., Burghuber, O.C., Stacher, G., Schwarz, W., Punzengruber, C., Graninger, W. *et al.* (1991): Efficacy of cyclosporin A in systemic sclerosis. *Clin. Exp. Rhematol.* **9**, 383–390.

Hamuryudan, V., Özyazgan, Y., Hizli, N., Mat, C., Yurdakul, S., Tüzün, Y., Senocak, M. & Yazici, H. (1997): Azathioprine in Behçet's syndrome. *Arthritis Rheum.* **40**, 769–775.

Hoffman, G.S. & Fauci, A.S. (1994): Emerging concepts in the management of vasculitis diseases. *Adv. Intern. Med.* **39**, 277–303.

Hoffman, G.S., Leavitt, R.Y., Kerr, G.S., Fauci, A.S. (1992): The treatment of Wegener's granulomatosis with glucocorticoids and methotrexate. *Arthritis Rheum.* **35**, 1322–1329.

Hoffman, G.S., Leavitt, R.Y., Kerr, G.S., Rottem, M., Sneller, M.C. & Fauci, A.S. (1994): Treatment of glucocorticoid-resistant or relapsing Takayasu arteritis with methotrexate. *Arthritis Rheum.* **37**, 578–582.

Kerr, G.S., Hallahan, C.W., Giordano, J., Leavitt, R.Y., Fauci, A.S., Rottem, M. & Hoffman, G.S. (1994): Takayasu arteritis. *Ann. Intern. Med.* **120**, 919–929.

Kremer, J.M., Alarcon, G.S., Lighfoot, R.W., Wilkens, R.F., Furst, D.E., Williams, H.J. *et al.* (1994): Methotrexate for rheumatoid arthritis. Suggested guidelines for monitoring liver toxicity. American College of Rheumatology. *Arthritis Rheum.* **37**, 316–328.

Lower, E.E. & Baughman, R.P. (1995): Prolonged use of methotrexate for sarcoidosis. *Arch. Intern. Med.* **155**, 846–851.

Mathew, T.H., for the Tricontinental Mycophenolate Mofetil Renal Transplantation Study Group (1998): A blind, long-term, randomised multicenter study of mycophenolate mofetil in cadaveric renal transplantation. *Transplantation* **65**, 1450–1454.

Mladenovic, V., Domljan, Z., Rozman, B. *et al.* (1995): Safety and effectivess of leflunomide in the treatment of patients with active rheumatoid arthritis. Results of a randomized, placebo-controlled, phase II study. *Arthritis Rheum.* **38**, 1595–1603.

Morgan, S.L., Baggot, J.E., Vaughn, W.H., Austin, J.S., Veicth, T.A., Lee, J.Y. et al. (1994): Supplementation with folic acid during methotrexate therapy for rheumatoid arthritis. A double-blind, placebo-controlled trial. *Ann. Intern. Med.* **121**, 833–841.

Neuwelt, C.M., Lacks, S., Kaye, B.R., Ellman, J.B. & Borenstein, D.G. (1995): Role of intravenous cyclophosphamide in the treatment of severe neuropsychiatric systemic lupus erythematosus. *Am. J. Med.* **98**, 32–41.

Nussenblatt, R.B., Palestine, A.G., Chang, C., Mochizuki, M. & Yancey, K. (1985): Effectiveness of cyclosporin therapy for Behçet's disease. *Arthritis Rheum.* **28**, 671–679.

Oddis, C.V. & Medsger, T.A. (1989): Current management of polymyositis and dermatomyositis. *Drugs* **37**, 383–390.

O'Dell, J.R. (1997): Methotrexate use in rheumatoid arthritis. *Rheum. Dis. Clin. North Am.* **23**, 779–796.

O'Duffy, J.D., Robertson, D.M. & Goldstein, N.P. (1984): Chlorambucil in the treatment of uveitis and meningoencephalitis of Behçet's disease. *Am. J. Med.* **76**, 75–81.

Pasero, G., Priolo, F., Marubini, E., Fantini, F., Ferraccioli, G., Magaro, M. et al. (1996): Slow progression of joint damage in early rheumatoid arthritis treated with cyclosporin A. *Arthritis Rheum.* **39**, 1006–1015.

Patanian, H., Graham, S., Sambrook, P.N., Browne, C.D., Champion, G.D., Cohen, M.L. & Day, R.O. (1988): The oncogenicity of chlorambucil in rheumatoid arthritis. *Br. J. Rhematol.* **27**, 44–47.

Pearson, D.C., May, G.R., Fick, G.H. & Sutherland, L.R. (1995): Azathioprine and 6-mercaptopurine in Crohn disease. A meta-analysis. *Ann. Intern. Med.* **123**, 132–142.

Ponticelli, C., Zucchelli, P., Passerini, P. et al. (1995): A 10 years follow-up of a randomized study with methylprednisolone and chlorambucil in membranous nephropathy. *Kidney Int.* **48**, 1600–1604.

Radis, C.D., Kahl, L.E., Baker, G.L., Wasko, M.C.M., Cash, J., Gallatin, A., Stolzer, B.L., Agarwal, A.K., Medsger, T.A. & Kwoh, K. (1995): Effect of cyclophosphamide on development of malignancy and on long-term survival of patients with rheumatoid arthritis. *Arthritis Rheum.* **38**, 1120–1127.

Ransom, J.T. (1995): Mechanism of action of mycophenolate mofetil. *Ther. Drug Monit.* **17**, 681–684.

Schreiber, S.L. & Crabtree, G.R. (1992): The mechanism of action of cyclosporin A and FK506. *Immunol. Today* **13**, 136–142.

Seimasko, K.F., Chong, A.S., Williams, J.W., Bremer, E.G. & Finnegan, A. (1996): Regulation of B-cell function by the immunosuppressive agent leflunomide. *Trasplantation* **61**, 635–642.

Silver, R.M., Warrick, J.H., Kinsella, M.B., Staudt, L.S., Baumann, M.H. & Strange, C. (1993): Cyclophosphamide and low-dose prednisone therapy in patients with systemic sclerosis (scleroderma) with interstitial lung disease. *J. Rheumatol.* **20**, 838–844.

Smolen, J.S., Kalden, J.R., Scott, D.L., Rozman, B., Kvien, T.K., Larsen, A., Loew-Friedrich, I., Oed, C., Rosenburg, R. & the European Leflunomide Study Group (1999): Efficacy and safety of leflunomide compared with placebo and sulphalazine in active rheumatoid arthritis: a double-blind, randomised, multicentric trial. *Lancet* **353**, 259–266.

Steinberg, A.D. (1993): Chlorambucil in the treatment of patients with immune-mediated rheumatic diseases. *Arthritis Rheum.* **36**, 325–328.

Steinberg, A. & Steinberg, S.C. (1991): Long-term preservation of renal function in patients with lupus nephritis receiving treatment that includes cyclophosphamide versus those treated with prednisone only. *Arthritis Rheum.* **34**, 945–950.

Takuda, M., Kurata, N., Mizoguchi, A., Inoh, M., Seto, K., Kinashi, M. & Takahara, J. (1994): Effect of low-dose cyclosporin A on systemic lupus erythematosus disease activity. *Arthritis Rheum.* **37**, 551–559.

Talar-Williams, C., Hijazi, Y.M., Walther, M.M., Linehan, W.M., Hallahan, C.W., Lubensky, I. et al. (1996): Cyclophosphamide-induced cystitis and bladder cancer in patients with Wegener granulomatosis. *Ann. Intern. Med.* **124**, 477–484.

Villalba, L. & Adams, E.M. (1996): Up-data on therapy for refractory dermatomyositis and polymyositis. *Curr. Opin. Rheumatol.* **8**, 544–551.

Weinblatt, M.E. (1995): Methotrexate for chronic diseases in adults. *N. Engl. J. Med.* **332**, 330–331.

Williamson, R.A., Yea, C.M., Robson, P.A., Curnock, A., Gadher, S. *et al.* (1995): Dihydroorotate dehydrogenase is a high affinity binding protein for A77 1726 and mediator of a range of biological effects of the immunomodulatory compound. *J. Biol. Chem.* **270**, 22467–22472.

Willkens, R.F. & Watson, M.A. (1982): Methotrexate: a perspective of its use in the treatment of rheumatic diseases. *J. Lab. Clin. Med.* **100**, 314–321.

Wu, J.C. (1994): Mycophenolate mofetil: molecular mechanisms of action. *Perspect. Drug Discovery Res.* **2**, 185–204.

Chapter 25

Immunomodulation by plasmapheresis and immunoadsorption for autoimmune neurological disorders in children

Carlo Antozzi

Department of Neuromuscular Diseases, Istituto Nazionale Neurologico 'C. Besta', via Celoria 11, 20133 Milan, Italy

Summary

Several autoimmune disorders involve the peripheral and central nervous systems, causing severe disability. The mainstay of treatment is always represented by immunosuppression, but plasma treatment, either as therapeutic plasma exchange (TPE) or more recent selective techniques, has been increasingly used with successful results. TPE has a definite role in the treatment of autoimmune disorders involving the peripheral nerves or the neuromuscular junction. On the contrary, the use and efficacy in disorders involving the central nervous system is still debated, but several lines of evidence suggest the need for controlled studies, particularly in severely compromised patients. In this regard, immunoadsorption with new selective techniques offers a considerable advantage over TPE and deserves further investigation.

Introduction

Our understanding of the pathogenesis, and hence the quality of care, of autoimmune neurological disorders has been considerably improved in recent years and the general criteria for treatment with corticosteroids and immunomodulating drugs have been established. Among the therapeutic options available, plasma treatment, either as therapeutic plasma exchange (TPE) or as removal of single plasma components, can be of great help in several autoimmune conditions involving the peripheral or central nervous systems.

TPE and more selective techniques such as IgG immunoadsorption allow the removal of pathogenic humoral factors. Their efficacy is not simply related to removal *per se* but also to the pathogenesis of the disease, to the features of the target organ and the clinical conditions of the patient. Therapeutic apheresis can be considered either as an 'acute' treatment in patients requiring a massive and rapid removal of a pathogenic factor, or as maintenance therapy in selected patients, particularly in case of failure of immunosuppressive drugs or of severe side effects requiring reduction of their dosage.

Therapeutic apheresis in children is technically similar to procedures performed in adults. However, the adequacy of vascular access, the extracorporeal fluid volume and the patients' compliance are major concerns in the application of apheresis to the small child. Moreover, controlled trials are lacking in children and indications and therapeutic decisions are derived from experience developed in the adult patient (Assessment of plasmapheresis, 1996).

Recently, selective techniques such as adsorption of IgG immunoglobulins have been used more widely in patients with autoimmune diseases. The general indication is the treatment of autoimmune disorders mediated by IgG autoantibodies. Immunoadsorption removes IgGs with a negligible interaction with other plasma components, it does not require any replacement fluid, and therefore allows the removal of greater amounts of immunoglobulins compared to TPE. Because of its efficiency, immunoadsorption can be a useful alternative to TPE in selected patients with chronic antibody-mediated autoimmune diseases. We will briefly review the current applications of apheretic techniques in autoimmune neurological disorders of paediatric interest.

Acute and chronic inflammatory polyneuropathies

Guillain-Barré syndrome (GBS) is an acute demyelinating inflammatory polyneuropathy characterized by symmetric motor impairment, variable sensory loss and areflexia; the disease is frequently preceded by an upper respiratory infection or gastrointestinal illness (Bradshaw & Jones, 1992; Hartung et al., 1998). Even though improvement and eventual recovery is the rule in the majority of patients, supportive care and early physiotheraphy are of primary importance in the management of GBS, particularly in bed-ridden patients. Two large controlled trials performed in adult patients established that TPE can shorten the recovery phase of the disease (Guillain-Barré Syndrome Study Group, 1985; French Cooperative Group on Plasma Exchange in Guillain-Barré Syndrome, 1991, 1992). TPE is usually performed every other day with removal of at least one plasma volume for each session, replaced with 5 per cent albumin. There is no standardization of treatment protocol; the results of the studies mentioned above suggested that five exchanges can be effective. Retrospective studies in children indicated that TPE diminished morbidity of the disease and shortened the time for recovery, as reported in adults (Epstein & Sladky, 1990; Khatri et al., 1990; Lamont et al., 1991; Jansen et al., 1993). TPE is generally recommended for patients with rapid progression of the disease, signs of bulbar involvement, and loss of ambulation. A therapeutic alternative is represented by high-dose intravenous immunoglobulins (IVIG), which were found to be at least as effective as TPE in adult GBS patients (Van der Meché et al., 1992; Sharar et al., 1990; Abd-Allah et al., 1997). The most widely used protocol consists of five consecutive daily infusions of 400 mg/kg of immunoglobulins. IVIG offer the considerable advantage of their ease of use, particularly when vascular access is difficult to obtain. Recently, the outcome of severe paediatric GBS has been retrospectively evaluated after immunotherapy or supportive care in 26 patients (Graf et al., 1999): the authors found that recovery times in each treatment group were similar, raising the question about the importance of disease severity in the evaluation of treatment, either retrospectively or prospectively.

TPE, as well as IVIG, has a place in the treatment options for chronic inflammatory demyelinating polyradiculoneuropathy (CIDP) in children (Nevo, 1998). The majority of children with CIDP are treated with corticosteroids and/or IVIG; TPE can be also considered for patients resistant to pharmacological therapy (Korinthenberg, 1999).

Autoimmune ion channel disorders

Autoimmune ion channel disorders are clinically different diseases sharing a common pathogenesis mediated by autoantibodies against different ion channels. They comprise myasthenia gravis (MG) caused by antibodies against the muscle acetylcholine receptor, and Lambert-Eaton myasthenic syndrome and neuromyotonia caused by antibodies against presynaptic voltage-gated calcium channels and potassium channels, respectively (Vincent, 1999). MG, even though more frequent in adults, shows similar features in children (Engel, 1994). The disease is treated with anticholinesterase drugs, prednisone and thymectomy. In severe cases other immunosuppressants can be considered. The prognosis of MG in children is good in the majority of patients. The introduction of TPE for MG patients since 1976 has considerably modified the natural course of the disease (Pinching et al., 1976). The procedure is effective in about 70 per cent of treated patients. Moreover, the effect is time-related to removal of plasma and therefore observable within a few days from the beginning of treatment. TPE is particularly helpful in rapidly improving the clinical condition of the patients and, since its introduction, has considerably reduced the incidence of respiratory insufficiency and admittance to the intensive care unit for assisted ventilation. The indications to TPE in children are similar to those in adults, and are based mainly on the severity of the disease. Patients with severe bulbar muscles involvement, myasthenic crisis, and deterioration of their clinical conditions at the beginning of steroid treatment are the main indications of TPE. There is no standardized protocol for TPE in MG. In our experience, two exchanges performed every other day, with removal of about one plasma volume, are effective in 70 per cent of patients. Such a schedule can be repeated in case of nonresponse, or of short-lasting improvement (Antozzi et al., 1991). The improvement lasts usually for a few weeks if plasma treatment is not associated with adequate immunosuppression. For the majority of MG patients TPE remains an 'acute' treatment option. However, periodic TPE can be of help in selected patients with severe forms of the disease, unresponsive to immunosuppression. In these rare patients, the chronic removal of a pathogenic humoral factor is recommended. Selective IgG immunoadsorption can be of considerable help in improving the patients' outcome. Immunoadsorption implies the removal of a single plasma component, namely IgG, selectively from plasma. The technique does not require any replacement fluid. Different ligands have been developed. We used staphylococcal protein A, derived from the bacterial cell wall, which has a very high affinity for subclasses 1, 2 and 4 of human IgG; variable, but limited binding of IgM and IgA has been observed. Moreover, protein A is remarkably stable with regard to changes in pH and temperature, can be covalently linked to a support matrix and easily regenerated for extensive re-use in the same patient (Gjorstrup & Watt, 1990). We obtained a dramatic clinical improvement in severely compromised MG patients unresponsive to ongoing immunosuppression (Antozzi et al., 1994; Berta et al., 1994). Interestingly, we obtained a positive response even after failure with TPE or IVIG. Due to its particular biochemical properties and to the continuous on-line regeneration, protein A allows the removal of unlimited amounts of IgGs from the patient's plasma; this feature probably explains the superiority of protein A immunoadsorption over TPE from a clinical perspective. However, due to the relative complexity from a technical standpoint, this procedure is indicated in severe patients requiring prolonged treatments. No side effects directly attributable to protein A have been noted. Therefore, it can be considered safe for its application in children.

As mentioned above for GBS, IVIG are an alternative to TPE and share the same indications (Howard, 1998). The dosage is similar to that used in inflammatory neuropathies. No controlled studies comparing TPE and IVIG are available in children. One randomized trial performed in adults concluded that IVIG are as effective as TPE in the short term (Gajdos et al., 1997). However, the onset of improvement does not seem to be as rapid as is observed with TPE. IVIG can be a very helpful alternative in children when TPE cannot be performed due to inadequate vascular access.

Autoimmune disorders involving the central nervous system

Several disorders are included under the general heading of autoimmune disorders of the central nervous system (CNS). A systematic classification of these diseases is beyond the scope of this review. We will consider those in which TPE or immunoadsorption have been investigated or might be considered on the basis of pathogenetic considerations.

Multiple sclerosis (MS) is an inflammatory demyelinating disease of the central nervous system (CNS). The cause of MS is still unknown but several lines of evidence strongly suggest that the immunopathological events responsible for the disease are autoimmune in nature, such as the morphological features of the MS lesion, T-cell studies, immunogenetic data and the relative response to immunomodulating therapies. Extensive investigation has been devoted to factors causing or involved in the process of demyelination. These include cytotoxic T-cells, proinflammatory cytokines and antibodies with demyelinating activity (Lassmann et al., 1998). Recently, elegant immunopathological studies led to the hypothesis that, at least in some patients and in some animal models, antibodies reacting with myelin oligodendrocyte glycoprotein (MOG) have a role in demyelination. The accepted issue that CNS inflammation is triggered by autoaggressive T-cells reacting with myelin antigens does not exclude that a humoral factor can be a further, and in some instances necessary, effector mechanism. This hypothesis has been suggested by studies performed in the marmoset model, the immunopathological and clinical features of which more closely resemble those of MS (Genain et al., 1999; Raine et al., 1999). Even though several questions are still open, these studies have set the basis for the concept of antigen-specific, antibody-mediated demyelination (Wekerle, 1999; McFarland, 1999). However, we do not know (a) whether these antibodies are actually an initial step in promoting demyelination, (b) whether they come from serum or spinal fluid, and (c) which is the influence of a disrupted blood-brain barrier on their occurrence within the CNS. Moreover, their presence and specificity is still controversial and deserves further investigation in large groups of patients (Reindl et al., 1999; Karni et al., 1999). Nevertheless, the concept of antibody-mediated demyelination in MS is new and can be of great importance on both pathogenetic and therapeutic grounds.

The issue that an antibody may be involved in demyelination suggests that its removal from plasma might be associated with clinical improvement; if this is the case, a clinical response can be considered an indirect, further proof of the pathogenic importance of antibodies as as effector mechanism in MS. Previous studies on plasma exchange in MS were not encouraging (Compston, 1998). However, Rodriguez and coworkers claimed that plasmapheresis can be useful in the treatment of fulminant CNS demyelination of different aetiology (Rodriguez et al., 1993). The same authors recently reported the results of a randomized, sham-controlled, double-masked study on plasma exchange in patients with a recent attack of inflammatory demyelinating disease unresponsive to high-dose intravenous corticosteroids (Weinshenker et al., 1999). They claimed that plasma exchange was effective in reducing neurological disability in a considerable proportion of patients. Other reports, even though anecdotal, indicated that plasmapheresis can be considered in selected cases after failure of conventional treatments (Takahashi et al., 1997). The above findings suggested that clinical improvement was associated with the removal of a pathogenic humoral factor. However, factors other than antibodies, such as complement components and pro-inflammatory cytokines involved in the pathogenesis of MS are actually removed by plasma exchange. Because of the lack of selectivity of plasma exchange, no further statement can be made on its mechanisms of action in responder patients. In this regard, IgG immunoadsorption should be investigated in MS and other demyelinating disorders, as suggested by recent preliminary observations (Schneidewind et al., 1998; de Andres et al., 2000). A selective technique such as immunoadsorption with protein A or other ligands might be considerably more effective than conventional TPE, and in case of efficacy, it would confirm the role of the still debated humoral component in the pathogenesis of the disease. Similar considerations can be made for acute disseminated encephalomyelitis (ADEM), a monophasic disease frequently preceded by an infectious illness or vaccination (Stuve & Zamvil, 1999). High-dose corticosteroids are used and considered effective, but immunomodulation with intravenous immunoglobulins or plasmapheresis has been considered and reported as successful in some patients (Stricker et al., 1992; Kanter et al., 1995; Dodick et al., 1998; Balestri et al., 2000).

The central nervous system can be also involved in patients with lupus, vasculitis and connective tissue disorders. In these diseases, immunosuppression is the treatment of choice, but plasmapheresis or immunoadsorption have been used with variable results. Again, anecdotal reports suggest the need for the investigation of new selective approaches, particularly in severely affected patients (Garcia-Consuegra et al., 1992; Wallace, 1999; Schneider et al., 1997; Gaubitz et al., 1998).

Rasmussen's encephalitis (RE) is a rare devastating disease characterized by childhood onset of partial and secondarily generalized seizures, often with epilepsia partialis continua (EPC) and recurrent status epilepticus, progressive dysfunction of one cerebral hemisphere and cognitive decline. From a pathological point of view, inflammatory changes, neuronal loss, laminar necrosis and glial scarring have been reported. Antiepileptic drugs are usually ineffective, and functional hemispherectomy is still the treatment of choice (Antel & Rasmussen, 1996; Aarli, 2000). The disease raised considerable interest after the observation that rabbits immunized with a fusion protein containing part of the extracellular domain of the glutamate receptor 3 (GluR3) developed seizures and histopatological features similar to those of RE. These findings suggested a possible role for antiGluR3 antibodies in the pathogenesis of the disease in the experimental animal and hence in humans. Moreover, immunoreactivity for GluR3 was found by immunoblot analysis of serum from three patients in which the diagnosis of RE was confirmed pathologically (Rogers et al., 1994). Subsequently, the same authors suggested that glutamate receptor antibodies were able to evoke currents in cultured neurons (Twyman et al., 1995). These observations, pointing to an autoimmune component in the pathogenesis of the disease, suggested the use of TPE that produced transient improvement in seizure frequency and neurologic function in some patients affected with RE (Rogers et al., 1994; Andrews et al., 1996). Since antiGluR3 antibodies are IgG, and RE is a severe chronic disorder, we evaluated the efficacy of long-term IgG immunoadsorption with protein A, as mentioned above for MG.

We obtained a significant improvement in both seizure frequency and neuropsychological deficit in a 16-year-old patient with RE (Antozzi et al., 1998). Interestingly, the selectivity of immunoadsorption supported once more the hypothesis of an autoimmune component in the pathogenesis of RE. We therefore suggested that IgG immunoadsorption can be considered for severe RE patients as adjunctive therapy at least to delay the need for functional hemispherectomy in selected cases (Antozzi et al., 1998).

A possible involvement of autoimmunity in the exacerbations of tics and obsessive symptoms after streptococcal infection has been postulated in children with obsessive-compulsive disorder (OCD) and tic disorders in childhood. It has been recently shown that TPE or IVIG were effective in reducing the severity of symptoms in children with infection-triggered OCD, suggesting the need for further investigation of immunomodulatory treatments in these diseases (Perlmutter et al., 1999).

References

Aarli, J.A. (2000): Rasmussen's encephalitis: a challenge to neuroimmunology. *Curr. Opin. Neurol.* **13**, 297–299.

Abd-Allah, S.A., Jansen, P.W., Ashwakn S. & Perkin, R.M. (1997): Intravenous immunoglobulin as therapy for pediatric Guillain-Barré syndrome. *J. Child. Neurol.* **12**, 376–380.

Andrews, P.I., Dichter, M.A., Berkovic, S.F., Newton, M.R. & McNamara, J.O. (1996): Plasmapheresis in Rasmussen's encephalitis. *Neurology* **46**, 242–246.

Antel, J.P. & Rasmussen, T. (1996): Rasmussen's encephalitis and the new hat. *Neurology* **46**, 9–11.

Antozzi, C., Gemma, M., Regi, B., Berta, E., Confalonieri, P., Peluchetti, D., Mantegazza, R., Baggi, F., Marconi, M., Fiacchino, F. & Cornelio, F. (1991): A short plasma exchange protocol is effective in severe myasthenia gravis. *J. Neurol.* **238**, 103–107.

Antozzi, C., Berta, E., Confalonieri, P., Zuffi, M., Cornelio, F. & Mantegazza, R. (1994): Protein A immunoadsorption in immunosuppression-resistant myasthenia gravis. *Lancet* **383**, 124.

Antozzi, C., Granata, T., Aurisano, N., Zardini, G., Confalonieri, P., Airaghi, G., Mantegazza, R. & Spreafico, R. (1998): Long-term IgG immunoadsorption improves Rasmussen's encephalitis. *Neurology* **51**, 302–305.

Assessment of plasmapheresis. Report of the therapeutics and technology subcommittee of the American Academy of Neurology (1996): *Neurology* **47**, 840–843.

Balestri, P., Grosso, S., Acquaviva, A. & Bernini, M. (2000): Plasmapheresis in a child affected by acute disseminated encephalomyelitis. *Brain Dev.* **22**, 123–126.

Berta, E., Confalonieri, P., Simoncini, O., Bernardi, G., Busnach, G., Mantegazza, R., Cornelio, F. & Antozzi, C. (1994): Removal of antiacetylcholine receptor antibodies by protein A immunoadsorption in myasthenia gravis. *Int. J. Artif. Organs* **11**, 603–608.

Bradshaw, D.Y. & Jones, H.R. (1992): Guillain-Barré syndrome in children: clinical course, electrodiagnosis, and prognosis. *Muscle & Nerve* **15**, 500–506.

Compston, A. (1998): Treatment and management of multiple sclerosis. In: *McAlpine's multiple sclerosis*, eds. A. Compston, G. Ebers, H. Lassman, I. McDonald, B. Matthews & H. Wekerle (3rd edn.), pp. 437–498. London: Churchill Livingston.

de Andres, C., Anaya, F. & Gimenez-Roldan, S. (2000): Plasma immunoadsorption treatment of malignant multiple sclerosis with severe and prolonged relapses. *Rev. Neurol.* **30**, 601–605.

Dodick, D.W., Silber, M.H., Noseworthy, J.H., Wilbright, W.A. & Rodriguez, M. (1998): Acute disseminated encephalomyelitis after accidental injection of a hog vaccine: successful treatment with plasmapheresis. *Mayo Clin. Proc.* **73**, 1193–1195.

Engel A.G. (1994): Acquired autoimmune myasthenia gravis. In: *Myology*, Vol. 2, eds. A.G. Engel & C. Franzini-Armstrong, pp. 1769–1797. New York: McGraw-Hill.

Epstein, M.A. & Sladky, J.T. (1990): The role of plasmapheresis in childhood Guillain-Barré syndrome. *Ann. Neurol.* **28**, 65–69.

French Cooperative Group on Plasma Exchange in Guillain-Barré Syndrome (1991): Role of replacement fluids. *Ann. Neurol.* **22**, 753–761.

French Cooperative Group on Plasma Exchange in Guillain-Barré Syndrome (1992): One year follow-up. *Ann. Neurol.* **32**, 94–97.

Gajdos, P., Chevret, S., Clair, B., Tranchant, C. & Chastang, C. (1997): Clinical trial of plasma exchange and high-dose intravenous immunoglobulin in myasthenia gravis. Myasthenia Gravis Clinical Study Group. *Ann. Neurol.* **41**, 789–796.

Garcia-Consuegra, J., Merino, R., Alonsa, A. & Goded, F. (1992): Systemic lupus erythematosus: a case report with unusual manifestations and favourable outcome after plasmapheresis. *Eur. J. Pediatr.* **151**, 581–582.

Gaubitz, M., Seidel, M., Kummer, S., Schotte, H., Perniok, A., Domschke, W. & Schneider, M. (1998): Prospective randomized trial of two different immunoadsorbers in severe systemic lupus erithemathosus. *J. Autoimm.* **11**, 495–501.

Genain, C., Cannella, B., Hauser, S. & Raine, C. (1999): Identification of autoantibodies associated with myelin damage in multiple sclerosis. *Nat. Med.* **5**, 153–154.

Gjorstrup, P. & Watt, R.M. (1990): Therapeutic protein A immunoadsorption. A review. *Transfus. Sci.* **11**, 281–302.

Graf, W.D., Katz, J.S., Eder, D.N., Smith, A.J. & Chun, M.R. (1999): Outcome of severe pediatric Guillain-Barré syndrome after immunotherapy or supportive care. *Neurology* **52**, 1494–1497.

Guillain-Barré Syndrome Study Group (1985): Plasmapheresis and acute Guillain-Barré syndrome. *Neurology* **35**, 1096–1104.

Hartung, H.P., van der Meche, F.G. & Pollard, J.D. (1998): Guillain-Barré syndrome, CIDP and other chronic immune-mediated neuropathies. *Curr. Opin. Neurol.* **11**, 497–513.

Howard, J.F. (1998): Intravenous immunoglobulins for the treatment of acquired myasthenia gravis. *Neurology* **51** (Suppl. 5), S30–S36.

Jansen, P.W., Perkin, R.M. & Ashwal, S. (1993): Guillain-Barré syndrome in childhood: natural course and efficacy of plasmapheresis. *Pediatr. Neurol.* **9**, 16–20.

Kanter, D.S., Horensky, D., Sperling, R.A., Kaplan, J.D., Malachowski, M.E. & Churchill, W.H. Jr (1995): Plasmapheresis in fulminant acute disseminated encephalomyelitis. *Neurology* **45**, 824–827.

Karni, A., Bakimer-Kleiner, R., Abramsky, O. & Ben-Nun, A. (1999): Elevated levels of antibody to myelin oligodendrocyte glycoprotein is not specific for patients with multiple sclerosis. *Arch. Neurol.* **56**, 311–315.

Khatri, B.O., Flamini, J.R., Baruah, J.K., Dobyns, W.B. & Konkol, R.J. (1990): Plasmapheresis in acute inflammatory polyneuropathy. *Pediatr. Neurol.* **6**, 17–19.

Korinthenberg, R. (1999): Chronic inflammatory demyelinating polyradiculoneuropathy in children and their response to treatment. *Neuropediatrics* **30**, 190–196.

Lamont, P.J., Johnston, H.M. & Berdoukas, V.A. (1991): Plasmapheresis in children with Guillain-Barré syndrome. *Neurology* **41**, 1928–1931.

Lassmann, H., Raine, C.S., Antel, J. & Prineas, J.W. (1998): Immunopathology of multiple sclerosis: report on an international meeting held at the Institute of Neurology of the University of Vienna. *J. Neuroimmunol* **86**, 213–217.

McFarland, H.F. (1999): The path to damage in multiple sclerosis. *Ann. Neurol.* **46**, 141–142.

Nevo, Y. (1998): Childhood chronic inflammatory demyelinating polyneuropathy. *Europ. J. Paediatr. Neurol.* **2**, 169–177.

Perlmutter, S.J., Leitman, S.F., Garvey, M.A., Hamburger, S., Feldman, E., Leonard, H.L. & Swedo, S.E. (1999): Therapeutic plasma exchange and intravenous immunoglobulin for obsessive-compulsive disorder and tic disorders in childhood. *Lancet* **354**, 1153–1158.

Pinching, A.J., Peters, D.K. & Newsom-Davis, J. (1976): Remission of myasthenia gravis following plasma exchange. *Lancet* **ii**, 1373–1376.

Raine, C.S., Cannella, B., Hauser, S.L. & C.P. Genain (1999): Demyelination in primate autoimmune encephalomyelitis and acute multiple sclerosis lesions: a case for antigen-specific antibody mediation. *Ann. Neurol.* **46**, 144–160.

Reindl, M., Linington, C., Brehm, U., Egg, R., Dilitz, E., Deisenhammer, F., Poewe, W. & Berger, T. (1999): Antibodies against the myelin oligodendrocyte glycoprotein and the myelin basic protein in multiple sclerosis and other neurological diseases: a comparative study. *Brain* **122**, 2047–2056.

Rodriguez, M., Karnes, W.E., Bartleson, J.D. & Pineda, A.A. (1993): Plasmapheresis in acute episodes of fulminant CNS inflammatory demyelination. *Neurology* **43**, 1100–1104.

Rogers, S.W., Andrews, P.I., Gahring, L.C., Whisenand T., Cauley, K., Crain, B., Hughes, T.E., Heinemann, S.F. & McNamara, J.O. (1994): Autoantibodies to glutamate receptor 3 (GluR3) in Rasmussen's encephalitis. *Science* **265**, 648–651.

Schneider, M., Gaubitz, M. & Perniok, A. (1997): Immunoadsorption in systemic connective tissue diseases and primary vasculitis. *Ther. Apher.* **1**, 117–120.

Schneidewind, J.M., Winkler, R., Ramlow, W., Tiess, M., Hertel, U. & Sehland, D. (1998): Immunoadsorption: a new therapeutic possibility for multiple sclerosis? *Transfus. Sci.* **19** (Suppl), 59–63.

Sharar, E., Murphy, E.G. & Roifman, C.M. (1990): Benefit of intravenously administered immune serum in patients with Guillain-Barré syndrome. *J. Pediatr.* **116**, 141–144.

Stricker, R.B., Miller, R.G. & Kiprov, D.D. (1992): Role of plasmapheresis in acute disseminated encephalomyelitis. *J. Clin. Apheresis* **7**, 173–179.

Stuve, O. & Zamvil, S.S. (1999): Pathogenesis, diagnosis, and treatment of acute disseminated encephalomyelitis. *Curr. Opin. Neurol.* **12**, 395–401.

Takahashi, I., Sawaishi, Y., Takeda, O., Enoki, M. & Takada, G. (1997): Childhood multiple sclerosis treated with plasmapheresis. *Pediatr. Neurol.* **17**, 83–87.

Twyman, R.E., Gahring, L.C., Spiess, J. & Rogers, S.A.W. (1995): Glutamate receptor antibodies activate a subset of receptors and reveal an agonist binding site. *Neuron* **14**, 755–762.

Van der Meché, F.G.A, Schmitz P.I.M. & the Dutch Guillain Barré Study Group (1992): A randomized trial comparing intravenous immune globulin and plasma exchange in Guillain-Barré syndrome. *N. Engl. J. Med.* **326**, 1123–1129.

Vincent, A. (1999): Immunology of the neuromuscular junction and presynaptic nerve terminal. *Curr. Opin. Neurol.* **12**, 545–551.

Wallace, D.J. (1999): Apheresis for lupus erithematosus. *Lupus* **8**, 174–180.

Weinshenker, B.G., O'Brien, P.C., Petterson, T.M., Noseworthy, J.H., Lucchinetti, C.F., Dodick, D.W., Pineda, A.A., Stevens, L.N. & Rodriguez, M.A. (1999): A randomized trial of plasma exchange in acute central nervous system inflammatory demyelinating disease. *Ann. Neurol.* **46**, 878–886.

Wekerle, H. (1999): Remembering MOG: autoantibody mediated demyelination in multiple sclerosis. *Nat. Med.* **5**, 153–154.

Chapter 26

New perspectives in the treatment of childhood rheumatic diseases

Marina Vivarelli and Alberto Martini

University Department of Paediatric Sciences, IRCCS San Matteo, Piazzale Golgi 19, 27100 Pavia, Italy

Summary

Chronic rheumatic diseases represent one of the most important causes of acquired disability in childhood. Despite available therapy, prognosis is still poor and new approaches, made possible by the advances in the understanding of the mechanisms underlying these diseases, are needed.

These new experimental approaches include: (1) Biological agents, targeting cells or molecules involved in the immune response or in inflammation, such as tolerance-inducing anti-CD4 antibodies, anti-adhesion molecule antibodies, anti-pro-inflammatory cytokine antibodies (anti-IL-1, anti-TNF, anti-IL-6), recombinant forms of soluble receptors for IL-1 and TNF and of IL-1Ra, or anti-inflammatory cytokines themselves (IL-10, IL-4). The transfer of genes coding for these agents into inflamed synovial tissue is also being attempted. (2) Other therapies, such as induction of tolerance to antigens present in the joints by their oral administration or, for the most severe cases, autologous stem cell transplant following intense myelo- and immunosuppression.

Introduction

Chronic rheumatic diseases affect about one in 1000 children; taken all together, they represent one of the most important causes of acquired disability in childhood (Martini, 1996). They are considered secondary, in genetically predisposed subjects, to an abnormal immune response to infectious agents. The infection would simply serve as trigger, and the abnormal immune response, which is thought to be also directed against endogenous antigens, would persist even after removal of the infectious agent.

The mechanisms leading to this autosensitization are unknown, and for this reason the therapeutic approach employed against these diseases is a general and unspecific inhibition of the immune response and of inflammation. Even though it is unspecific, this approach has significantly improved the prognosis of many rheumatic diseases. Nonetheless, the most severe forms of these diseases are scarcely sensitive to this type of treatment, and next to the possible multiple organ failures due to a poor control of the disease itself, the noxious effects of prolonged treatment (stunted growth, osteoporosis, atherosclerosis, sterility, etc.) have become increasingly relevant.

More recently, considerable advances in the understanding of the mechanisms underlying immunity and inflammation have suggested new and potentially more effective therapeutic approaches.

Evidence-based medicine in paediatric rheumatology

The efficacy of any new drug has to be assessed according to the criteria of evidence-based medicine (Feldman & Giannini, 1996). Data obtained from trials in adults, although potentially of interest, are not applicable to children due to potential age-related differences in toxicity and especially due to the fact that very often rheumatic diseases in childhood are different from those affecting adults. However, controlled studies in children present two main problems: (1) the lack of standardized criteria, universally accepted, for a reliable assessment of improvement related to therapy; (2) the rarity of these diseases.

In the last few years the international community has made many important efforts to address these issues; these efforts have led to the organization of a Consensus Conference in Pavia in May 1996, in which: (1) an internationally acknowledged definition of improvement for juvenile idiopathic arthritis (JIA) has been established (Giannini *et al.*, 1997); (2) a European network of paediatric rheumatology centres (Paediatric Rheumatology International Trial Organization or PRINTO) has been set up; its main purpose is to perform controlled clinical trials in paediatric rheumatic diseases.

New therapeutic perspectives

The search for new, more effective therapies for chronic rheumatic diseases is based on new approaches and also on the employment, with new indications, doses and/or associations, of already available drugs. The vast majority of these studies has been performed in adults with RA resistant to common forms of treatment.

Old drugs

Methotrexate (MTX) is the only second-level drug whose effectiveness in the treatment of JIA has been proved by a controlled trial (Giannini *et al.*, 1992). Controlled studies involving other drugs of proven efficacy in adult RA, are lacking. Recently a controlled study has shown the effectiveness, but modest tolerability, of sulphasalazine in the treatment of polyarticular forms of JIA (van Rossum *et al.*, 1998).

A number of controlled studies have been performed in adult RA to verify whether the association of more than one second-level anti-rheumatic drug (so-called combination therapy) was more effective that their individual use. The results up to now have been disappointing (Verhoeven *et al.*, 1998) except for two studies. Tugwell *et al.* (1995) have observed that a combined therapy of MTX and cyclosporin is more effective than MTX alone in RA patients with partial response to MTX. O'Dell *et al.* (1996) have compared the association of MTX, sulphasalazine and hydroxychloroquine with the association of sulphasalazine and hydroxychloroquine and with MTX alone and have found that patients respond better to triple therapy. As mentioned above, the relevance of these studies in JIA is yet to be proven.

New drugs

Cycloxygenase inhibitors

Non-steroidal anti-inflammatory drugs (NSAIDs) are the first-line drugs in all forms of JIA. Their effectiveness stems from their ability to inhibit cyclooxygenase and consequently the synthesis of pro-inflammatory prostaglandins. The inhibition of cyclooxygenase, however, is also the cause of their side effects.

Until a few years ago it was thought that a single enzyme, constitutively expressed in all tissues (now called cyclooxygenase 1 or COX1) were responsible for all prostaglandin synthesis. Recently however a new isoform of cyclooxygenase (cyclooxygenase 2 or COX2) has been discovered; normally present in negligible amounts in non-proliferating cells, it is induced by pro-inflammatory cytokines, such as interleukin-1 (IL-1) and tumour necrosis factor (TNF), and by all conditions causing cell proliferation. Therefore, COX1 would seem responsible for the basal synthesis of prostaglandins involved in physiological processes, while COX2 would seem responsible for prostaglandin synthesis only during inflammation. The pharmaceutical industry is trying to synthesize NSAIDs targeting specifically COX2 without significantly inhibiting COX1 (de Brum-Fernandes, 1997). In theory these drugs, because of their marginal effect on COX1 and thus on basal prostaglandin production, should be associated with a lower incidence of side effects.

New immunosuppressive drugs

New immunosuppressive drugs, some of which already employed clinically in organ transplants, are about to be investigated also in chronic rheumatic diseases (Yocum, 1996).

Two of these, FK-506 (tacrolimus) and rapamycin (sirolimus) are, as cyclosporin, derived from fungi and they also work principally by inhibiting the activation of T-lymphocytes through cytokine synthesis inhibition (FK-506) or through cytokine signal transduction (rapamycin). While use of rapamycin in experimental arthritides has up to now proven disappointing, FK-506 has proven effective in the treatment of experimental collagen-induced arthritis.

Mofetil (mycophenolate) by inhibiting purine synthesis has an anti-proliferating effect which is stronger on lymphocytes than on other rapidly-dividing cells. It has proven effective and well-tolerated in adjuvant-induced experimental arthritis. Data on patients is still very limited.

Leflunomide is another new immunosuppressor that works by reversibly inhibiting lymphocyte proliferation through a mechanism involving the suppression of cytokine signal transduction. It has proven effective in numerous animal models of arthritis and, more recently, even against placebo in a study conducted on RA patients (Mladenovic et al., 1995).

Biological agents

Biological agents are molecules produced by cells belonging to the immune system and are mainly represented by monoclonal antibodies or by recombinant forms of natural cytokine inhibitors; their specific targets are cells or molecules involved in the immune response or in inflammation.

The rationale suggesting the use of biological agents stems from a more detailed understanding of the mechanisms underlying the pathogenesis of joint inflammation. Synovial inflammation is thought to be triggered by the induction of a T-lymphocyte response directed against one or more antigens or auto-antigens that are yet to be identified. CD4[+] lymphocytes, thus sensitized, by activating macrophages induce release of cytokines, in particular of IL-1 and TNF. These cytokines are powerful pro-inflammatory agents on a vast array of mesenchymal and endothelial cells. In particular, they induce: (a) the release of collagenase and stromelysin which degrade connective tissue thus causing articular damage; (b) the expression, on endothelial cells, of adhesion molecules which promote the migration of inflammatory cells, thus perpetuating inflammation.

In the absence of an aetiological therapy the use of biological agents works by blocking specific links of this chain of events, in the hope of obtaining a form of treatment which is more effective and with fewer side effects. The main strategies involve: (a) the removal or tolerance of activated T-cells; (b) the inhibition of migration across the endothelium and towards the synovium of lymphocytes and phagocytes; (c) the inhibition of pro-inflammatory cytokines (Moreland et al., 1997; Kalden et al., 1998).

T-lymphocytes

Initially, therapies employing monoclonal antibodies directed against different cell surface markers (including CD4) present on T-lymphocytes aimed at eliminating this cell type. The results of this approach have been disappointing, despite an important peripheral lymphocyte depletion. The reasons for this failure are probably at least in part due to the inability to effectively deplete T-lymphocytes in the synovium.

The discovery in the last 10 years that anti-CD4 antibodies which do not destroy lymphocytes are able to induce tolerance (Waldmann & Cobbold, 1998) has refueled interest in the use of these antibodies to reprogram the immune system in autoimmune diseases. The mechanisms underlying this effect are not yet well understood, but they seem to involve an 'immune-deviation'. Recently, encouraging preliminary results have been obtained in the treatment of RA with anti-CD4 antibodies which do not determine cellular depletion; this suggests that functional modulation rather than cellular depletion may be the relevant therapeutic mechanism.

Adhesion molecules

One of the functions of endothelial cells during inflammation is to mediate the migration of white blood cells from the bloodstream to peripheral tissues; this phase is crucial both for initiation and for perpetuation of the inflammatory process. Pro-inflammatory cytokines (especially IL-1 and TNF) induce endothelial cells to express on their surface adhesion molecules which bind the corresponding counter-receptor present on the surface of leukocytes. This bond causes first adhesion of leukocytes to the endothelial surface and subsequently their migration to peripheral tissues. There are as yet few studies on the use of anti-adhesion molecule antibodies in the treatment of RA and up to now results have been quite disappointing.

Cytokines

Cytokines are a heterogeneous group of proteins with intercellular regulatory functions that play a very important role in the immune response and in inflammation. Some of them, such as IL-1, TNF and interleukin-6 (IL-6), are pivotal in the inflammatory process.

As mentioned above, numerous experimental pieces of evidence suggest that IL-1 and TNF may play a relevant role in the pathogenesis of adult RA. Cytokines work by interacting with specific cell membrane receptors; the extracellular portion of the receptors for IL-1 and TNF can be released from the membrane, thus creating soluble receptors which maintain their ability to bind their respective cytokines and thus prevent interaction of these with their cellular receptor. Furthermore, IL-1 has a natural inhibitor (IL-1 receptor antagonist or IL-1Ra) which competes with IL-1 in binding the cell surface receptor but which does not possess agonistic activity, or in other words is not capable of activating the receptor. Biological agents capable of inhibiting the activity of IL-1 and TNF are represented, in addition to monoclonal antibodies, by recombinant forms of these soluble receptors and of IL-1Ra.

The treatment of adult RA with IL-1 soluble receptors has not proven effective, while that with IL-1Ra has shown a certain efficacy (Bresnihan et al., 1998). Very positive results have been obtained by inhibiting TNF with a chimeric anti-TNF monoclonal antibody (Elliott et al., 1994) or with a fusion protein in which the TNF soluble receptor is bound to the constant portion of an IgG immunoglobulin (Moreland et al., 1997).

The results obtained in RA therapy by inhibition of TNF, though very interesting, present some drawbacks: this type of treatment is symptomatic, requires continuous administration, and the long-term side effects of prolonged use are as yet unknown. Furthermore, the effectiveness of this approach in other autoimmune diseases has yet to be assessed. In experimental lupus, for example, TNF appears to be protective rather than noxious while IL-10 (see below), whose effect is anti-inflammatory in experimental arthritis, appears to increase disease activity in murine models of lupus. Data obtained by animal experimentation have indeed shown that single cytokines play different roles in different animal models of arthritis (Kalden et al., 1998).

The importance of data on TNF inhibition for the treatment of JIA has yet to be established. Preliminary results of a study conducted by Pediatric Rheumatology Collaborative Study Group (PRCSG) on polyarticular forms of JIA seem to confirm the results obtained in adults (Lovell et al., 1999). On the contrary, the only patient presenting the systemic form of JIA yet treated with anti-TNF antibodies has shown no improvement of the articular symptoms (Elliott et al., 1997). This last observation is in agreement with data indicating that the central cytokine in the pathogenesis of systemic JIA is IL-6. In this form, in fact, circulating and synovial levels of IL-6 are much higher than those measured in other forms of JIA and in adult RA (De Benedetti et al., 1994) and these elevated levels appear to explain practically all the manifestations of this disease (De Benedetti & Martini, 1998), including chronic anaemia (Cazzola et al., 1996) and stunted growth (De Benedetti et al., 1997). Data on the possible effectiveness of therapeutic IL-6 inhibition in patients with systemic JIA are not yet available.

Another possible approach in the treatment of rheumatic diseases is the use of anti-inflammatory cytokines, such as interleukin-10 (IL-10) and interleukin-4 (IL-4). Both of these cytokines are in fact capable of inhibiting the release and effect of pro-inflammatory cytokines (such as IL-1, TNF and IL-6), of inhibiting production of metalloproteinases (enzymes that are able to degrade collagen), and of stimulating the secretion of natural cytokine inhibitors, such as IL-1Ra and soluble TNF-receptor. Both IL-10 and IL-4 are currently being employed in experimental therapeutic protocols in adult RA (Kalden et al., 1998).

Other experiments that are being conducted attempt to increase expression of anti-inflammatory molecules (such as IL-10, IL-4, IL-1Ra or the soluble receptors of IL-1 or TNF) in the inflamed synovial tissue by gene therapy. The transfer of genes has been attempted in laboratory animals using both viral and non-viral (liposomes, complexes that bind DNA, etc.) vectors. Target cells can be exposed to the vectors *in vivo*, i.e. *in situ*, or they can be removed, treated with the vector and subsequently returned to the host (*ex vivo*). However, there are many problems to be resolved for this approach to be implemented, such as the transitory expression of the gene, the immune reaction against the virus or its by-products, and security issues connected mainly with the use of retroviral vectors (Evans & Robbins, 1997). Human experimentation is still at a very preliminary stage.

Other therapies

Orally induced tolerance

Orally induced tolerance is a well-known phenomenon in which the oral administration of an antigen is capable of inducing, by mechanisms which are only partly understood, a systemic tolerance towards the administered antigen (Weiner, 1997). It is thought that this system may have evolved to prevent immune reactions against dietary proteins. A vast number of studies has proved the effectiveness of oral administration of the antigen responsible for the disease in numerous experimental models of autoimmune diseases, such as experimental autoimmune encephalomyelitis, collagen-induced arthritis and non-obese diabetic mice. The process appears to be at least partly determined by an active immune suppression operated by T-lymphocytes which, having originated in intestinal lymphatic tissue, subsequently migrate to other tissues. What makes this oral tolerization mechanism interesting even in diseases such as chronic arthritides, in which the responsible antigen is unknown, is the existence of a phenomenon known as bystander immune suppression, i.e. suppression extended to nearby cells: suppressor lymphocytes responsible for orally induced tolerance are in fact known to act non-specifically by releasing anti-inflammatory cytokines in the surrounding microenvironment. Thus, induction of oral tolerance to an antigen present, for example, in the joint may determine a suppression of articular inflammation if the sensitized lymphocyte migrates to the joint and, following contact with the specific antigen, releases suppressive cytokines. The first antigen that has been tested for the treatment of adult RA and of a limited number of patients with JIA is type II collagen; however, results have up to now been quite disappointing (Kalden & Sieper, 1998).

Autologous transplant of stem cells

Immunosuppressive therapy has considerably improved the prognosis of some rheumatic diseases, such as systemic lupus erythematosus and necrotizing vasculitides. An even more aggressive treatment than the one currently employed could theoretically be more effective but is made impossible by the risks related to severe immunosuppression and bone marrow toxicity. A possible solution to this problem would be to replenish the bone marrow after completion of therapy using autologous stem cells (autologous stem cell transplant). This therapeutic approach, which associates an intense myelo- and immunosuppression to an autologous stem cell transplant and which is vastly employed in onco-haematologic diseases, has recently been proposed as a form of treatment for the most severe forms of autoimmune diseases (Martini, 1997). The rationale backing this approach is based upon the following observations: (a) data in animals shows that adjuvant arthritis or experimental autoimmune encephalomyelitis can be cured by total-body irradiation followed by syngeneic or autologous bone marrow transplant; (b) there have been some cases in the literature in which an autologous transplant employed to treat a neoplastic disease was followed by prolonged remission of the coexisting autoimmune disease; (c) the use of stem cells harvested from peripheral blood and of cellular growth factors, which allow a faster replenishment of the bone marrow, has led to a decrease in mortality due to the auto-transplant to values beneath 3 per cent, which is an acceptable margin of risk in patients with a very severe form of autoimmune disease. The implementation of this therapeutic approach, reserved for the time being to very severe forms which do not respond to other types of treatment, is entirely preliminary and thus, notwithstanding anecdotic successful cases (Wulffraat *et al.*, 1999; Martini *et al.*, 1999) it is not yet possible to draw conclusions regarding its effectiveness.

References

Bresnihan, B., Alvaro-Gracia, J.M., Cobby, M., Doherty, M., Domljan, Z., Emery, P., Nuki, G., Pavelka, K., Rau, R., Rozman, B., Watt, I., Williams, B., Aitchison, R., McCabe, D. & Musikic, P., (1998): Treatment of rheumatoid arthritis with recombinant human interleukin-1 receptor antagonist. *Arthritis Rheum.* **41**, 2196–2204.

Cazzola, M., Ponchio, L., De Benedetti, F., Ravelli, A., Rosti, V., Beguin, Y., Invernizzi, R., Barosi, G. & Martini, A. (1996): Defective iron supply to erythropoiesis and adequate endogenous erythropoietin production in the anemia associated with systemic-onset juvenile chronic arthritis. *Blood* **87**, 4824–4830.

De Benedetti, F. & Martini, A. (1998): Is systemic juvenile rheumatoid arthritis an interleukin-6 mediated disease? *J. Rheumatol.* **25**, 203–207.

De Benedetti, F., Massa, M., Pignatti, P., Albani, S., Novick, D. & Martini, A. (1994): Serum soluble IL-6 receptor and IL-6/soluble IL-6 receptor complex in systemic juvenile rheumatoid arthritis. *J. Clin. Invest.* **93**, 2114–2119.

De Benedetti, F., Alonzi, T., Moretta, A., Lazzaro, D., Costa, P., Poli, V., Martini, A., Ciliberto, G. & Fattori, E. (1997): IL-6 causes growth impairment in transgenic mice through a decrease in insulin-like growth factor-1: a model for stunted growth in children with chronic inflammation. *J. Clin. Invest.* **99**, 643–650.

de Brum-Fernandes, A.J. (1997): New perspectives for nonsteroidal antiinflammatory drugs. *J. Rheumatol.* **24**, 246–248

Elliott, M.J., Maini, R.N., Feldmann, M., Kalden, J.R., Antoni, C., Smolen, J.S., Leeb, B., Breedveld, F.C., Macfarlane, J.D., Bijl, H. & Woody, J.N. (1994): Randomised double-blind comparison of chimeric monoclonal antibody to tumour necrosis factor α (cA2) versus placebo in rheumatoid arthritis. *Lancet* **344**, 1105–1110.

Elliott, M.J., Woo, P., Charles, P., Long-Fox, A., Woody, J.N. & Maini, R.N. (1997): Suppression of fever and the acute-phase response in a patient with juvenile chronic arthritis treated with monoclonal antibody to tumor necrosis factor-alpha (cA2). *Br. J. Rheumatol.* **36**, 589–593.

Evans, C.H. & Robbins, P.D. (1997): Getting genes into human synovium. *J. Rheumatol.* **24**, 2061–2063.

Feldman, B.M. & Giannini, E.H. (1996): Where's the evidence? Putting clinical science into pediatric rheumatology. *J Rheumatol.* **23**, 1502–1504.

Giannini, E.H., Brewer, E.J., Kuzmina, N., Shaikov, A.S., Maximov, A., Vorontsov, I., Fink, C.W., Newman, A.J., Cassidy, J.T. & Zemel, L.S. (1992): Methotrexate in resistant juvenile rheumatoid arthritis. Results of the U.S.A-U.S.S.R., double blind, placebo-controlled trial. *N. Engl. J. Med.* **326**, 1043–1049.

Giannini, E.H., Ruperto, N., Ravelli, A., Lovell, D.J., Felson, D.T. & Martini, A. (1997): Preliminary definition of improvement in juvenile arthritis. *Arthritis Rheum.* **40**, 1202–1209.

Kalden, J.R. & Sieper, J. (1998): Oral collagen in the treatment of rheumatoid arthritis. *Arthritis Rheum.* **41**, 191–194.

Kalden, J.R., Breedveld, F.C., Burkhardt, H. & Burmester, G.R. (1998): Immunological treatment of autoimmune diseases. *Adv. Immunol.* **68**, 333–418.

Lovell, D.J., Giannini, E.H., Lange, M., Burge, D. & Finck, B.K. (1999): Safety and efficacy of ENBREL® (Etanercept) in the extended treatment of polyarticular-course JRA. *Arthritis Rheum.* **42**, S117 (Abstract).

Martini, A. (1996). *Reumatologia pediatrica*. Turin: UTET.

Martini, A. (1997): Il trapianto autologo di cellule staminali emopoietiche nel trattamento delle malattie autoimmuni severe. *Riv. Ital. Pediatr. (IJP)* **23**, 776–778.

Martini, A., Maccario, R., Ravelli, A., Montagna, D., De Benedetti, F., Bonetti, F., Viola, S., Zecca, M., Perotti, C. & Locatelli, F. (1999): Marked and sustained improvement two years after autologous stem cell transplant in a girl with systemic sclerosis. *Arthritis Rheum.* **42**, 807

Mladenovic, V., Domljan, Z., Rozman, B., Jajic, I., Mihajlovic, D., Dordevic, J. & Popovic, M. (1995): Safety and effectiveness of leflunomide in the treatment of patients with active rheumatoid arthritis. Results of a randomized, placebo-controlled, phase II study. *Arthritis Rheum.* **38**, 1595–1603.

Moreland, L.W., Baumgartner, S.W., Schiff, M.H., Tindall, E.A., Fleischmann, R.M., Weaver, A.L., Ettlinger, R.E., Cohen, S., Koopman, W.J., Mohler, K., Widmer, M.B. & Blosch, C.M. (1997): Treatment of rheumatoid arthritis with a recombinant human tumor necrosis factor receptor (p75)-Fc fusion protein. *N. Engl. J. Med.* **337**, 141–147.

Moreland, L.W., Heck, L.W., Jr. & Koopman, W.J. (1997): Biologic agents for treating rheumatoid arthritis – Concepts and progress. *Arthritis Rheum.* **40**, 397–409.

O'Dell, J.R., Haire, C.E., Erikson, N., Drymalski, W., Palmer, W., Eckhoff, P.J., Garwood, V., Maloley, P., Klassen, L.W., Wees, S., Klein, H. & Moore, G.F. (1996): Treatment of rheumatoid arthritis with methotrexate alone, sulfasalazine and hydroxychloroquine, or a combination of all three medications. *N. Engl. J. Med.* **334**, 1287–1291.

Tugwell, P., Pincus, T., Yocum, D., Stein, M., Gluck, O., Kraag, G., McKendry, R., Tesser, J., Baker, P. & Wells, G. (1995): Combination therapy with cyclosporine and methotrexate in severe rheumatoid arthritis. *N. Engl. J. Med.* **333**, 137–141.

van Rossum, M.A.J., Fiselier, T.J.W., Franssen, M.J.A.M., Zwinderman, A.H., ten Cate, R., van Suijlekom-Smit, L.W.A., van Luijk, W.H.J., van Soesbergen, R.M., Wulffraat, N.M., Oostveen, J.C.M., Kuis, W., Dijkstra, P.F., van Ede, C.F.P. & Dijkmans, B.A.C. (1998): Sulfasalazine in the treatment of juvenile chronic arthritis. A randomized, double-blind, placebo-controlled, multicenter study. *Arthritis Rheum.* **41**, 808–816.

Verhoeven, A.C., Boers, M. & Tugwell, P. (1998): Combination therapy in rheumatoid arthritis: updated systematic review. *Br. J. Rheumatol.* **37**, 612–619.

Waldmann, H. & Cobbold, S. (1998): How do monoclonal antibodies induce tolerance? A role for infectious tolerance. *Ann. Rev. Immunol.* **16**, 619–644.

Weiner, H.L. (1997): Oral tolerance: immune mechanisms and treatment of autoimmune diseases. *Immunol. Today* **18**, 335–343.

Wulffraat, N., van Royen, A., Bierings, M., Vossen, J. & Kuis, W. (1999): Autologous stem-cell transplantation in four patients with refractory juvenile chronic arthritis. *Lancet* **353** (9152), 550–553.

Yocum, D.E. (1996): Cyclosporine, FK-506, rapamycin, and other immunomodulators. *Rheum. Dis. Clin. N. Am.* **22**, 133–154.

Chapter 27

Interferon beta and glatiramer acetate in multiple sclerosis

Giancarlo Comi and Bruno Colombo

Multiple Sclerosis Centre, Department of Neurosciences, Istituto Scientifico H San Raffaele, via Olgettina 60, 20132 Milan, Italy

Summary

Recent successes in the treatment of relapsing-remitting multiple sclerosis with interferon beta (1b/1a) and glatiramer acetate have raised hopes and expectations both in patients and in the medical community for a more effective and complete control of this disease. Data derived from different clinical trials are in agreement with a more aggressive approach to early treatment of multiple sclerosis. Although interferons and glatiramer acetate cannot be considered as a cure and much clinical research is still needed to better understand their different mechanisms of activity, it seems possible to consider these drugs as a strategy to delay neurological deterioration. The two drugs are characterized by different mechanisms of action, so that each of them can be considered as an alternative treatment when the other one fails. There is accumulating evidence that these therapies mantain their efficacy even after 5 or more years of administration. Therapy has to be tailored to the patient considering his/her clinical history and magnetic resonance imaging findings. Side effects should be carefully monitored.

Introduction

The advances in understanding the pathogenesis of multiple sclerosis (MS) according to immunological and pathological evidence highlights the T-cell-mediated inflammatory autoimmune process as the factor responsible for the patchy central nervous system (CNS) demyelination (Steinman *et al.*, 1996). Depending on these immunological concepts, various non-specific immunosuppressive agents have been tested in clinical trials from the 1970s. They all demonstrated marginal or no benefits on the course of the disease and sometime relevant short- and long-term adverse effects (Polman *et al.*, 1995).

Beta interferons

Interferon beta 1b was the first therapeutic intervention shown to alter the natural history of multiple sclerosis (MS). Since publication in 1993 of results of a double blind, placebo-controlled trial in outpatients with relapsing-remitting multiple sclerosis (RR-MS) (The IFNB MS

Study Group, 1993; Paty et al., 1993) and subsequent acquisition of United States and European product licenses for use in RR-MS, the management of the disease seems to be transformed from simply symptomatic treatment to providing a sort of pharmacological partial prophylaxys against further attacks.

Four different interferons are actually available: natural interferon beta and three other molecules of recombinant interferon. The clinical utilization of the former is nowadays reduced because of impurity growing during preparation and leading to frequent side effects. Avonex and Serobif are produced in Chinese hamster ovary and share an identical chemical structure. Interferon beta 1b (Betaferon) is produced by a different recombinant DNA technology, in *Escherichia coli*, is not glycosylated in the asparagine residue at position 80, lacks the N-terminal methionine and has a serine residue substitution for cysteine at position 17 to prevent disulphide bond formation.

A little confusion about the activity of different beta interferons was generated by the original titration in biological units, referred to the viral growth inhibition. More recently, due to a new approach in titration, it was realized that 6 MIU of Rebif correspond to 22 µg of active product.

According to Redlich (Redlich et al., 1991), the peptide 32-56 should be regarded as responsible for interferon biological effects. From a molecular point of view one should consider the possibility of aggregation for interferon beta 1b due to lack of glycosylation. Therefore, in order to obtain the same biological activity, more molecules of interferon beta 1b are requested if compared to interferon beta 1a (in 1:8 ratio). Although not proven, this observation could raise speculation about the hypothetical relationship between the higher number of molecules injected, the possibility of greater immunogenicity and the more frequent production of anti-interferon antibodies.

A recent study compared the pharmacokinetics and pharmacodynamics properties of Rebif and Avonex given in healthy volunteers respectively at a dosage of 60 µg s.c. or i.m. for Rebif and 60 mcg i.m. for Avonex. After administration, serum concentrations were not different and pharmacodynamics of different interferons were fully superimposable (Munafo et al., 1997). However in another study (Salmon et al., 1996) the biological activity of Avonex administered i.m. was higher and more persisting than the same dose of Rebif administered s.c. The contradictory results of these two studies remain unexplained. Anyway, serum levels of interferons do not seem predictive of biological effects (Salmon et al., 1996).

The pivotal North-American multicentre clinical trial showed that interferon beta 1b (Betaferon) reduced the exacerbation rate in patients with RR-MS if compared with placebo and decreased the activity of disease in the brain as demonstrated by magnetic resonance imaging (MRI). Although the impact on disability scores did not reach a statistical significance, the total brain MRI lesion load during the three-year period of the study was strongly decreased in patients treated with interferon beta 1b as compared with patients who received placebo.

More recently, two other phase III clinical trials have demonstrated that both interferon beta 1a (Avonex) administered intramusculary once a week and interferon beta 1a (Rebif), administered subcutaneously three times a week, significantly reduced the frequency of clinical attacks and the progression of disability in RR-MS. Once again the positive effects of clinical markers were supported by the effects on brain MRI parameters: reduction of the number of active lesions and of the T2 lesion load (Jacobs et al., 1996; PRISMS Study Group, 1998).

The results of a large multicentric trial (718 patients enrolled in 32 different centres) demonstrated that interferon beta 1b (Betaseron) has an efficacy on the secondary progressive (SP) form of the disease. The study was stopped by the External Advisory Board before the three-year scheduled period due to demonstrated efficacy of the drug. The time of confirmed progression was increased in a statistically significant way and the proportion of worsened patients was decreased if compared with placebo-treated patients (38.9 per cent and 49.7 per cent respectively). Interestingly, these results were reached both on patients who complained of neurological attacks and on patients who were free of relapses during the treatment period. Furthermore, a reduction of 31 per cent in relapse frequency was demonstrated. More data are necessary to properly understand if the reduction in progression of disease in patients free from attacks is due to a beneficial effect on subclinical activity of disease (reduction of new MRI lesions) or to other putative mechanisms (remyelinization processes enhanced?). All MRI end-points were also significantly reached; in particular the number of active lesions decreased in treated patients compared to the placebo group.

Based on the results of the performed clinical trials it would be important to compare efficacy, safety and tolerability of the three different Interferons, however, such a comparison must be interpreted with great caution because of differences among the population included in the studies. Tables 1 and 2 summarize the clinical and MRI findings observed in the three major clinical trials. In another study (Pozzilli *et al.*, 1996), two different doses of interferon beta 1a Serobif (3 MIU and 9 MIU 3 times a week) were compared to placebo in a single crossover study. A significant reduction of the number of T1-enhancing lesions was observed with both doses when compared to placebo; there was a trend for a higher effect of the high dose compared to low dose, but the difference was statistically not significant. Finally in a recent trial the results of weekly injections of 22 µg and 44 µg of Rebif were compared to placebo in a frequent MRI study, of 48 weeks duration (OWIMS, 1999). The median number of active lesions decreased of 29 per cent for low-dose and 53 per cent for high-dose Rebif, during the first 6 months of treatment; only the high-dose results achieved statistical significance. Data at 48 months showed a significant reduction in the total PD/T2 lesion activity in both treated groups, but with a stronger effect for 44 µg qw than for 22 µg qw compared to placebo.

Table 1. Interferon beta in RR-MS: results of Phase III trials. MRI parameters

	Avonex	Betaseron	Serobif LD	Serobif HD
Active lesions: % decrease vs. placebo	−75	−59	−81	−88
% change of T2 lesion load	−13.2	− 9	− 1.2	− 3.8
	(−6.5)*	(+15)*	(+10.9)*	(+10.9)*

*Results in placebo group are reported in parentheses.

Table 2. IFN beta in RR-MS: results of phase III trials. Clinical parameters

	Avonex	Betaseron	Serobif LD	Serobif HD
Exacerbation reduction (%)	24	33	29	32
% of patients exacerbation free	38 (26)* +47**	31 (16)* +93**	26 (15)* +73**	32 (15)* +113**
% of patients progression free	21 (33) −37**	20 (28) −29**	30 (39)* −23**	27 (39)* −31**

*Results in placebo group are reported in parentheses.
**Difference between active treatment and placebo group.

Considering all these suggestions derived by clinical and MRI data, a sort of not proportional dose-related efficacy seems to be evidenced as far as interferon beta treatment is concerned. The frequency of administration for interferon beta is still under debate. After a single dose of interferon beta 1a, the values of two proteins inducted by the drug (neopterin and beta2 microglobulin) rise to a high level which is maintained for at least 4–5 days. Other cytokines are otherwise influenced for a shorter time. There is experimental evidence about the pharmacodynamic response to interferon beta 1a administered s.c. once or three times a week. The effect in terms of production of neopterin and *in vitro* mitogen-induced cytokine secretion was much more sustained by more frequent administration. No comparative data are available for same dose s.c. administration of interferon beta 1a and interferon beta 1b (Munafo *et al.*, 1998). There are no clinical studies comparing the effects of different frequency of administration. An indirect comparison is however possible for Rebif: such a comparison suggests that when the drug is injected subcutaneously the same dose administered three times a week determines better results than when administered once a week.

Glatiramer acetate

In addition to beta interferons, two double-blind, placebo controlled studies established the efficacy of glatiramer acetate in RR-MS: relapse rate was reduced by about one-third, and moreover the number of active lesions and the MRI disease burden were also significantly decreased (Johnson *et al.*, 1998; Comi *et al.*, 1999). Glatiramer acetate (Copaxone) is a mixture of random synthetic polypeptides composed of four aminoacids: L-alanine, L-glutamic acid, L-lysine and L-tyrosine and was originally synthesized as an immunochemical mimic of myelin basic protein (MBP), a putative autoantigen in MS. Its biological activity seems to be mediated via production of specific T-suppressor cells, cross-reacting with myelin basic protein (MBP) and mediating a sort of 'bystander suppression' (Arnon, 1996).

The Food and Drug Administration has approved the use of interferon beta 1a (Avonex), interferon beta 1b (Betaseron) and glatiramer acetate (Copaxone) for selected RR-MS patients, whereas the European Agency for the Evaluation of Medicinal Products (EMEA) licensed Betaseron, Avonex and Rebif for the same kind of patients. Moreover, both drug agencies approved Betaseron for SP-MS patients.

Public health systems have generally followed the inclusion and exclusion criteria used in the quoted clinical trials as a parameter for reimbursing patients. This means that in many countries it is possible to prescribe Avonex to RR-MS patients with an Expanded Disability Status Scale (EDSS) score below 4 whereas the use of Betaseron is possible in RR-MS patients with an EDSS score between 1 and 5.5.

The impulse in basic research on the pathogenesis of MS derived from the results of these studies (involving about 1000 patients affected by RR-MS) and the need for patients to be assessed in a more complete and positive way particularly during therapy with interferons and glatiramer acetate was the key point for setting up more specialized MS centres all over the world. Moreover, since many patients and their families have expressed great interest in obtaining information about interferons and glatiramer acetate, MS centres throughout America and Europe have developed specific training programmes, and nurses were specifically taught to educate patients and their families about drug administration, side effects and management.

Candidates for treatment

All patients with a diagnosis of clinically definite or laboratory-supported definite MS in an active phase of the disease are candidates for treatment potentially modifying the disease course. However, the decision to treat should be individualized according to a careful evaluation of clinical and paraclinical variables and a deep discussion with the patient and her/his family. Patients with relapsing-remitting, progressive-relapsing and secondary-progressive courses may benefit from interferon beta (IFNß) treatment; moreover RR-MS patients may also benefit from copolymer 1 treatment. In RR-MS patients who already accumulated some degree of disability the clinical evidence of disease activity requires immediate treatment. Patients with a benign course or anyway with long-lasting disease inactivity should be treated if they start to have recurrent attacks. The decision is more difficult in non-disabled RR-MS patients who present an attack after a long period of clinical inactivity. It is reasonable not to treat these patients immediately, unless the brain MRI shows multiple enhancing lesions or the recovery from the attack is incomplete: a further brain MRI should be performed 4–6 months later to test the presence of new active lesions: the presence of new lesions will indicate to start the treatment.

Brain MRI is of the utmost importance in evaluating when to start treatment in MS. It reveals disease activity with a sensitivity ten times superior to the clinical evaluation (Redlich *et al.*, 1991). The presence and number of active lesions is predictive of the short-term clinical and MRI disease activity (Munafo *et al.*, 1997; Pozzilli *et al.*, 1996). The predictive value decreases over time and is lost after 2 years (Salmon *et al.*, 1996). The lesion load, too, is predictive of the future disability (Lassmann *et al.*, 1995). From a practical point of view, patients with a high brain MRI lesion load and/or multiple active lesions should be considered candidates for treatment.

The European Study on IFNß 1b in secondary progressive MS (Hughes, on behalf of the PRISMS Rebif Study Group, 1997) showed that the treatment is effective both in patients with progression without relapses and in patients with progression and superimposed relapses. Because in patients without relapses it will require time to detect the neurological deterioration prospectively, it could be judicious to start treatment anyway. In patients with severe disability it could be useful to start treatment with low doses, because of the risk of increased spasticity and fever.

To date there is no convincing evidence that any treatment may be beneficial in patients with primary progressive (PP) course. These patients have disease onset at an older age, disability mostly related to spinal cord involvement, infrequent cognitive dysfunction and low brain MRI lesion load. These aspects suggest that pathogenetic mechanisms may be at least partially different in RR and PP multiple sclerosis and consequently the therapeutic approach may also be different.

In patients with clinically isolated syndromes (CIS) suggestive of MS, the presence of typical brain MRI findings and intrathecal IgG synthesis is predictive of the conversion to clinically definite (CD) MS: about 50 per cent of the cases in five years (Munafo *et al.*, 1998); moreover the number of brain MRI lesions at clinical presentation is predictive of the disability at 5 and 10 years (Qu *et al.*, 1998). Ideally CIS patients with typical brain MRI and positive CSF examination should be treated because they have MS and are in an active phase of the disease.

However about 20 per cent of them will not accumulate a significant disability in the following 15 years and a further 5 per cent will probably never relapse. At present CIS patients should not be treated until they evolve to CD-MS. This indication could change in the near future, if the results of two ongoing clinical trials testing the efficacy of IFNß 1a in CIS is positive. In fact, there is a rationale for an early treatment in MS and also some clinical evidence seems to support this strategy.

The rationale for early use of immunomodulatory drugs in RR-MS patients could be explained on a pathophysiological basis (Table 3). Treatment may lead to down-regulation of antigen-specific T-cells (effector cells) and may inhibit epitope spreading at an early stage of the immune pathological processes (Tuohy et al., 1997). Moreover, the potent inhibition of TNF alpha production and the increased expression of cytokine IL10 by activated peripheral blood monocytes are likely to play an important role even in early therapeutic effects of interferon beta in MS patients (Neuteboom et al., 1997; Rudick et al., 1997).

Table 3. Rationale for an early treatment in MS

- Antigen spreading
- Longitudinal changes of immunopathology
- Prevention of irreversible pathological damage
- To reduce disease activity in the early phases (prognostic implications)
- Evidence of a better response to immunoactive therapies in patients with:
  – less disability at entry
  – younger age at entry

Recent MRI studies have focused on early occurring axonal damage in normal appearing white matter (Fu et al., 1998). Immunomodulatory treatment could help in reducing axonal injury, providing a protection against further clinical manifestations. Furthermore, MS gives patients a measurable cerebral atrophy that increases yearly, and considering that disability progression could be delayed until a threshold of tissue injury is exceeded it seems reasonable to prevent these events by starting treatment in the early phases of the disease.

Conclusions

For the first time two types of treatments, beta interferons and copolymer 1, have been approved as therapies able to modify the disease course in MS. Patients with RR, SP and PR courses may benefit from these treatments and ongoing clinical trials will clarify in a short time if such therapies can be useful also for patients with PP-MS. The available immunogical, clinical and pathological data suggest that the early treatment of RR-MS with immunomodulatory drugs with a safe profile could be advantageous compared to late treatment. Ideally treatment should be started at clinical presentation; however, we must await the results of ongoing clinical trials in CIS to define if such early treatment has substantial advantages compared to postponed treatment.

The classical limitation of at least two relapses in the last 2 years, applied in most countries by private or public insurance companies for treatment reimbursement, does not meet the clinical criteria for such a decision, but merely reflects the inclusion criteria used in clinical trials performed so far. There is no evidence that the level of response to treatment is related to the frequency of relapses in the pre-treatment period. MRI reflects the dynamics of MS better than clinical variables: which makes the technique a powerful complement to clinical data in the selection of appropriate candidates for treatment. Future studies will clarify if genetic and immunological markers may play a role in this decision.

In deciding whether to start treatment to modify the disease course, even in the presence of clear clinical indications, the physician should consider all possible physical, psychological and social implications. Most patients feel worse right after starting therapy, particularly with beta interferons and, even if these adverse effects are usually short lasting, they may have a deep impact on the patient's quality of life. Side effects tend to diminish as treatment is continued, and simple management strategies are successfully used to minimize these reactions, including patient education. Patients under treatment have to be followed by an expert clinician who can take care of them during the entire treatment period, to assure a continuous and accurate overview. This has to be particularly stressed during the first period of therapy.

References

Arnon, R. (1996): The development of Cop 1 (Copaxone), an innovative drug for the treatment of multiple sclerosis: personal reflections. *Immunol. Lett.* **50**, 1–15.

Comi, G. *et al.* (1999): The effect of glatiramer acetate (Copaxone) on disease activity as measured by cerebral MRI in patients with relapsing-remitting multiple sclerosis: a multi-center, randomized, double-blind, placebo-controlled study extended by open-label treatment. *Neurology* **52** (Suppl. 2), A289.

Fu, L. *et al.* (1998): Imaging axonal damage of normal-appearing white matter in multiple sclerosis. *Brain* **121**, 103–113.

Hughes, A.C. on behalf of the PRISMS Rebif Study Group (1997): interferon beta 1a (Rebif) in the treatment of relapsing-remitting multiple sclerosis: the clinical results of a large multicentric study. *Multiple Sclerosis* **3**, 269 (Abstract).

Jacobs, L.D. *et al.* (1996): Intramuscular interferon beta 1a for disease progression in relapsing multiple sclerosis. The Multiple Sclerosis Collaborative Research Group (MSCRG). *Ann. Neurol.* **39**, 285–294.

Johnson, K.P. *et al.* (1998): Extended use of glatiramer acetate (Copaxone) is well tolerated and mantains its clinical effect on multiple sclerosis relapse rate and degree of disability. Copolymer 1 Multiple Sclerosis Study Group. *Neurology* **50**, 701–708.

Lassmann, H. *et al.* (1995): Are current immunological concepts of multiple sclerosis reflected by the immunopathology of its lesions? *Springer Seminars in Immunopathology* **17** (1), 77–87.

Munafo, A. *et al.* (1997): Pharmacodynamic response to IFN beta 1a administered subcutaneously once a week or three times a week over 1 month. *Multiple Sclerosis* **3**, 226.

Munafo, A. *et al.* (1998): Comparative pharmacokinetics and pharmacodynamics of recombinant human interferon beta-1a after intramuscular and subcutaneous administration. *Eur. J. Neurol.* **5**, 187–193.

Neuteboom, B. *et al.* (1997): Pharmacological studies with recombinant human interferon beta 1a (Rebif): control of TNF alpha secretion. Presented at the 7th meeting of the European Neurological Society, 14–18 June 1997, Rhodes.

OWIMS, The Once Weekly Interferon for MS Study Group (1999): Evidence of interferon β-1a dose response in relapsing-remitting MS. *Neurology* **53**, 579–586

Paty, D.W. & Li, D.K.B. for the UBC MS/MRI Study Group, the IFNB MS Study Group (1993): Interferon beta 1b is effective in relapsing-remitting multiple sclerosis. II. MRI analysis results of a multicenter, randomized, double-blind, placebo-controlled trial. *Neurology* **43**, 655–661.

Polman, C. *et al.* (1995): The treatment of multiple sclerosis: current and future. *Curr. Opin. Neurol.* **8**, 200–209.

Pozzilli, C. *et al.* (1996): Magnetic resonance imaging changes with recombinant human interferon beta 1a: a short-term study in relapsing-remitting multiple sclerosis. *J. Neurol. Neurosurg. Psychiatry* **61**, 251–258.

PRISMS (Prevention of Relapses and Disability by Interferon beta-1a Subcutaneously in Multiple Sclerosis) Study Group (1998): Randomized double-blind placebo-controlled study of interferon beta 1a in relapsing/remitting multiple sclerosis. *Lancet* **352**, 1498–1504.

Qu, Z.X. *et al.* (1998): All-trans retinoic acid potentiates the ability of interferon beta 1b to augment suppressor cell function in multiple sclerosis. *Arch. Neurol.* **55** (3), 315–321.

Redlich, P.N. *et al.* (1991): Antibodies that neutralize human beta interferon biologic activity recognize a linear epitope: analysis by sinthetic peptide mapping. *Proc. Natl. Acad. Sci. USA* **88**, 655–661.

Rudick, R.A. *et al.* (1997): Management of multiple sclerosis. *New Engl. J. Med.* **337**, 1604–1611.

Salmon, P. *et al.* (1996): Pharmacokinetics and pharmacodynamics of recombinant human interferon beta in healthy male volunteers. *J. Interf. Cytokine Res.* **16**, 759–764.

Steinman, L. *et al.* (1996): A few autoreactive cells in an autoimmune infiltrate control a vast population of nonspecific cells: a tale of smart bombs and the infantry. *Proc. Natl. Acad. Sci. USA* **93**, 2253–2256.

The IFNB MS Study Group (1993): Interferon beta 1b is effective in relapsing-remitting multiple sclerosis. I. Clinical results of a multicenter, randomized, double-blind, placebo-controlled trial. *Neurology* **43**, 655–661.

Tuohy, V.K. *et al.* (1997): Diversity and plasticity of self recognition during the development of multiple sclerosis. *J. Clin. Invest.* **99**, 1682–1690.